Eat Well

For your Self,
For the World

Linda Bacon, PhD

Disclaimer: *Eat Well* is a work in progress and is not as well edited or comprehensive as I intend. I'm writing as fast as I can so my students at City College of San Francisco can have written material to support what they are learning. This incomplete work is being made available to meet present demand; visit www.LindaBacon.org, to purchase additional copies or find information about publication of a final draft.

Invitation: *Eat Well* is a living, growing book, and I welcome your advice and suggestions. My writing always develops as I learn more about what readers are interested in and motivated by. Do you have any questions that I neglected to address? Evidence that contradicts anything in the book? Were parts of *Eat Well* confusing or unhelpful? Please let me know by sending an e-mail to Linda@LindaBacon.org. Advice, criticism and comments are greatly appreciated. If you would like to be notified when a completed work is available, please send an e-mail requesting to be on the mailing list. Thank you.

lbacon@ccsf.edu
okan.pekgil@gmail.com

Eat Well

For your Self,
For the World

For information:
Linda Bacon, PhD
Box S-80
City College of San Francisco
50 Phelan Street
San Francisco, CA 94112
lbacon@ccsf.edu

Date of Publication: December 15, 2008.

Contents

Acknowledgements

Thanks to my students at City College of San Francisco (CCSF) for guiding the content and tone of the book. It could not have been written without their feedback, support and inspiration.

Personal experience has shown me that challenging commonly-held beliefs is threatening - both to those who accept the commonly-held beliefs and to those who question them - and carries consequences that potentially inhibit academic integrity. I am very fortunate to have found a supportive community of thoughtful individuals who are committed to engaging in academic debate and are willing to question the status quo, keeping the pursuit of learning as the focus. I'd like to express my appreciation to those friends and colleagues; your support helped me tremendously in many ways, including weathering some resistance. I also want to acknowledge Chancellor Phillip Day, who has been instrumental in nurturing intellectual challenge and academic freedom within the CCSF community.

Thanks also go to Smiley Curtis and CCSF's Graphic Communications Department for facilitating the cover art.

I am also grateful to my friends and colleagues in the Health at Every Size community. Our ongoing "Show Me the Data" listserve dialogue and our Bay Area "HAES Think Tank" in particular helped to inform my views and provided much needed support. Thanks also to my friends and colleagues working on issues related to sustainability for similarly informing my views and providing support.

Many reviewers are helping along the way, providing commentary on parts or all of the text. Thanks especially to Shoshi Bacon, Barbara Altman Bruno, Anne Coyle, Jack Norris, Michele Simon, Marilyn Wann, and Meg Webster for their contributions.

Special appreciation to my life partner, Anne Coyle, for providing the safe haven which makes everything possible; to our son, Isaac Bacon Coyle, who is living proof that eating in a way that is health-enhancing and environmentally-friendly can be a natural and joyful experience; and to my parents, Janet and Bob Bacon, for their ongoing love and confidence in me.

Preface

When I started teaching nutrition, I had no intention of writing a textbook. I reviewed all the textbooks, looking for the best resource for my students. What I found was that all were remarkably consistent in promoting conventional government recommendations regarding nutrition, even when those guidelines conflicted with scientific research. They all offered pro-industry analyses of controversial topics and rarely even mentioned concerns expressed by consumer advocates or environmentalists. And they all promoted a "food-negative" approach – food was something to be feared and its calories monitored and controlled to prevent "excess" weight. They also spent too much time espousing theory, with little effort made to help readers understand the everyday applications. While I found many excellent popular press books that didn't suffer from these same deficiencies, none provided a comprehensive view of nutrition.

For lack of a better option, I started using a conventional textbook, and supported my students in getting what they could from it. I encouraged my students to approach it critically, so that they could move beyond the book's limitations.

Over time I realized that the disparity between the conventional approach and the awareness I wanted to cultivate in my students was too confusing and contradictory. Exposing them to the textbook reinforced the food-negative, body-negative, environmentally and socially short-sighted message endemic to our culture, and was contributing to an increasing discomfort around food. Perhaps worse, the students complained of being bored by the textbooks, which they attributed to the lack of practical applicability.

I started to generate written materials that would provide an alternative view and better support the material discussed in class. This book is the result of that ongoing process.

My largest complaint with the conventional textbook approach to nutrition (and I levy this complaint against most academic and nutrition books) is that authors don't acknowledge their personal bias, but instead present their information under the pretense of objectivity. Scientific ideas are never the result of objective "knowing." What we believe to be true is heavily influenced by our culture and preconceptions. When bias is not acknowledged, I believe this indicates that the author is reflecting the values of the status quo.

I am concerned that much of what we believe to be true about nutrition has been heavily influenced by private industry (such as the food, agriculture, pharmaceutical, beauty and health care industries). As we all have to eat, there is a huge market for food – and tremendous profit to be made by those who can influence the cultural paradigm around food. Those working in private industry are well aware of this and have successfully exploited it. The distinctions between private industry, science, government, and medicine have become blurred, as have the distinctions between promoting health and making a profit.

Private industry has not only transformed our understanding of nutrition, but also our attitude toward food, and even our taste preferences. There is nothing inevitable about what you like to eat. It has been shaped by a complex interplay of biological, cultural, psychological and economic forces.

What you choose to eat is not without consequences. The foods that carry the largest profit margin are also those that are most damaging to our health, both personal and planetary. There is little profit to be made from marketing the foods that are most health-promoting nor making them appealing or accessible. It is no surprise that fast food tastes so good to many people, while vegetables, beans and whole grains hold less appeal.

There is substantial scientific evidence that our current eating and agricultural practices can't be sustained: food and weight preoccupation, disordered eating, and nutrition-sensitive diseases are rampant, environmental damage is spiraling out of control, and the social consequences of inequitable access to safe, healthy food are increasingly damning. We have swung too far in the direction of corporate profits, with too few protections for consumer, environmental and community health and well-being, and too little attention to giving us the full range of pleasure from our food.

I believe that a large part of the problem is consumer ignorance. We eat food everyday without giving it much thought, unaware of why we are drawn to particular foods or the ramifications of our purchases. We rarely consider how the food was grown or made. It is difficult to understand the consequences of our food choices when we are so distanced from them in the grocery store or fast food restaurant. We tend to not connect supermarket meat and produce to water pollution or global warming. We don't consider the conditions of the pig's life or that of the slaughterhouse worker when we buy our packaged sausage. Nor are we aware of the chronic diseases that may be developing in our bodies, in the moment, from our eating practices. The effects are out of sight.

Without knowing the true cost of our food - or having been exposed to its full range of possibilities and pleasures - many people have unknowingly acquiesced to allowing their tastes, food choices, and attitudes to be molded by industry.

I didn't begin my career as a nutrition professor with the ideas expressed in this book. Rather, they grew as a direct result of my education and ongoing research. I believe that education and active engagement can change the course of our future. Indeed, increasing consumer awareness is already having an impact. I am encouraged by the enthusiasm of my students, the changes they report in their own eating and buying habits as a direct result of increased knowledge, and the possibilities and realities expressed by the growing consumer rebellion.

My goal is to present a new framework for understanding how food choices affect you and our shared world. I want to encourage you to dump the short-sighted messages we've been fed by others and honor your own expertise in knowing how best to take care of yourself.

The best nutritionist you will ever know lives right inside your skin. Within each one of us dwells a source of guidance that will lead us toward whatever will help us, in all our uniqueness, survive and thrive.

Is body wisdom the one and only resource we need to preserve and promote our health? These days, especially when we're making choices about the food we'll eat, most of us need more than our inner knowing to guide us. As you'll learn throughout this book, the industrialization of food production puts our dinner plate smack dab in the middle of the consumer economy. The industries producing and processing food have every incentive to manipulate what and how much food we consume by tricking the body wisdom that speaks to us through taste, appetite, hunger, and the sensation of having eaten enough.

If we can't rely entirely on the body wisdom we're born with, what's a person to do? We can gather the best information on nutrition that science can provide.

While the science of nutrition can offer general guidelines, each person is biologically unique and variable. Your nutritional requirements change from day to day, season to season, year to year. They vary according the level of stress in your daily life, how much you exercise, how many hours of sleep you get. What's more, attempting to make your food choices based solely on nutritional information tends to make eating an intellectual exercise, diminishing the bodily pleasures you richly deserve.

What's a person to do? When it's bewildered by the faux flavors and biochemical tricksters embedded in processed food, your intuitive body wisdom can't totally be trusted. Nutritional information can offer evidence-based pointers but rarely specific guidance particular to any one person at any one moment in time.

This book offers you the best of both worlds, intuitive and scientific. Here you'll learn many methods for fine-tuning your body-wise capacity for making health-promoting food choices. At the same time, you'll find sound scientific information you can use to make healthy choices even when your body wisdom is subject to the food processing industries' trickery.

The substance of your body is a gift of soil, sunlight, and water. Your body is, in truth, the portion of planet Earth that you carry around with you. As this book will demonstrate, when you make the food choices that promote your personal health, you also help preserve the planet which sustains you.

You can reclaim or strengthen your ability to identify and enjoy nutritious and sustainable food – and know that you are doing your part to ensure a viable world for future generations. You hold tremendous power in your fork.

Why do you choose the foods you do?

Before you continue reading, take some time to become more conscious of why you make food choices by completing the following survey. Below are some of the many reasons that people make food choices. In each row, put an X in the box to the right of the statement that best describes you. Next, in the first column, use the numbers 1 through 5 to rank the five that are most important to you. (For example, if "appeals to my senses" is your most important consideration, put a "1" in the first column (called "Rank"), and if "is inexpensive" is your second most important consideration, put a "2" in the "Rank" column before "is inexpensive.")

Use this as an opportunity to get to know yourself better. Try not to be judgmental or choose answers based on what you believe you "should" value.

It is important to me that the food I eat on a typical day:

Rank		not at all important	a little important	moderately important	very important
	Satisfies my physical hunger.				
	Appeals to my senses (tastes, smells and looks good)				
	Is nutritious and has a positive impact on my health.				
	Results in my having stable or good moods.				
	Gives me comfort or cheers me up.				
	Is environmentally friendly.				
	Is convenient to buy, eat or prepare.				
	Supports my religious values or reflects my culture.				
	Is inexpensive.				
	Will help me to lose, maintain or gain weight.				
	Attracts approval/does not attract disapproval from others.				
	Is a respectful choice in terms of minimizing world hunger.				
	Doesn't contribute to animal cruelty.				
	Is shared with others socially.				
	Is organic.				

Rank		not at all important	a little important	moderately important	very important
	Has not been genetically modified.				
	Has not been irradiated.				
	Is locally grown.				
	Is low risk for contamination in ways not specified above (e.g. harmful bacteria, viruses, or prions)				
	Other:				

The purpose of this exercise was to help make your values more conscious. Did you learn anything about your value system for choosing food from completing this survey? Many people find that while taste plays a primary role in their food choices, their desire for good tasting food gets mediated by other concerns. For example, it is common for people to balance their desire for pleasurable food with their perception of the impact it will have on their weight.

What values you hold and how important each one is to you determines whether you choose a rich cup of hot cocoa made from chocolate and whole milk, a water-based hot cocoa with an artificial sweetener, some gradation in between, or whether you eschew processed foods and/or dairy products entirely. It also determines whether you experience your choice as guilt or pleasure.

This book helps you to better understand the issues that underlie these values. Perhaps your values and food choices will change with a little more education!

Introduction

Everyone eats – giving food the powerful characteristic of uniting us all. **Nutrition** is a very broad field which describes the ramifications of eating foods. Its definition encompasses not only *the science of how the body uses food* (including the relationship to health and disease), but also *the implications of food production, manufacturing and eating*. It includes all of the statements on the "Why We Choose Foods" list, although not all of them may be important to you as an individual.

It is a fundamental principle of this book that your fork is among the most powerful tools available to improve the quality of your own life and that of our world community (or your chopsticks or fingers, depending on your culture). This book will discuss the relationship between food and:

- personal health, well-being and emotional state;
- the health and sustainability of the environment; and
- food security and social welfare throughout the world.

My goal in presenting this information is ambitious: I want to help you define and clarify what is important to you, to help you understand the relationship between your food choices and those values you hold, and to give you the tools to make satisfying food choices that support your values.

The checklist reappears at the end of this book so that you can see whether increased nutrition knowledge changes your "food values" and food choices.

Is tasty food a priority for you?

If "appeals to my senses" topped your list of reasons you choose food, you are not alone – and I hope this is a value that you will continue to honor and respect. Food can taste delicious and give us great pleasure. This is not an accident. If we didn't enjoy food, we wouldn't be as driven to eat, and without eating, of course, we would die. That food activates pleasure centers in our brain, biologically motivating us to eat, makes sense. It maintains the viability of our species.

Our need for food, water and air connects us to our planet and makes us part of an intricate web of interconnections in which every organism is dependent on and affecting one another. Plants, for example, capture energy from the sun, which allows them to transform carbon dioxide and water into chemical energy (that they can use and store) and oxygen (necessary to sustain human life). When we eat plants, we capture their stored energy and can use it to fuel ourselves or store it for another time. The plants, in turn, rely on animals for pollination or spreading seeds, and on microorganisms for creating nutrient-rich soil from dead waste.

As humans have increased in number and our technologies have an increasingly dramatic impact, we are profoundly changing how the planet works. The foods we eat can nourish or poison us, and the act of growing and processing them has a similar impact on our planet. It has become increasingly important that we take responsibility for our food choices, from the perspective of both individual and planetary health and survival.

What's in our Food?

There are many substances contained in foods. Some are necessary for survival and classically considered to be **nutrients**, including carbohydrates, proteins, fats, vitamins, minerals, and water. Of course, there are other compounds in food, such as phytochemicals, flavor chemicals, color chemicals and caffeine.

One of the main reasons we need to eat is because some nutrients supply us with *energy*. Without energy to fuel us, we die. It is that simple. You can't drive a car on an empty tank. (We do of course differ from cars in several important ways – not the least of which is that you can refill the car's fuel tank and get it to start up again; a person would die if their fuel tank were completely emptied.)

Carbohydrates[a], proteins and fats, called macronutrients, provide us with energy when they are digested and absorbed into our bodies.

Of course, we need more than just energy from our food. Even after our initial growth during childhood, the human body is constantly being broken down and reassembled. Many cells have a short life span and need to be replenished frequently. Skin and blood cells, for example, regenerate every 10-30 hours. Some cells in your digestive system last only a few hours. Every time you digest your foods, you also digest (break down) part of the inner layer of cells in your digestive tract!

Food, therefore, has to do more than just supply our energy needs. We also need nutrients that are **building blocks** for making and maintaining cells, and for making compounds such as hormones, antibodies and enzymes. Other nutrients help to **regulate body functions**, and without them, our health will be compromised. For example, our bones may become fragile and break, we may lose our vision, and our blood may not be able to efficiently carry oxygen to our cells.

The nutritional content of food varies. All food provides energy. But not all foods come with extra nutritional benefits such as phytochemicals, vitamins, minerals, essential amino acids, essential fatty acids, or fiber – all of which support our survival and good health.

The term **"nutrient density"** compares the content of beneficial nutrients to the amount of energy (number of calories). Nutrients are analyzed in relationship to how much they "cost" you, in terms of calories. An **"empty calorie"** food provides energy but few or no other nutrients. From a health perspective, it is in our best interests to **maximize nutrient density**: in other words, get the biggest bang (helpful nutrients) for the buck (calories).

We can describe a food's nutrient density in general, or we can discuss its nutrient density in relation to a specific nutrient. For example, vegetables on the whole are nutrient dense, especially when compared to candy. Spinach is nutrient dense in terms of protein, while potatoes are not. (For a better idea of the nutrient density of specific foods, see the Nutrient Density comparison in the Appendix.)

Another way that foods differ greatly from one another is in their environmental and social impact. Some types of agricultural practices deplete our natural resources, pollute our air and water, and release carbon and other greenhouse gases faster than the earth can re-absorb them. And sometimes growing foods endangers workers' lives, or government subsidies and free trade agreements between countries contribute to devastating starvation in less developed countries. Our food choices are one of the most potent ways we can ensure the sustainability of our planet and a more compassionate world.

"Sustainable agriculture" refers to a way of producing food that respects the environment, respects workers, and is humane to animals. When foods are sustainably grown, we nurture the earth and our community, and can continue these growing practices in the future. Unsustainable practices, on the other hand, damage our community and can't be sustained in a way that allows for the viability of future generations.

Fortunately, nutrient density and agricultural sustainability are perfectly compatible: the same food choices support both. What's good for the planet and our peoples is good for you!

Another term that will be helpful to know throughout the book is "essential nutrient." The word "essential" has a very specific meaning for nutritionists, which is different from its lay definition. An **essential nutrient** is a nutrient that: 1) we have to get from our diet as the body can't manufacture it; and 2) without it, our health will be compromised. Most vitamins and minerals are essential, as are several amino acids (parts of proteins) and at least two fatty acids (types of fat).

In this introductory section, let's get started with basic descriptions of some nutrients so we can use the terms. We'll go into each in more depth throughout the book.

---

[a] Fiber, a type of carbohydrate, is an exception. (Will be discussed in more depth in the carbohydrates chapter.)

Macronutrients

The term "**macronutrient**" describes compounds that the body needs in large quantities: protein, fat and carbohydrates. In addition to hydrogen and oxygen, all macronutrients contain carbon, which is found in all living entities. They are therefore called "organic" compounds, which literally means "alive." (This differs from use of the term "organic" in farming, where "organic" refers to food grown without manufactured pesticides and fertilizers. Don't get confused by this. As an example of the differing usage of the term, carbohydrates are organic compounds, but some are grown with non-organic farming methods.) Protein contains an additional element: nitrogen.

There are two types of *carbohydrates*: **simple** (otherwise known as sugars) and **complex**, and complex carbohydrates are further broken down into two categories, **starch** and **fiber**. Sugars and starch are in large part used as sources of energy for our body. Little fiber is absorbed into your body and so it does not supply you with energy. Fiber does, however, provide numerous health benefits.

Lipids (fats and oils) also supply energy, in addition to serving as an energy reserve on our body. They give structure to cell membranes; provide insulation and cushioning; carry certain vitamins and other compounds; and provide starting material for some hormones.

We'll be discussing different types of lipids, including **saturated fatty acids** (predominantly found in animal products), **unsaturated fatty acids** (predominantly found in plant products), **cholesterol** (only found in quantity in animal products), and **trans fatty acids** (which predominantly result from the commercial processing of fat).

While we are able to extract energy from *protein*, our body prefers to use it for other purposes. For example, the amino acids contained in protein provide the main structural building blocks of the body and help to regulate body processes.

Food Sources of the Macronutrients[†]

Most foods are mixtures of different macronutrients as well as different types of each of the macronutrients. When we refer to bread as a carbohydrate or fish as a protein, we are saying that it is rich in that nutrient, not that it exclusively contains that nutrient. Bread actually contains water, a trace of fat, a little protein, and some vitamins, minerals and phytochemicals in addition to its carbohydrate. Fish contains water, fat, vitamins and minerals in addition to its protein.

Get acquainted with which macronutrients are found in different foods. Use this list as a guide, and supplement your learning by reading food labels.

Carbohydrates
Simple Carbohydrates (also known as "sugars"): fruit*, milk and milk products, sweets and candies
Starches (a type of complex carbohydrate): vegetables*, grains*, and beans*
Fiber (another type of complex carbohydrate): Everything with an * also has **fiber**, when in its whole form. Fiber is additionally found in nuts and seeds.

Fats (lipids)
Saturated Fat: animal foods (meat, poultry, dairy) except fish and shellfish
Unsaturated Fat: plant foods (vegetable oils, nuts, seeds, beans) and fish and shellfish
Cholesterol: animal foods

Proteins
Animal sources: meat, fish and shellfish, poultry, dairy
Plant sources: beans, nuts, seeds, vegetables, grains

[†]These are provided as general categories, although there are many exceptions.

Beyond Energy

Of course, there is more to food than its energy content. Food also contains water and **micronutrients** (compounds needed in smaller quantities) - such as vitamins, minerals, and phytochemicals.

You can survive without the energy-containing nutrients for a short while, getting subsistence levels of nutrients by digesting your own body parts. It may not be an enjoyable experience, but it's possible. **Water**, however, is different. Without it, you die within days. This is because water is a solvent, meaning that it dissolves other substances and can carry nutrients and other materials throughout the body. It also helps with temperature regulation.

Micronutrients

A **vitamin** is an organic compound (meaning that it contains carbon) that your body requires to help regulate functions within cells. Most vitamins are essential, although a few can be synthesized by your body. They affect a wide variety of functions in your body, such as promoting good vision, forming healthy blood cells, creating strong bones and teeth, and ensuring good functioning of your heart and nervous system. While they don't supply energy, some of them help you extract the energy from the macronutrients.

Minerals come from the earth, and in contrast to vitamins, they are inorganic (don't contain carbon). They are absorbed into water and taken up by plants through the water or soil, and transfer to animals that consume the mineral-laden plants and water. Humans get minerals through drinking water or eating plants or animals that contain them.

Minerals help with many vital body functions, such as bone formation or effective functioning of the heart, nervous and digestive systems.

A **phytochemical** is a health-promoting compound found in plants that is not a vitamin, mineral or macronutrient. Though phytochemicals promote good health, they are not essential for life. Phytochemicals protect plants against the elements, and confer these benefits on to us when we eat them. For example, sulforophane glucosinolates found in broccoli protect against macular degeneration, high blood pressure, and several cancers. And the resveratrol found in ginger and grapes (and yes, wine) can help combat cancer.

Anti-Oxidants

Micronutrients serve many varied functions. I'd like to give one example here, so that we can use it as a basis for understanding many health-related issues later in the book. Some micronutrients function as antioxidants, compounds that protect our body from insult and disease. Examples include Vitamin C, Vitamin E, the mineral selenium, or phytochemicals called polyphenols).

To understand antioxidants, it is helpful to appreciate the role of oxygen in our world and our bodies. The external environment contains oxygen. We inhale it, filter it through our lungs, and then our circulatory system delivers it to the cells in our body, each of which requires oxygen for survival. Without the presence of oxygen, a human couldn't survive for more than a few minutes.

Yet oxygen is a double-edged sword; though it gives us life, it also slowly takes it away, by a process known as **oxidation**, the process by which all things decay and humans "return to dust." Almost every substance on earth is subject to attack and decay from oxygen. Oxidation is the human form of rusting.

How does oxygen play both these roles? Most of the oxygen in the air is in the form of O_2, two oxygen atoms bonded together. A single oxygen atom is unstable due to its electrical charge; however, when two oxygen atoms bond they can share electrons, helping to stabilize one another.

Oxygen in its unstable form is called a free radical, or an oxidant. We'll use the terms "free radical" or "oxidant" throughout the book so that we can discuss more than just oxygen, but keep in mind that oxygen is one of the most active of all of the free radicals in our body.

A **free radical** is any unstable, destructive molecule. They come in a variety of forms, but what they share in common is that in their effort to gain stability they can attack and damage other molecules, rendering them as unstable free radicals, ready, in turn, to attack another molecule, starting a chain reaction of destruction in your body. In other words, a free radical is like a loose cannon, crashing into other cells in a quest to find an electron and gain stability. These highly reactive molecules attack cell membranes as well as the constituents of cells (such as DNA), wreaking widespread damage.

Other molecules (the oxygen singlet and hydrogen peroxide), termed "free oxygen species" behave similarly to free radicals, though they are constructed differently and don't technically meet the definition of a free radical. For the sake of simplicity we will consider these to be free radicals as well.

This process of damage inflicted by free radicals, called oxidation, is one of the leading causes of illness and aging, having been implicated in over 200 diseases, among them cancer and cardiovascular disease. Many aspects of aging and disease can be thought of as the oxidation of our bodies.

While scientists often focus on the damage done by free radicals, some free radicals also serve a useful purpose, allowing you, for example, to fight inflammation, kill bacteria, and maintain proper muscle tone in your blood vessels. The key is balance, making sure that free radicals don't exceed your needs. We will see that this delicate balance is out of whack in most people.

We generate free radicals in our body on a regular basis; they are a normal result of metabolism, so you can't avoid them entirely. Free radicals are also created through processing fats and chemicals, such as drugs, food additives, and preservatives; and by cigarette smoke, pesticides and other pollutants, sunlight, radiation, and emotional stress. Poor nutritional habits, including consumption of fried, processed, and denatured foods, as well as consumption of fats and oils which are oxidized through improper storage and exposure to light and heat, also results in ingesting damaging free radicals.

To understand the impact of free radicals better, let's look at how oxidation causes damage and disease. If you put some skin cells on a plate and gave them all the nutrients they needed, they would grow. Each cell would divide in two, and those two cells would grow and divide again, and this process would repeat over and over. At some point, however, the cells would lose their ability to reproduce[1]. The amount of times they can reproduce is biologically predetermined, although the time between one division and the next can be quickened or slowed.

Now suppose those skin cells are exposed to oxidants which overwhelm your body's counterbalancing mechanisms. The oxidants would damage the cells and you could use up your cell's capacity to replace themselves quicker than would occur in the absence of damage.

This occurs during aging. Aging actually has little to do with the passage of time. Compare the skin on your face to the skin near your underarm. The skin near your underarm has less exposure to the sun, and keeps its smoothness and youthful appearance longer. Sun-damaged skin, on the other hand, has a more weathered look; its cells are nearer the end of their life span.

So how do you protect yourself from this damage? First, you can minimize your exposure to oxidants. While this is encouraged, there is clearly no way to avoid oxidants completely. You can't avoid the sun entirely – nor would you want to – and your cells are always generating free radicals from normal metabolism anyway. If you did not have a way to neutralize free radicals, you would self-destruct.

If, on the other hand, there were a way to protect yourself from oxidation, your cells would need to replace themselves less frequently and would retain their vitality for longer.

Fortunately, you do have that capacity. **Antioxidants** neutralize free radicals and block the oxidation that would otherwise occur. The body can generate antioxidants – and we can also get antioxidants from our foods. They work by allowing themselves to be attacked by free radicals, so that the cell itself is not damaged.

Antioxidants partially explain why consumption of whole plant foods such as fruits, vegetables, beans, nuts, seeds and whole grains, seem to help protect against almost every disease from Alzheimer's and cancer to heart disease, diabetes and stroke: they are rich in antioxidants which help squelch free radical damage. Eat a carrot and the beta-carotene enters the cells of your body, knocking out the free radicals that would age the skin, damage your heart, or spark cancer.

It makes sense that plants are rich in antioxidants. They are constantly exposed to sunlight, and need defenses against the sun's damaging rays. As the sun shines, free radicals form in the plants just as they do on your skin – but the plant's beta-carotene neutralizes the free radicals before they do damage. (To test this theory, one scientist developed a plant that lacked beta-carotene; when the plant was exposed to light and air, it died[2].)

We'll talk more about oxidation and antioxidants throughout the book. This was just intended to give you a taste for the power of micronutrients, and allow us to use these terms while we build the basis for understanding them in more depth later in the book.

There are a few other vocabulary terms that will be useful to know. Human beings were designed to be able to eat a wide variety of foods from both animal and plant sources. The term **omnivore** is used to describe someone who chooses to eat food from both plant and animal sources ("omni" means everything). The word **carnivore** is sometimes used interchangeably ("carn" refers to meat), although carnivore technically refers to an animal that only eats meat. (A handy term when discussing dinosaurs, but perhaps less useful for humans!)

Some people make the choice not to eat animals, and they are called **vegetarians**. (Contrary to popular conceptions, a vegetarian does not eat fish, which is an animal!) Vegetarians may eat food that is derived from animal sources (such as milk, eggs, or other dairy products), but they don't eat the animals themselves.

A **vegan** (pronounced vee-gin, with a hard "g"), on the other hand, chooses not to eat animal foods *and* any products derived from animals. (Many people define the term vegan even more strictly to describe someone who lives a lifestyle free of animal products. For example, some vegans choose not to wear leather shoes as leather comes from a cow.)

Action Tips...

Most chapters in this book will include "action tips," which will be a quick summary of steps you can take to incorporate the information from the section into your life. If you want to get started maximizing your antioxidant defenses and limiting the oxidative damage to your body, here are some good tips.

Nutrition suggestions
- Eat whole, nutrient-dense foods (such as vegetables, fruits, beans and whole grains) as these will provide you with antioxidants.
- Minimize consumption of processed foods as these are more likely to be oxidized. (Fats are particularly vulnerable to oxidation. The food categories section provides advice for finding less oxidized fats.)
- Minimize exposure to pollutants such as pesticides.

Non-nutrition suggestions

- Get moving! Light or moderate-intensity activity will boost your body's ability to make antioxidants.
- Protect yourself from sun damage.
- Minimize your exposure to pollutants such as cigarettes.

Food Politics

We have an overly abundant food supply in the United States, which sets the stage for dramatic competition for our money within the food industry. Since our population isn't growing substantially, in order to increase profits, **the food industry employs two practices: encouraging us to eat more food in general and to eat more processed food**.

The more we eat, the more money stands to be made. If we only eat when we are hungry, and if we stop when we are full, it would be bad for business! The food industry is clearly not interested in supporting us in paying attention to our body's needs. They have a vested interest in getting us to live above the chin.

They have to sell the idea that food, rather than being consumed to meet physical needs, can successfully meet other needs, such as emotional caretaking, prestige and status, or as a sign of love and caring. Advertising tugs at our heart and ego, enticing us to pay less attention to our hunger and fullness. Buy this pie… to recapture romance in your relationship. Purchase this cereal… if you care about your child. Drink this soda… and others will think you're cool. Depressed? Don't worry; there's always chocolate. Scrape your knee? This ice cream will make you feel better.

"Eat More!"

Part of how they entice us to eat more is obvious when you consider the "super-sizing" trend. Americans think we're savvy consumers and we're always looking for a bargain. The food industry has discovered a neat way to capitalize on this. The cost of food itself is low relative to labor and other factors involved in production. In other words, giving us more food doesn't cost them proportionately more money. So they make larger portions "better buys," enticing us to buy more food and spend more money. A large portion of McDonald's french fries, for example, is 40 percent cheaper per ounce than a small.

The larger portions attract consumers because we want more for our money, and it's hard not to get suckered in. How can you buy the small fries, knowing you are spending 40 percent more per ounce? Though a small order might be enough to satisfy our appetite, we tend to think of waste in terms of money. While it is clear that the choice of whether to buy the large or small is ultimately the consumer's, it certainly is hard to choose the more expensive option. You have to be pretty courageous to make good choices in the current environment. The typical result is that you behave exactly the way the food industry wants you to, and come to believe that you are doing it out of personal choice.

Sure it's a better financial deal per burger to get a Triple Whopper at Burger King, but who benefits from your eating the four beef patties its stacked with? Of course, that seems small compared with Burger King's "Meat 'Normous," a breakfast sandwich that the company pitches with the slogan: "A full pound of sausage, bacon and ham. Have a meaty morning." And are you really saving financially when you're buying food that you don't need?

And I'm certainly not enthused about the marketing campaign that links eating more to manhood. In their ad campaign for Whoppers, a man ditches his female date at an upscale restaurant, complaining that he's "too hungry to settle for chick food." Pumped up on Whoppers, a swelling mob of men shake their fists, punch one another, toss a van off a bridge and chant, "I am hungry. I am incorrigible. I am man."

"Eat More Processed Food!"

Food processing is also very profitable to the food industry. Potatoes themselves are cheap, and there is little profit to be made in selling them. But put a little (cheap) labor into transforming the potatoes into potato chips, and there is much more profit to be made. The industry calls this "added value." Potatoes in their raw form, for example, sell for about 50 cents per pound. Once transformed into potato chips, on the other hand, they sell for about $4.00 a pound. Of course the labor and packaging costs are much less than the additional $3.50 that they are sold for!

Because of this profit incentive, the food industry plays a large role in promoting overeating and eating processed foods, which typically are much less-nutrient dense than unprocessed foods. One of the ways they do this is by creating confusion about what is a healthy diet, and trying to get us to believe that their foods are health-enhancing when they are not. Although an obvious way they do this is through their advertising, their impact is far more insidious and powerful than this. They also act behind the scenes to influence media, non-profit organizations, health care and nutrition professionals, researchers, and government agencies, to promote their message.

Let's start to examine this by putting their advertising budget into perspective. Advertising costs for any *single*, nationally distributed food product often far exceed (often by 10-50 times) government spending on *overall* nutrition education[3]. For example, the average advertising budget for a nationally advertised candy bar is $50 million, and for a nationally advertised soft drink is $100 million. (PepsiCo spent $145.2 million in advertising Pepsi and Diet Pepsi in 1998.) Even a relatively small product like Altoids mints sinks a lot of money into advertising: $10 million annually. Want to know how much the government spends on their overall nutrition education campaign to promote fruits and vegetables? Two million dollars!

No wonder we're getting the message loud and clear that soft drinks are cool, while we hear relatively little about the fun possibilities of fruits and vegetables! Of the money spent on advertising, only 2.2 percent goes to fruits, vegetables, grains or beans, in contrast to the 70 percent spent on convenience foods, candy and snacks, alcohol and soft drinks and desserts[4].

That there is enormous financial clout behind advertising is, I'm sure, of no surprise to anyone. I expect we're all a little tired of the constant drone that tells us how cool we'll be if we eat certain products or how other products will magically melt our pounds away. Perhaps we are distrustful of the ads (although it is clear that they do have their influence). But few of us are aware of what goes on behind the scenes. In fact, advertising is just a small part of the influence the food industry holds on our tastes and ideas. Most nutrition information for the general public either comes directly from or is influenced by food manufacturers. Let's examine how this occurs.

First, consider the media (newspapers, magazines, television, radio, Internet, etc.). The media require *news*. I used italics to emphasize the word "new." There is very little new news about nutrition - the research about what constitutes a healthy diet has remained remarkably consistent for 50 years.

Eat your fruits and veggies is old news but a story about the benefits of chocolate, on the other hand, can be provocative and entertaining. Which do you think will hit the press?

It is not surprising that researchers found a healthful compound in chocolate[5]. There are so many compounds in food that it is inevitable that something can be found in almost every food that promotes health, even if it is surrounded by numerous other compounds that promote disease. Do enough research about any product and you're bound to find some good stuff for the media to eat up!

Check out the example of the media attention towards promoting red wine. Yes, the resveratrol in wine promotes health, but there is also extensive research which documents that when consumed in excess, alcohol kills brain cells, damages the liver, suppresses the immune system, and otherwise wreaks havoc on our society through poor judgment and alcoholism. Given the extraordinarily negative consequences that also come with drinking wine regularly, should we really promote it? (Of course, moderation – not excess – is promoted.) Note that it's not just the media promoting it, but also nutrition professionals.

And why not mention that resveratrol's benefits are equally abundant in the grapes themselves – where they are bundled with fiber and other beneficial nutrients not found in wine?

All that hype about chocolate and wine, but this headline, significantly more important to our health and better documented by research, never hit the popular press: Prevent Breast Cancer - Eat Broccoli! It just wouldn't sell papers to discuss a study showing that young women who eat just a single stalk's worth of broccoli per week were 40 percent less likely to develop breast cancer than others[6]. Yet research consistently documents that a diet rich in whole plant products can dramatically reduce your risk for many chronic nutrition-sensitive diseases. Clearly, a diet rich in unprocessed plant foods has a much larger health-promoting impact than chocolate or wine can ever have.

Now imagine if a drug had the powers of broccoli – and without any nasty side effects? There would be regular media reports and some drug company would be raking in the millions. Well, here's the good news: broccoli is available to all – and without a prescription. Check out your local farmers' market or grocery store. But you won't find the press hawking it!

To avoid misunderstanding here, I want to be clear: there are health-promoting benefits to a wide range of foods, including wine and chocolate, and I don't dispute their role in the overall context of a health-promoting diet. My concern is more about the sensationalism. It's a lot easier for the media to highlight our "guilty indulgences" than the dietary habits that play a more significant role in health, but don't provide juicy headlines.

Another important point to recognize is that many stories in the media are actually written directly by the public relations departments of private industry. I woke up to this fact when I was a graduate student. I had conducted research that was being published in professional journals, and thought it important to get the word out to the general public. So I called several newspapers to tell them about the research and suggest an article. The response was consistent: I was told to write an article and send it in.

When I repeated this to my advisor, she was not surprised – in fact, she directed me to my university's public relations department, which routinely writes articles of this nature. When we did write the article and send it to the papers, several reproduced it verbatim. They didn't bother to contact me or fact check – and of course no one credited me as the author. The pretense was that it was generated by the paper.

Private industry is of course savvy to this. Their public relations departments routinely write articles which are sent to the media, who often publish it verbatim; television news programs often air videos similarly created and distributed by industry. These processes occur without attribution. Time-pressed journalists appreciate receiving prepackaged news that can easily be turned into copy. The media present it as news, not the advertising that they actually are. I'm not just describing the small, less-respected media outlets here. I'm talking about NBC and the New York Times as well. Much of what we read and hear today is marketing, created by those trying to sell us something.

Why do the media give us a singular message about certain products or research? Because the public relations firms target the wire services, which then send it to individual media outlets. A Gallup poll in 1990 found that "the most prevalent sources of medical news on television are the wire services and network feeds used by 98 percent of all TV news directors." So the result is that not only do we get the industry message masked as "objective news," but we get the same message reiterated everywhere. It's not so surprising that we accept it as fact.

Even the well-respected academic journals are looking for headlines in the popular media and try to control the spin. JAMA (the Journal of the American Medical Association), for example, spends $1 million annually on its media and communications program. Half goes to packaged video interviews, which TV reporters use in their stories. The other half is used to run the communications office, hold press conferences and prepare press releases, which reporters receive before the studies are published so that news articles can be timed to match publication.

It's also interesting to observe what happens when you follow the money behind published research. Industries with a stake in the outcome often fund nutrition studies. Statistics clearly show that when industry funds research, what gets published is more likely to show beneficial effects than research conducted without industry funding[7].

Maybe you are generally cynical and the above doesn't come as a surprise. Perhaps you know the media are not to be trusted. Maybe you turn instead towards the non-profit health agencies for advice. You figure they shouldn't have a vested interest and can give us the truth, right? Well, not always! It is not uncommon for the major health organizations to sell their name to the highest bidder. The food industry is well aware that their "legitimacy" is enhanced (or created) if they can get a respected non-profit organization to advocate on their behalf[8].

The American Diabetic Association (ADA) provides a good example. They routinely send out information about Nestle products to their members and others seeking advice. While the details of their sponsorship arrangement are not publicly available, it is public knowledge that Nestle contributed more than $100,000 to the ADA in the fiscal year ending June of 2003[8]. Nestle is not known for making products that are kind to diabetics, but this affiliation with ADA sure provides them with a positive spin!

And when the American Heart Association (AHA) launched their FRESH Steps Initiative, the Chief Executive Officer of Subway stood at their side[b]. According to the AHA, Subway has given the AHA $4 million since 2002, and will give an additional $7 million through 2007. In exchange, Subway can use the AHA "fighting heart disease and stroke" logo on its materials.

Do you really think Kellogg's Cocoa Frosted Flakes is "heart-healthy" while the Post equivalent is not? No, it's because Kellogg's paid for AHA's endorsement – the AHA heart-healthy label - while Post did not[b]. No need to worry about finding "heart-healthy" cereals for your kids as they abound: Kellogg's Frosted Flakes and Fruity Marshmallow Krispies, Malt-O-Meal Frosted Mini Spooners, and General Mills Count Chocula all carry the AHA stamp of approval.

AHA sure makes a hefty sum selling its endorsement label. The Center for Science in the Public Interest estimates that AHA received over $2 million for use of the "heart-healthy" label in 2002[8].

One last example: the American Academy of Pediatric Dentistry (AAPD) accepted $1 million from Coca-Cola in 2003[8]. A little surprising? An organization ostensibly concerned about children's teeth taking money from a soda company? AAPD President David Curtis defended the acceptance of this money, stating that "Scientific evidence is certainly not clear on the exact role that soft drinks play in terms of children's oral disease." A slight twist from the group's previous stance: "…frequent consumption of sugars in any beverage can be a significant factor in the child and adolescent diet that contributes to the initiation and progression of dental caries." Wonder what caused the shift?

My point is not to tell you that the American Diabetic Association, the American Heart Association, or others are corrupt organizations. In fact, I believe that in general many non-profits with these conflicts of interest conduct excellent work and provide important services. These examples were given to support the bigger point – that we need to be critical of *all* the information we hear. Even most non-profits are financially beholden to the interests of private industry, and don't always provide bias-free information to support consumer health. Using non-profits is a great technique for private industry to gain the pretense of legitimacy.

Also disturbing is that even the nutrition professionals have been co-opted by industry. Take the example of the American Dietetic Association (ADA), the largest, most well-respected organization of food and nutrition professionals. Their website proclaims that "ADA serves the public by promoting optimal nutrition, health and well-being. ADA members are the nation's food and nutrition experts, translating the science of nutrition into practical solutions for healthy living[9]."

Dietary advice provided by the ADA is consistently supportive of private industry[3]. They apparently will partner with any food company or trade organization, regardless of the nutritional quality of the products they provide. For example, they have in the past collaborated with McDonald's, and still routinely carry a page of nutrition "news" that is compiled by the Sugar Association.

Go to an ADA conference – which most nutritionists do - and the funding is obvious: any major corporation that manufactures food is likely to be found here. They apparently find attendees useful conduits to market their products.

Blurring of advertising/dietary advice is evident in their Nutrition Fact Sheets, which are provided in quantity to member nutrition professionals free of charge. The fact sheets are easy-to-read informational handouts written for the general public, graphically appealing and well-designed. Nutritionists can personalize them so that it appears that they were generated by their office. Many nutritionists give them to clients; it makes them look good to provide professional-looking documents.

Here is one example, the ADA Fact Sheet on Chocolate. Let's jump right to the conclusion: "Chocolate is no longer a concern for those wary of saturated fat, and... in fact, chocolate can be part of a heart-healthy eating plan." Sponsor? Mars, manufacturer of Mars Chocolate Bars, among many other candies. While I'm not disputing that chocolate can have its place in the context of an otherwise nutrient-dense diet, should the ADA allow Mars to educate nutritionists about chocolate, in the name of the ADA?

The ADA takes a surprisingly soft stance on soft drinks. From their fact sheet called "Straight Facts on Beverage Choices": "Regular carbonated soft drinks contain calories; milk and juice contain calories, vitamins and minerals – all beverages can have a place in a well-balanced eating pattern"[10]. That the fact sheet was paid for by a grant from the National Soft Drink Association may make one wary, however – particularly since the Soft Drink Association in turn conveniently uses statements from the ADA as proof that soft drinks can be part of a healthy diet.

Or check out this statement from the ADA Fact Sheet on canned foods: "recipes using canned ingredients are as nutritious as recipes prepared with fresh or frozen ingredients." Sponsor? The Steel Packaging Council. Do you trust that?

McDonald's sponsors the fact sheet on "Nutrition on the Go," while Ajinomoto, the maker of MSG, sponsors the fact sheet on "Food Allergies and Intolerances." In reality, the fact sheets typically are written by corporate public relations departments or firms, intended to improve the image of certain products or practices[8].

Indeed, co-opting professionals is an important corporate strategy. Corporations routinely provide money and information to academic and research institutions and professional organizations, and support meetings, conferences and journals. It is hard to "excel" and get recognition as an expert in most fields without corporate ties. (This is not to say that accepting corporate money necessarily makes one compromise one's integrity, but to make the point that private industry has a hand in academia.)

Check out this example. University of California, Berkeley, has a deal with Novartis, a large biotech company, which is said to be worth about $50 million over five-years. Dr. Ignacio Chapela, a professor at UCB, publicly criticized these ties, citing the obvious potential of conflicts of interest and corporate control of research. Dr. Chapela has also published research which reported a danger of biotechnology (contamination of non-genetically modified Mexican corn by genetically modified corn and the subsequent threat of loss of biodiversity). Dr. Chapela was well-respected among students and his colleagues, approved for tenure (a permanent position) 32 to 1, and unanimously approved by the Campus Ad-hoc Committee. This is ordinarily a call for rubber-stamping his tenure. Despite this, the budget committee denied him tenure. "This case sends a clear message that faculty who challenge the dominant paradigm are not welcome, especially if they don't accept corporate funding" comments Ethnic Studies Professor Carlos Munoz.

Chapela appealed this decision and I'm happy to report that two years later the decision was reversed and he was granted tenure. (No doubt, student and community uproar played a role in this reversal, showing that change can happen when individuals speak up and exercise their power!)

That industry co-opts academic researchers - and that this is commonly accepted practice - was flagrantly obvious in a survey by Harvard researchers, which was distributed to all U.S. accredited medical schools to evaluate the standards that exist between researchers and sponsors[11]. Half the schools said they would allow pharmaceutical companies and makers of medical devices to draft articles that appear in medical journals, and a quarter would allow them to supply the actual results.

Which professionals do most Americans look to for nutrition advice? Physicians – which could be a dangerous mistake. Nutrition training of doctors is not just inadequate, it is practically nonexistent. In fact, a nutrition course is not even a required part of their training (although some individual medical schools do include it). A report by the National Research Council found that physicians received an average of 21 classroom hours of nutrition education throughout their entire education, and the majority of schools actually taught less than that[12]. (Those 21 hours could include topics like tracing the biochemical reactions involved in nutrient metabolism rather than the applied elements of nutrition.)

Even more concerning is where this minimal education is coming from. Many medical schools use the curriculum provided by a Nutrition in Medicine program and the Medical Nutrition Curriculum Initiative[13]. Who are some of the organizations supplying this educational material? The Egg Nutrition Board, The Dannon Institute, National Cattleman's Beef Institute, National Dairy Council, Nestle Clinical Nutrition, Wyeth-Ayers Laboratories, Bristol-Meyers Squibb Company, Baxter Healthcare Corporation. Do you think a coalition of people who sell animal foods or pharmaceuticals will present an unbiased approach to nutrition? No wonder little emphasis is given to encouraging plant foods in our diets, and that pharmaceuticals are so frequently prescribed in situations where lifestyle changes have proven effective!

Do not assume that your physician has any more knowledge about nutrition than you do. What little education they receive is likely to have come from private industry.

Well now that I've taken on the media, non-profit organizations, professional organizations, academia, nutritionists and physicians, who is left to challenge? Let's address the problems with the government.

Suppose there were a food that:

- Contains as much saturated fat and cholesterol as red meat, both of which are strongly linked to increased risk for cardiovascular disease when consumed in quantity;
- Is highly associated with increased risk of ovarian cancer[14-17];
- Contains a protein that *may* (research is inconclusive) trigger type 1 diabetes in genetically susceptible children[15, 18-20];
- Contains a hormone (IGF-1) that is strongly linked to increased risk of breast[21] and prostate cancer[22-24b];
- Promotes gas, stomach cramps, bloating and/or diarrhea in most people, particularly people of color (70 percent of blacks and Native Americans, >90 percent of Asian Americans)[25];
- Is contaminated with ammonium perchlorate[26], a component of rocket fuel, at a level 5 times over the Environmental Protection Agency's standard for safety[27].

Would you make it a required product for all children in the federal lunch programs? (School districts actually lose their federal funding if they don't include it in every menu!) Would you

---

[b] Note that IGF-1 is a protein hormone and many suggest that it should be broken down during normal digestion. However, there have been several studies documenting that IGF-1 levels are boosted in people that drink milk. See the Food Categories chapter for more details.

recommend that every child drink three glasses of it daily? Would you allow Donna Shalala, at that time the Secretary of Health and Human Services, to appear in advertisements[28]?

Well, that describes milk – and it's precisely what our government does! Makes the slogan "Milk – it does the body good," sound a little hollow, doesn't it? And the picture of the head of Health and Human Services sporting a milk moustache makes a dramatic statement.

Would you believe that there is no evidence to support the commonly held belief that milk builds stronger bones[29]? When scientists reviewed all the studies that examined the relationship between dairy consumption and bone health published between 1985 and 2000 and narrowed it down to those that were well controlled and provided strong data, they found that *57 percent showed no significant relationship between the two*, while 29 percent showed a favorable relationship and 14 percent showed that dairy consumption was actually detrimental to bone health[30]. This is hardly convincing evidence to back the standard claim!

One of the largest studies, for example, the Nurses' Health Study, investigated 78,000 women and found no evidence that higher intakes of milk reduced bone fracture incidence or osteoporosis[31]. In fact, they found higher risk of hip fracture for women drinking two or more glasses per week compared to women who drank one or less per week!

It is true that milk contains calcium, an important component of bone strength, but it also contains acidic amino acids which cause your body to excrete calcium, which may partially explain why people who eat large quantities of dairy products don't have decreased rates of osteoporosis. Reducing calcium loss may play a larger role in promoting strong bones than calcium consumption. Milk is also low in some nutrients that promote calcium absorption.

I grew up believing that consuming dairy products is essential for a strong and healthy body, and that every child should drink milk daily. I now know these to be myths; they are promoted by health officials primarily because the National Dairy Council is extremely powerful at lobbying. They are also smart marketers: the Dairy Council is one of the leading suppliers of materials used to teach nutrition education in the schools. In this way, the Dairy Council shapes our beliefs under the guise of public service.

My point here is not that milk is poison and to be avoided – just that it doesn't do the job it is promoted for. If our government wants to promote a certain food, there are others that could do a better job of supporting the health of a broader spectrum of our population. Politics dictate dairy promotion and our staunch, almost religious, belief in its health-promoting qualities, not scientific data supporting its value.

Currently, most child nutrition programs (such as the National School Breakfast Program and the National School Lunch Program) require that milk be offered. Not only does the government mandate its inclusion in programs and promote milk, but it also hugely subsidizes the industry, essentially guaranteeing that dairy owners will make a profit[32]. Whenever the market price for milk falls below a government set standard, the government actually pays the dairy producers to make up for the deficit. This is in large part due to the very strong lobbying efforts by the dairy industry, which is one of the most influential industries in Congress[32].

One reason why the government is so vulnerable to industry influence is explained by a conflict of interest within the primary governmental body responsible for public nutrition education, the United States Department of Agriculture (USDA). Note the *Agriculture* in their name: another purpose of this agency is to promote agriculture, and its recommendations are in part to support agribusiness. These dual roles sometimes present a conflict of interest, and the result is that public nutrition education is often a compromise between what is best for industry and what is best for the consumer.

For example, the USDA halted publication of the 1991 Eating Right Pyramid after meat and dairy trade groups objected to placement of their products in the pyramid. They then issued a watered down version – the Food Guide Pyramid – revised to take into consideration industry's objections[3].

It would be pretty difficult for the government to give a recommendation like "eat less meat," which is advice well accepted by those who study nutrition, without offending a powerful industry. The word choice in the Food Guide Pyramid is more palatable to the meat industry: "choose lean meats," though less scientifically meaningful.

The USDA runs the National School Lunch Program and the School Breakfast Program. The good news about these programs is that they allow millions of low-income students to receive a free or reduced-price lunch or breakfast every day. The bad news? The nutritional quality of those meals. The USDA buys millions of pounds of surplus beef, pork and other meat products to distribute to schools, but it does not subsidize more nutritious alternatives. That poses a tough dilemma for schools on a tight budget. It can cost a school district more than twice as much to provide a veggie burger instead of a hamburger. As a result, the government's own School Nutrition Dietary Assessment Study has found that an astonishing 80 percent of schools serve too much artery-clogging food in the lunch line to comply with federal guidelines. (But imagine how the pork industry would squeal if it couldn't off-load its excess to the USDA to redistribute to schools.)

One consequence of this conflict of interest became painfully clear when the Humane Society released an undercover video showing horrific slaughtering practices. But while violently forcing disabled cows to their feet prior to slaughter in order to supply the School Lunch Program may nauseate the public, the role of the USDA in this process is even more unconscionable. It was not until after the horrific video was released to the media that the embarrassed USDA withdrew its inspectors from the plant, thereby forcing the company to issue the recall. It was the largest recall in our country's history, 143 million pounds of beef dating back two years. More than 25 percent of the recalled beef had been distributed free of charge through the USDA's commodity food program to about 150 school districts across the nation. Undoubtedly, at the time of the recall most of this potentially tainted beef had already been eaten by the 30 million children who participate in the National School Lunch Program every day.

The recall raises the obvious and shocking question of why the onsite USDA inspectors didn't stop the illegal practices before they were secretly filmed and publicly exposed. It seems apparent that the USDA is incapable of ensuring the safety of the food produced by the industrial agricultural system that it exists to support.

The revolving door between the USDA and private industry has done much to inhibit sound nutrition policy. President Bush, for example, has appointed more than 100 top officials who were once lobbyists, attorneys or spokespeople for the industries they oversee[33]. In many cases, former industry advocates have helped their agencies write, shape or push for policy shifts that benefit the industries they used to work for[33].

(Here's what is meant by the term "revolving door": Lobbyists give public officials campaign contributions and solicit their vote. The public officials are often influenced by the money to vote in favor of the lobbyists' platform. When the public official loses an election or otherwise decides to leave public office, they often take well-paying jobs as lobbyists. In their new job as lobbyists they now have easy access to the public officials they used to work with. Of course, lobbyists can also leave their positions to obtain a job in public office, and then directly vote on policies favorable to the industries they used to represent.)

Even if they are not officially in public office, members of the agricultural industry serve on government committees that help to draft nutrition policy. Suppose you need accurate information about the health impact of cigarette smoking. Would you call a tobacco company? Not a chance, right?

Should the committee that helps the government draft nutrition recommendations be dominated by people who work within or have financial ties to the food industry? Of course not, right?

But that is what happens. The USDA and Department of Health and Human Services (HHS) formulate the Dietary Guidelines for Americans – which includes the Food Pyramid and other guidelines which form the basis for all federal food programs, including the National School Lunch Program. More than half the committee's members have extensive ties to the meat, dairy, sugar, processed food, egg and supplement industries. Including scientists that work for Proctor & Gamble, the Cattleman's Beef Association, the National Dairy Board, M&M Mars, and the American Egg Board among the federal government's most trusted advisors on nutrition policy is not much different than letting food companies themselves write the guidelines!

Clearly, no government agency has the funds to research or promote dietary recommendations in competition with the food industry. Government agencies are highly influenced by the food industry. Food companies have been able to obtain laws and manipulate government dietary recommendations in ways that act in their favor at the expense of public health.

Disease Manipulation

So I hope you're convinced now: When you hear a nutrition tip, it's likely that some industry is making lots of money off that nutrition "fact." The same is true when you consider nutrition-sensitive diseases. The importance of cholesterol wasn't very well known until the pharmaceutical companies wanted to sell billions of dollars worth of statin drugs. But of course, now everyone is all too familiar with the dangers of high cholesterol levels (though this is disputable by scientific evidence). The marketing of dairy products, calcium pills, and hormone replacement therapy led to osteoporosis becoming a household word. GERD (gastroesophageal reflux disease) is now familiar to many thanks to the antacid industry. Fear-mongering about disease supports industry interests.

What to do?

Calorie consumption has increased dramatically in the last few decades[34], and much of the increase is attributed to processed foods[35]. It is not a coincidence that these foods are most profitable to the food industry.

While it is clear that our food choices are a matter of personal responsibility, it is important to recognize that we do not make our choices in a vacuum. We select our foods in an environment in which billions of dollars have been spent to convince us that certain foods are health-enhancing when they are not, that nutrition is confusing, that eating healthfully is impossible, and that there's no point to trying. Which foods are accessible to us has also been severely controlled by private industry – who get little benefit from selling more nutrient-dense foods. In other words, our tastes have been shaped by a very powerful food industry.

The most important advice I have is to relax. You don't have to leap from your seat every time a new carcinogen or miracle food is hyped. Be cynical about the fads, headlines - and even the latest research findings.

Develop your "media literacy" skills so that you are less likely to be suckered in. Next time you encounter nutritional advice, ask the hard questions: Who benefits by me knowing this information? Where did the story come from? Was it planted by a public relations department (much of today's news is). Who paid for the research? Who is paying the experts that are cited? Are the conclusions supported by the data? Did the study design ensure a fair outcome? Is this sensationalizing a small issue? Is there another way to tackle a problem that doesn't involve consumerism? Following the money trail will go a long way to helping you discern what is meaningful.

And I want to end this section with optimism. There is no reason to feel like the rug has been pulled out from under you and there is no one to trust. One goal of this book is to help you learn the science behind nutrition and to become educated consumers, so that you are less vulnerable to the myths and disinformation which are more commonly available. You will see that the science of nutrition is not nearly as confusing as we are led to believe.

You can learn the tools necessary to rely on yourself and to make better choices. Moreover, you will learn that the real expertise won't come from the media or professionals, but from your lived experience about how your food choices make you feel.

Get informed...

Note that I may not endorse any of these individuals or organizations whole-heartedly (in this section or other sections of the book). In the spirit of this section, I encourage you to be a critical reader!

- Check out *Appetite for Profit: How the Food Industry Undermines our Health...and How to Fight Back*, by Michele Simon, and *Food Politics* by Marion Nestle.
- *The China Study*, by T. Colin Campbell, also has some particularly interesting insider information.
- Peruse the website of the Center for Informed Eating: www.informedeating.org.
- The Center for Science in the Public Interest (CSPI) maintains a database that catalogues the financial relationships between non-profits, academic researchers, and private industry: www.IntegrityInScience.org.
- The Physicians Committee for Responsible Medicine (www.pcrm.org) also educates on these issues.

Action Tips...

- Disturbed by how we get manipulated by the food industry, and how inept our government is at protecting us? There are several organizations working to protect our rights. For example, check out the Center for Informed Food Choices at www.informedeating.org or the Center for Science in the Public Interest at www.cspinet.org/.
- Trust your body to help you to make decisions, as opposed to doing what is encouraged by the food industry. For example, you don't have to purchase larger portions than feel comfortable to eat, just because they are better deals financially. And you can recognize that ice cream may not be nearly as effective as a good friend can be at cheering you up.
- Learn the science of nutrition so that you are less vulnerable to the nutrition myths. (Keep reading this book!)
- Improve your "media literacy" skills so that you can discern fact from fiction. Think critically when confronted with ideas about nutrition.
- Don't fall for media sensationalism, single nutrient hype, or get lured by gratuitous endorsements. Always remember that when it comes down to it, food is just food. Individual encounters rarely have the ability to significantly transform your health or overall well-being. You are much better served by attention to overall dietary patterns rather than smaller considerations in food choices.

Eating in a Disordered Culture

The goal of this chapter is to help you put nutrition into perspective, as our culture tends to give it much more power than it deserves – with devastating results. It is certainly clear that many of us are affected by nutrition-sensitive diseases. It is also clear that the average weight of our population has been creeping up over the last few decades (until a recent leveling off), that many people are concerned about obtaining or maintaining a low weight, and that food and its relation to body weight is a painful issue for many people.

Despite the media sensationalism, however, life expectancy has increased dramatically during the same time period in which our weight rose (from 70.8 years in 1970 to 77.3 years in 2003)[36]. Meanwhile, heart disease rates have plummeted and many common diseases emerge at older ages and are less severe. We are simply not seeing the catastrophic consequences predicted to result from the "nutrition transition" and the "obesity epidemic."

Eating disorders and body image distress are also at epidemic proportions, a fact that often gets overlooked when considering nutrition. Whether our concern is about weight, our physical or emotional health, the environment, or social justice, most of us suffer from a "high-fact" diet, and are more burdened by what we know than comforted.

We spend so much time considering the fat content, carbohydrate content, or antioxidant abilities of foods, that it has become extremely difficult to navigate a healthy relationship with food, to truly enjoy eating and to allow our food to nourish us. Instead of eating for pleasure, we count calories and are riddled with guilt after we eat. We worry that that we eat too much, that we're not eating the right foods or that we're missing out on the latest life-extending "miracle food." Food has become a battleground.

The painful irony is that our concern with eating isn't producing the weight dividends it was intended to evoke: the more obsessed we have become with "healthy eating" and weight loss, the worse our eating habits and the fatter we have become!

To understand this, let's examine the context for eating. The over-eating and eating foods low in nutrient density that is promoted and encouraged by the food industry take place in a cultural milieu marked by an obsession with thinness. We get conflicting messages: eat more (and particularly eat more low-nutrient processed foods) and eat less. Many people feel an intense fear of being fat and a disturbing preoccupation with the effect that food has on their weight. Instead of eating for the enjoyment and physical nurturance that food can provide us with, we view food as our enemy, a test of our resolve and willpower, even our moral superiority.

Culturally, we believe that healthy eating entails "watching our diets" and fighting our desires. Controlling and restricting our food intake is viewed as a positive quality. Indeed, dieting, whether it is for weight control or health, is so strongly part of our culture that it is experienced as normal and appropriate by most people, and encouraged by health professionals – even though almost all dieters fail to reap the rewards that dieting is said to provide.

Contrary to almost everything we hear, watching your diet or calorie counting is not an effective way to improve your health or to lose weight. Instead, I believe that it is the hallmark of our cultural eating disorder. If you are among the majority of our population who struggles with a fear of food and the impact it will have on your weight, health or other concerns, the solution to healthy eating isn't limiting yourself to salads and skinless chicken breasts: it's eating normally.

What do I mean by "normal eating?" **Normal eating** is about responding to internal body cues that tell us we're hungry and full, rather than our ideas of appropriate foods and amounts. Our internal drive to eat well is comparable to our drive for temperature control: just as our body has very effective internal mechanisms for maintaining appropriate body temperature despite ongoing differences in external climates, it can also help us choose foods and amounts supportive of a healthy body.

Our job is to support our bodies: we put on a sweater when our body sends us "cold" signals, we eat when we get hunger signals, and we stop eating when we get satiety signals. Instead of fighting our body and trying to control our drives, we honor and respect them. As this process becomes second nature, it allows us to make food choices that make us feel good, honoring our health, environmental concerns, or other values, along with our taste buds. After eating, we feel satisfied, not guilty.

There is a presumption in our culture that the critical aspect of food's influence on health and longevity has to do with its nutrient content, but this is unlikely to be true. Eating health-promoting food is only part of the equation. Being able to properly digest, absorb and assimilate it is another. Anytime you are stressed, anxious or rushed, you activate physiologic changes which interfere with these abilities. The health impact of eating is much more than the nutrients our foods contain or lack, but also includes components such as the pleasure you derive from eating, your emotional state, who surrounds you when you eat, and the ambiance in which food is consumed.

As an example, the American attitude towards food contrasts with a much more pleasure-oriented attitude among the French[37]. The French consume a diet much higher in fat, and only 4 percent eat in a way that meets our saturated fat recommendations[38]. From a nutrient intake perspective, then, one would expect the French to have higher rates of cardiovascular disease. To the contrary, however, cardiovascular disease rates are much lower in France than the U.S. Scientific explanations for this so called "French Paradox" have focused almost entirely on finding protective compounds (e.g. red wine)[38], but little has been paid to differences in attitude[37]. The French put a premium on savoring their food. Perhaps this is the missing link?

I want to support you in lightening up on your fear of food. Food is clearly one of our greatest sources of pleasure. Thinking too much about the long-term consequences of your food choices will take away from your enjoyment of foods – and the fear may make disease a self-fulfilling prophesy. As you study the science of how food affects your body and our planet, I hope you won't lose sight of this. I want to support you in shifting your focus to discovering the joys of food, rather than fearing its consequences.

There's one nutritional concept that seems to make a healthy relationship with food particularly difficult, and that's the idea that some foods are good while others are bad.

It is clear that certain foods will enhance health, both personal and environmental, while others will detract from it. However, much of our discomfort with eating is related to the consequences of assigning moral value to food. While foods do have differing effects, no food is *morally* good or bad. When you consider a food as bad, it relegates you to being a bad person for eating it. So you either heap on the guilt and shame when you eat the "bad" foods that compel you, or you sentence yourself to a miserable low-calorie diet or unsatisfying foods. This clearly isn't helpful.

Food itself – like other objects - is neutral. You can use a knife to chop your garlic or to slit someone's throat; it is *you* that gives the knife its character. I believe this distinction is of utmost importance if we wish to have a happy relationship with food and a well-nourished body.

Labeling a food good or bad also denies that dosage is important. Food rarely has the ability to change lives in a single encounter. A daily diet of chocolate glazed donuts has very different implications than eating a donut as an occasional treat. A breakfast of steak and eggs will not permanently and irreversibly raise your blood cholesterol. A serving of broccoli and tofu stir-fry does not guarantee protection from breast cancer.

Labeling a food good or bad also stops you from questioning and discovery. If you label a Twinkie as bad, you don't have to observe its effects on you, and you lose the opportunity to learn from it. On the other hand, if you maintain a neutral attitude, you can watch your response to that Twinkie.

You can be more perceptive to its flavor, noticing whether it really tastes good to you or if it was just the idea that tasted good. Perhaps you learn that it doesn't satisfy your craving – that there was something else you really wanted that the Twinkie can't provide. Perhaps you become more sensitive to your taste buds toning down after the first few bites, making the next bites less pleasurable. Or perhaps you notice that half an hour after indulging in that Twinkie, your energy crashes and you start craving sugar again. This information will ultimately affect your taste for Twinkies in the future.

Is eating that Twinkie good or bad? It all depends on how frequently you eat it, how much you eat, what else you eat it with, whether you were attentive to it... Rather than eliminating these variables, we need to listen to them. By staying connected to your body, some foods may lose their appeal or you may no longer feel driven to over-indulge.

So, in answer to the question, "Is [fill in the blank] bad?," the response is, "Of course not." We simply need to respect it. Let it teach us whether or not we want to indulge or when enough is enough.

Of course, the food industry has a vested industry in having consumers believe that there is no such thing as a "good food" or a "bad food" as this suggests that no advice to restrict any product is warranted. "No good food/ bad food" has now become the standard rallying call of the food industry, and has bled into the recommendations delivered by nutritionists. While a generally good principle, it also has its limitations, as it may mask the dangers hidden in some foods or distract people from qualitative differences.

If there is no such thing as a good food or a bad food, yet certain foods are clearly better or worse for our health or other concerns, how do we make decisions about what to eat? As we become more attentive to the total experience of our food, we increase our body knowledge. And as our body knowledge increases and we additionally become more educated regarding the non-physical impact of our choices, our tastes change. We no longer fight our desires; our desires become compatible with helping us to feel good.

If we know the Twinkie is not going to really cure our depression, it becomes less appealing to us. Perhaps we will be motivated to talk to a friend instead. If we expect that eating the Twinkie could make us feel tired and less able to concentrate during an upcoming seminar, we'll search for a food that will give us more sustained energy instead. But if that Twinkie presents in the context of a fun indulgence with friends, and doesn't conflict with other values at the time, eating the Twinkie (guilt-free!), is entirely reasonable and appropriate. There is plenty of room for Twinkies in the context of an overall healthy diet and lifestyle.

In the taste section, we're going to learn about how our tastes get formed, and you'll see that the food industry has manipulated our tastes so that many of us are drawn to their highly profitable (but typically nutrient-poor) processed foods. The food industry and the culture play a huge role in what foods you like – influencing which foods are available to you, what they cost, your belief system about their value, and even the biology of how you perceive flavor.

But you'll learn that you have power. If you find that you are drawn to foods that conflict with your values, you can cultivate new tastes. Wouldn't it be nice if you craved garbanzo beans and asparagus?

Of course, this isn't a simple process. Nutrition education alone is rarely sufficient to change tastes. It takes active rebellion to disengage from your culture and reclaim your own ability to nourish yourself and to find delicious food choices that support your values.

This is a book about nutrition, and we'll take nutrition seriously, but I want to encourage you to keep nutrition – and health, eating and weight issues - in perspective, and to shift your emphasis from the weight/food obsession so common in our culture, to nurturing yourself, and being happy and healthy. Nutrition alone does not have the magic power to transform your life – although it can certainly have its impact as part of a much larger context. Good nutrition is just one small aspect of a healthy lifestyle, which includes such aspects as: feeling good about yourself and others, living actively and fully, and… eating well.

Let me give a quick run-down about my perspective on those areas.

What does it take to feel good about who you are? First, recognize that being a good person is about your core being, not the package it comes in. Imagine how the world could be different if we took all the energy that was wasted on trying to change our bodies, and transformed it into trying to better the planet! There are many important ways to have your mark on the world, but I suspect that the most important stems from the love and compassion you generate.

Feeling good about yourself also includes feeling good about your body, although this is very difficult for anyone to achieve in our thinness-obsessed culture. However, humans come in all sizes and shapes, as does beauty, and I want to encourage you to find a way to enjoy and appreciate the beautiful body you have. Throw out those narrow cultural definitions. Current beauty standards are neither healthy nor attainable by most people - and leave most of us feeling inadequate.

And I'm not going to let anyone get away with rationalizing the drive to be thin or re-shape your body as a health imperative. The information in the weight regulation section should convince you that this is a myth. Genetics, eating and activity behaviors are much larger determinants of good health than weight, and people can be healthy regardless of their size. You'll feel lighter once you drop the load of shame and find self-acceptance - and that will allow you to move on and make positive changes.

Next on my list of a healthy lifestyle is extending that openness to others. Challenge your stereotypes of "fat" people and move beyond the limiting cultural definitions of beauty. Respect and appreciate the diversity (including size and shape) and special qualities we all have.

Live actively is yet more feel-good advice. Move for fun - not just because it's the healthy thing to do or because it has a sought effect on weight. Be more active as a normal part of your everyday life. Five minute walks or climbing a flight of stairs can be great ways to perk up your mood (and health).

Live fully is my next piece of advice. Too many people put their lives on hold, waiting until they accomplish weight goals or other superficial aims. Body-acceptance and self-acceptance don't mean complacency or giving up – they're about moving on. They give you the power to make more nurturing choices. After all, we take good care of things we like.

Lastly, I want to encourage you to eat well. If your diet doesn't conform to your values, explore new foods and preparations. You can discover healthful choices that you love – and that support your values. Food should be tasty, nurturing and enjoyable. Savor every bite, and you'll find that your attentiveness can lead to making nourishing choices.

To re-emphasize my point about keeping perspective, I want to encourage you to remember that good nutrition is just one component of healthy eating. I hope that your knowledge of nutrition will play a role in your food choices... but it doesn't need to control them. Good nutrition comes more naturally when you allow yourself to enjoy food - rather than focusing on calories or vitamin content - and when you have a healthy relationship with your body.

One of the difficulties posed by reading about nutrition or learning nutrition in an academic setting is that you may increase your knowledge to a greater extent than you increase your practical skills in applying the new-found information. We can't take trips to supermarkets, farmers' markets or your kitchen. So you've got your work cut out for you beyond this book! But I encourage you to do it – and put your knowledge to good use. Your reward will be an increased enjoyment of food – which is likely to lead you to making better choices.

May you discover the pleasures of eating well!

Pleasure and Taste

The human body is hard-wired to make us want to eat (as well as to want other things, like exercise, sex, social interaction…); good food turns on pleasure centers in our brain. Some of life's greatest pleasures come from biting into a raspberry, experiencing bittersweet chocolate melting over your tongue, or having that first sip of coffee in the morning. That we like good food is not just about fun: it's about survival. If we didn't like food, we wouldn't eat it. We'd waste away and our species would die off. Not surprising that nature built in a reward system for eating.

Let that hot fudge sundae roll over your tongue and what mouth sensations do you experience? Mmmm …sweet, creamy, cold - with the slightly bitter richness of chocolate as you close your mouth to swallow and the aroma wafts up into your nasal passages. Those are complicated sensations, so let's get started in this chapter with a discussion of why food tastes the way it does and why certain tastes are appealing to us.

Taste

Although we commonly use the word 'taste' to mean "flavor," in the strict sense it is applicable only to the sensations arising from specialized taste cells in the mouth.

Taste buds are onion-shaped structures that contain taste cells, each of which has fingerlike projections called microvilli that poke through the taste pore, an opening at the top of the taste bud. Chemicals from food dissolve in saliva and contact the taste cells through the taste pore. There they interact either with proteins on the surfaces of the cells known as taste receptors or with pore-like proteins called ion channels. These interactions cause electrical changes in the taste cells, triggering the release of chemical signals which travel to the brain. Taste neurons often respond to texture and temperature stimuli as well.

We have the ability to perceive five taste qualities: saltiness, sourness, sweetness, bitterness, and umami, although some researchers are still skeptical that umami constitutes a fifth major taste as significant as sweet, sour, salty and bitter. Umami results from eating the amino acids that comprise certain proteins (glutamates); it is often translated from its Japanese roots to refer to a meaty and savory taste. It's hard to describe, as it can be found in these disparate foods, among others: Parmesan and Roquefort cheese, fish sauce, soy sauce, walnuts, grapes, broccoli, tomatoes and mushrooms.

Similar taste buds are to some degree grouped together on your tongue (sweet at the tip; salty not far behind and flanking the sides near the tip; sour at the sides; bitter at the back, near the throat), although the classic taste map is an over-simplification. Sensitivity to all tastes is distributed across the whole tongue and to other regions of the mouth where there are taste buds (epiglottis, soft palate), but some areas are more responsive to certain tastes than others.

Each food contacts different numbers and combinations of each of these taste receptors, allowing foods to taste different from one another. A particular apricot, for example, may predominantly activate numerous sweet receptors, but also a fair amount of bitter receptors, and a few sour receptors, making it taste very different from chocolate, which perhaps activates more salt receptors than the apricot.

Some foods change your sensitivity to others, allowing food combinations to taste different than the individual foods they are composed of. Monosodium glutamate (MSG), for example, works by exciting receptors which are found in taste cells. Then, far less of a particular taste is required to cause the further excitation necessary to fully activate the taste receptor. MSG is therefore known as a taste enhancer (meaning that it intensifies the taste of other flavors in the food, as opposed to providing a strong taste on its own). (MSG also excites the umami receptors.)

Also interesting is that your taste buds tone down after initial exposure to a specific taste (over a short period of time), a process called negative allesthesia. (Most people are not aware of this because they eat too fast and without fully tasting their food. However, eat slowly and attentively and you will notice that the first few bites of a food trigger a much more robust taste response than subsequent bites.)

Combining certain foods can short-circuit your taste buds' ability to identify flavors correctly. For example, eat cheese before wine. The wine will taste smoother (less acidic) because the cheese's fat and protein molecules coat your taste receptor cells and the acidic molecules can no longer connect as easily. As another example, artichokes contain compounds (chlorogenic acid and cynarin) that suppress sour and bitter taste receptors. As a result, it makes any food you eat afterwards taste sweeter.

The average person has 2,000 to 5,000 taste buds, while some have as many as 10,000 and have a super sense of taste. Interestingly, women generally have more taste buds than men. Perhaps food takes on different meaning to men and women in part due to this biologic fact.

Your taste buds are initially set at birth to prefer just one taste: sweet. Children tend to be very drawn to sweets, but genetic programming turns down this taste a bit as we age (for most people), and other taste buds materialize.

Why do we have taste buds? Most likely it is about self-protection. We acquired the sense of taste as a way to get the nutrients we need and avoid being poisoned. Edible plants often taste sweet, and deadly plants generally taste bitter. Interestingly, the bitterness in broccoli and other cruciferous vegetables is due to tiny amounts of natural toxins that repel insects or other attackers[39]. (The toxin is not harmful to humans.)

Of course, not all bitterness is due to toxins. For example, the bitterness in grapefruit developed as an accident. The grapefruit came into existence when an orange was crossed with a pomelo. This breeding created naringin, a bitter compound that slows your liver's ability to eliminate chemicals from your bloodstream. (One result: eat a grapefruit and your morning caffeine buzz lasts longer!)

The evolution of various cuisines and specific food combinations has helped humans to deal with dangers in our food supply. For example, the dangers of eating raw fish are lessened by consuming it with wasabi, which is a potent antimicrobial. Similarly, the strong spices found in many cuisines in tropical climates, where food is quick to spoil, have antibacterial properties. And the meso-American practice of cooking corn with lime makes the corn's niacin more absorbable.

Aroma

Contrary to popular belief, your **taste buds play a very small role in the flavor you perceive in foods. Flavor is largely formed by aroma** (approximately 70-90 percent), as anyone with a head cold can testify. Eyes blindfolded and nose pinched, you are unlikely to be able to tell the difference between a grated onion and a grated apple. Try smearing chocolate syrup under your nose and check out how your hot dog tastes. And you'll find it's not so appealing to sit near someone exuding strong cologne when you're eating your pizza!

How does aroma translate into flavor? When you drink or chew a substance, it releases volatile gases. The gases flow to nerve cells called the olfactory epithelium, located at the top of the nose, right between the eyes. Additional nerve cells then deliver the aroma messages to your brain.

Some foods, like coffee, are so complex that their aromas may be composed of gases from nearly a thousand different chemicals. The smell of a cherry, less complex, comes from the interaction of several hundred different chemicals.

Interestingly, aroma and memory share neighboring space in our brains. Because there are so many cross-linkages, smells can readily evoke memories. Some foods may evoke comforting associations from childhood. As adults, we are drawn to these "comfort foods" without always being conscious of the reason.

Other senses

Other sensory systems also contribute to the flavor you perceive, transmitting information about the appearance, temperature, and texture of food. For example, split pea soup that looks like vomit may appeal to a blindfolded taster, but taste distinctly like vomit when that same person eyes a bowlful. In fact, research shows that people rate brightly colored foods as tasting better than bland-looking foods, even when the flavor compounds are identical!

Cold soda may be less cloyingly sweet than the same components served warm. And a soggy burrito is not nearly as sensually satisfying as a fresh one, despite containing the same ingredients.

Ever wonder what gives foods their crunch? When you chomp a pretzel or celery stick, you're popping open hundreds of tiny cells of air, and the crunch is the result of these tiny explosions. An apple's crunch comes from breaking cells filled with water.

Context matters!

How you respond to food is also strongly influenced by the context in which you eat. An ice cream sundae will be much more enjoyable as part of a happy birthday celebration than if it's eaten stealthily in the middle of the night. A Chianti sipped with your sweetheart on a romantic Tuscany hillside will please your palate in a way that may never be reproduced when gulped at your kitchen table while spoon-feeding your infant.

Flavor

Your brain grabs all your sensory information, combines it with the stored information in your memory and the information from the present context, and processes all of it as a unit. It receives so many messages that it can't process them all, and winds up filtering out certain messages, protecting itself from overload.

If you live next to a fast food restaurant that's constantly spewing strong smells and your friend comes for dinner, the smell over-rides the sensations from the food itself, and your friend can't properly appreciate your cooking. You, on the other hand, are so accustomed to the local smells that your brain automatically tunes them out[40], and you can be more sensitized to the flavor chemicals emanating from the food itself. (This also explains why people usually can't smell their own bad breath.)

After receiving this complex and detailed information, your brain sends back a simple message: this is what the food tastes like.

Cultural Influence

Because humans have been somewhat open-minded about trying new foods, we have been able to populate many disparate areas on our planet. Many other animals depend totally on one food source for their energy, and this limited diet restricts where they can live to locations that provide the type of food they need.

How do we end up with tastes that vary across different cultures? One researcher persuaded a group of people raised on Chinese food to try out a ripe stilton cheese, and a group of gourmet cheese lovers to try a Chinese delicacy known as a "Thousand Year Old Egg," a preserved fermented raw duck egg. Both groups, trying these tastes for the first time, found them repulsive. In other words, our taste preferences are in part learned, as a result of cultural experiences.

A delicacy like candied grasshoppers may not be highly valued outside of Mexico, nor would termite-cakes be as appreciated as they are in Liberia. And how many Americans relish roast dog, a traditional favorite in Samoa?

Taste Genes

Can you inherit a sweet tooth? No doubt about it! In fact, about one fifth of your taste preference is genetic. Your food preferences are a result of the combined influence of biology (genetics) and environment (what you were exposed to).

To see an example of the genetic influence on taste preferences, take this quiz[c]:

- Do you prefer your coffee with cream and/or sugar?
- Do you dislike cabbage and brussels sprouts?
- Do you find grapefruit exceedingly bitter?
- Do you find some sweets just too sickeningly sweet?

If you answered a definitive "yes" to most of those questions, you are a PROP super-taster.

PROP tasters also responded "yes" to most of the questions, but perhaps not so vehemently.

PROP non-tasters have minimal reactions to strong flavors and responded "no" to most questions.

PROP is a gene marker, an abbreviation for a chemical compound called 6-n-propylthiouracil. If you can detect it, you are more sensitive to many tastes. Sugar seems sweeter to you, and grapefruit and broccoli seem more bitter. Fatty foods taste too strong.

If neither biological parent gave you the PROP taster gene, you are a "non-taster." Bitter tastes don't bother you. In fact, you probably enjoy brussels sprouts and grapefruit.

If you got two PROP genes, you are a super-taster. Brussels sprouts are repulsive to you.

About half of Caucasians are PROP tasters. One quarter are super-tasters, and one quarter are non-tasters. People of African or Asian heritage are more likely to be prop tasters than Caucasians. (About 25-30 percent of Mediterranean peoples are non-tasters; 3 percent of West Africans; and 2 percent of Navajos. In Asia, 43 percent of Indians are non-tasters, and 7 percent in Japan[41].)

Extensive research has been conducted on PROP. In one study, researchers made two oil and vinegar dressings, one 10 percent oil and the other 40 percent oil. Non-tasters could not tell the two apart; tasters could tell them apart and preferred the lower oil version.

In another experiment, students were given various sugar water solutions. PROP tasters hated the more sugary mixes.

In general, PROP tasters are people with sensitive taste buds, so they are more alert to different flavors and need less intensity to get good flavor. The advantage to this is that they may not be as drawn to sweets and high-fat foods. A disadvantage is that they may also turn away from vegetables and fruit.

Being a PROP taster is not inherently good or bad, but one lesson that can be learned from the PROP research is that everyone has individual tastes, and there is no such thing as an objectively good- or bad-tasting food. It may be helpful to learn about your taste preferences so you can use them to your best advantage.

For example, PROP tasters may want to put extra energy into finding fruits and vegetables that they like, or experiment with different methods of preparation to cut the bitterness they perceive. Surprisingly, a sour taste, like lemon juice, can eliminate the bitterness of vegetables, so a sprinkle of lemon juice may make vegetables more appealing.

PROP non-tasters could put energy into recognizing subtle differences and limiting themselves to foods that really taste good. For example, they could develop their sensitivity to negative allesthesia.

Interestingly, PROP tasters not only have more sensitive taste buds, but are more sensitive in other ways too. For example, research shows that they react to medicines at a lower dose, have a lower tolerance for pain, are more introverted, and seek less stimulus. It may be that genes for those traits are frequently linked to PROP genes.

---

[c] Adapted from Neal Barnard's *Turn off the Fat Genes.*

Also interesting, is that couples and groups of friends are often similar in their taste patterns. Food may play such a large role in our lives that we are (unconsciously) drawn to people with similar taste preferences.

Environment rules!

Though genetics play a role in forming your taste preferences, environment is the stronger influence. Food preferences start to get formed in utero, progress in infancy, and change as we interact with family, friends, and the larger culture. Your food preferences are in large part formed and most strongly developed during the first few years of your life (like your personality).

Toddlers can learn to enjoy anything, from raw fruits and vegetables, to hamburgers and fries, depending on what people around them eat and like. (Don't expect your kid to like vegetables if you don't regularly eat and enjoy them!)

Most of us get stuck in these food preferences, but others increase their exposure to different foods and change their tastes over time. Fortunately, we have a remarkable ability to learn to love the taste of almost anything, on repeated exposure. You can change your tastes over time.

Flavoring in Food

When you eat a freshly picked, ripe strawberry, there are hundreds of natural compounds in the strawberry that combine to give you the flavor that you perceive. Since many flavor compounds are fragile, the quicker a ripe strawberry gets from the plant to your mouth, and the less it is handled and altered along the way, the more flavorful it is likely to be. That explains why freshly picked produce from your garden or the farmers' market often tastes so much better than produce from the supermarket, or produce in its frozen or canned state.

Food Processing

As citizens in a modern world, few of us grow and prepare our own food. Instead, we rely on a gigantic and hugely profitable food industry to provide it for us, and many of us are unaccustomed to the flavors of food in its original form.

The term **"processed foods"** is used to describe foods that have undergone some type of "process" or alteration from their original form. Examples of food processing include the addition of preservatives, flavorings or colorings, or techniques such as dehydrating, freezing, pre-cooking, or canning.

About 90 percent of the money Americans spend on food goes towards processed food. It is one of the ironies of modern life that as people become wealthier, their foods become less naturally flavorful and nutritious.

To understand the flavoring of foods, let's take a closer look at what happens to the food before it gets to our plate. We'll use a French fry as an example, following a potato through the factory and restaurant, and eventually to your palate. (The following was drawn from *Fast Food Nation*, written by investigative journalist Eric Schlosser.)

- Potatoes are grown, harvested, loaded on trucks, and delivered to manufacturing plants.
- Trucks dump the potatoes onto spinning rods, which let the small potatoes, rock and dirt fall to the ground and hold onto the larger potatoes.
- The rods lead to a rock trap, which is a pond of water in which the potatoes float and the remaining rocks fall to the ground.
- Water currents are manipulated so that potatoes of the same size float into different areas.
- The potatoes are transferred to conveyor belts and blasted with steam for 12 seconds, which boils the water under their skins and then explodes their skins off.

- A high pressure hose shoots the potatoes at a speed of 117 feet per second through a grid of sharpened knife blades, creating perfectly sliced french fries.
- Video cameras scrutinize the fries from different angles, looking for flaws.
- When a fry with a blemish is detected, a sorting machine uses compressed air to knock the fry onto another conveyor belt where tiny automated knives remove the blemish. The fry is then returned to main conveyor belt.
- Sprays of hot water blanch the fries.
- Gusts of hot air dry them.
- The fries are dropped in boiling oil until they are just slightly crispy.
- Air cooled by compressed ammonia gas quickly freezes them.
- The potatoes are then sealed in bags and loaded (by robots) onto wooden pallets, then delivered to a freezer until they are ready for delivery to a fast food restaurant.

Amazing process, huh? Particularly when you consider that there is no human involvement along the route – all manipulation is done by stationary machines and robots.

There are only a few french fry manufacturing companies that supply the french fries to most of the fast food eateries. They all use the same types of potatoes, the same basic technology for processing them, yielding virtually identical end products. However, the french fries taste different at many of these eateries. What accounts for the taste difference?

First, remember that flavor chemicals are very fragile. As a result, most of the flavor from the original potato has been lost through processing, leaving the end product with little or no taste. This is actually beneficial to the manufacturers, who are looking for consistency in their products (obviously not provided by nature). If the potatoes had taste remaining, they would have to treat each batch differently to make sure the final product was flavored appropriately. If on the other hand, they have a blank palette to work with, they can just add the same flavoring each time and don't have to adjust their recipe.

The final taste is created by the purchasers - the fast food restaurants - who buy these fries from the manufacturing plants. They add flavor chemicals to oil, and then deep-fry them before selling them to you, which imparts a flavor to the otherwise bland potatoes. It is the flavoring chemicals in the oil that distinguishes the restaurants.

Let's take a few steps back and examine what is meant by flavor chemicals. As discussed earlier, foods naturally contain hundreds of different compounds that ultimately contribute to its flavor. Eat a freshly baked potato, and your senses get hit by those molecules. The flavor messages contained in the molecules get summed along with nerve responses from any associations you might have and other responses – and that turns into your perception of the potato's flavor.

After a food manufacturer has processed a potato, however, many of the potato flavor compounds have been damaged. To reintroduce that flavor into their final product, the food manufacturers turn to chemists. Good flavor chemists can do wonders with re-creating tastes. A little chemical manipulation and even this book can be made to taste like a french fry.

Sometimes chemists extract all the flavor chemicals from an unprocessed product, concentrate them, and use them in flavoring other products. Though ideal, making this "natural flavor extract" is an expensive process, so it is not regularly conducted.

Another option is to identify the dominant compounds that give the potato its flavor and reproduce only those. This is much more commonly conducted. So "potato flavoring" is much more intense than the flavoring in the actual potato and does not contain all of the original potato's subtlety and complexity.

There are many different ways to make the flavor chemicals once they are identified, and flavor laboratories are big business (annual revenues of about $14 billion). How do they actually make the flavors?

One method uses a solvent to extract particular compounds from the original product. For example, you can add a particular solvent to bananas to remove the amyl acetate, which is the flavor chemical that dominates in the banana's flavor. Another option is to distill flavor compounds from the original product. A third way is to find a particular bacteria or yeast that can ferment a particular compound when given a particular food.

Natural and Artificial Flavors

Many consumers believe that natural is "healthy," as opposed to anything made or processed by humans, which is inherently evil and harmful. So we look for "natural flavor" on labels, and willingly spend more money than we would for "artificial flavor." However, the legal definition of the word "natural" is deceptive.

In simple terms, a "natural flavor" is legally defined as a substance derived from plant or animal matter. This means that any of the above methods could be used. "Natural apple flavor" may be made from ingredients that have never been on an apple tree. In fact, "natural flavor" rarely refers to extracting and concentrating the flavor essence from the original product, which is a costly process. It most often refers to the compounds created as a result of bacterial fermentation.

In fact, a "natural flavor" doesn't even need to come from the very food it is flavoring. For example, the amyl acetate which is often used to make "natural banana flavor" is typically derived from peach pits.

In reality, "natural flavors" are usually the result of laboratory manipulation – and rarely have much to do with the product they are designed to resemble.

Consider "natural smoke flavor." This is made by charring sawdust (a plant product, so it's "natural") and capturing the released aroma chemicals. This smoke is then turned into a liquid with a solvent and bottled. Many restaurants use "natural smoke flavor" and paint on grill marks to give the illusion that the food was cooked over an open fire.

An artificial flavor, on the other hand, is defined by the Food and Drug Administration (FDA) as any substance that does *not* fit the definition of a natural flavor. As an example, amyl acetate (banana flavoring) can be made by mixing vinegar with amyl alcohol and adding sulfuric acid as a catalyst. By this (cheaper) method, the amyl acetate would be considered an "artificial flavor." The end product – the amyl acetate - is identical regardless of the process used, and once you have amyl acetate you have no way of knowing how it was derived, making the distinction between natural and artificial seem a little absurd.

Furthermore, you can't make the assumption that artificial products are bad while "natural" ones are good. Nature hides some unfriendly chemicals in our foods. The amygdalin found in "natural" apricot and peach pits, for example, contains traces of cyanide, the lethal gas that has been used to execute convicted criminals (but obviously not in a high enough dose to knock you off). Mix oil of clove and a banana flavor and you get the exact same almond flavor without the poison – but by this method its "*artificial* almond flavor."

Also, remember that the majority of flavor that you perceive in foods comes from its aroma. Most aromas are made from the same basic process: culturing bacteria in a lab so that they generate aroma chemicals. Flavor companies work simultaneously for many industries in addition to the food industry, as the basic science behind the taste of your frozen dinner is identical to that of the scent in your shampoo.

How do you know if a product contains added flavoring chemicals? Check the ingredients list. If it says the word "flavor," regardless of whether it reads "natural flavor" or "artificial flavor," it is a sure sign that chemists were involved.

Because flavor compounds are so potent, they are only present in minute amounts. One drop of the flavor compound that predominates in bell peppers, for example, could flavor five average-sized swimming pools[42]! So don't be surprised that flavor chemicals are the last ingredient on ingredients lists; though they are in small quantity, they still have a potent effect. (Ingredients lists are written in descending order of weight.)

While manufacturers are generally required to list all ingredients on an ingredients list, flavoring compounds provide an exception, and the specific ingredients found in flavor compounds are not required to be listed on nutrition labels. Many consumers report that they avoid products with long ingredients lists. Don't be deceived: if it says "natural flavor" it is likely that there are many chemical compounds that are part of that "natural flavor" but not listed. In fact, many flavor chemicals contain more ingredients than the foods they are contained in.

Laws regarding coloring compounds are similarly lax, with manufacturers not required to list the included ingredients. This shelters us from knowing some rather bizarre ingredients. For instance, the pink, red or purple color in many foods such as some strawberry yogurt, many fruit bars, fruit fillings, and some juice drinks, is called carmine, derived from the dried, ground bodies of insects who fed on red cactus berries. (Vegetarians, be wary: if your food has added flavor or color compounds, regardless of whether they are natural or artificial, there is no guarantee that it is animal-free.)

Who Owns Your Tastes?

I hope that you are now reading food labels, and more attuned to the word "flavor" appearing on the ingredients list. Whether the label says "natural flavor" or "artificial flavor," this is an indication that the taste you perceive is likely to have come from a laboratory cocktail as opposed to real food – and one is not necessarily better or worse for you than the other.

Now let's consider the implications of what we've learned. First, remember that little is objective about the taste of food: the flavor you perceive is in part mediated by your subjective experience, with surprisingly little unaltered information emanating from the food's flavor compounds. This means that you – and others – have extraordinary power to manipulate what foods are appealing to you.

Next, let's put this in the context of the extent to which modern food processing pervades our lives. As mentioned earlier, 90 percent of the money we spend on food goes towards processed foods. This means that we are much more accustomed to added "flavoring" than to the actual taste that is part of "real" foods. Added flavoring is much more intense than a food's original flavor and lacks its complexity. (Food processors tend to rely on simple intensity, like sweet and salt, and rarely bring in other taste sensations.)

Our tastes and physiology adapt to the foods we eat, and we come to expect this intensity. When processed foods are your regular diet – like most Americans – you come to need them to get good "flavor" from foods as you have lost your ability to perceive (and enjoy) a wide range of taste sensations.

Since most people are much more accustomed to "raspberry flavor" than to raspberries, they may be disappointed when they taste a real raspberry. It lacks the intense sweetness they have come to associate with raspberries, and their tastes are no longer sensitive to all the marvelous complexity of the fruit. Cook's Magazine, for example, recently found that in a blind taste test, chefs preferred vanilla flavoring to actual vanilla. Our industrial diet has dulled our taste for the "real" qualities of foods.

Check out food labels on the foods you commonly eat. How many products contain "natural flavor" or "artificial flavor," giving you the illusion that you are tasting food? Are you less drawn to unprocessed foods, like whole fruits and vegetables?

It is not surprising if you like to eat french fries at McDonalds and you find broccoli boring. Your tastes have been manipulated by a very powerful food industry. They have shaped your attitude, and even influenced changing the biology of how you perceive flavor to get you hooked on their processed foods. This is of course much more income-generating to the food industry than if you liked whole foods.

Is Processed Food Addictive?

The idea that junk food is addictive is a popular concept. A number of studies in rats show that sugar stimulates the release of opiates[43, 44], which make you feel good. Opiates in turn stimulate your appetite for more sugar. In high quantities, sugar has addictive qualities in rats. For example, when rats were fed a concentrated sucrose solution, they started to self-select more sugar, and they exhibited abstinence symptoms when it was withdrawn and anxiety when given an opiate blocker[45].

Studies on high-fat foods show a similar opiate response. It would not be surprising if all good-tasting food elicited similar results, though most other foods have not been as well studied. In fact, research in rodents shows that the absorption of calories in general is enjoyable. Further research indicates that even artificial sweeteners, such as aspartame and saccharin, trigger a pleasure response without any calories.

A drug called naloxone blocks opiate receptors in the brain. Inject some naloxone and you won't get a buzz from narcotics like morphine and heroin. Same thing happens when researchers injected human subjects with naloxone after being fed various sugar-fat mixtures like chocolate, cookies and ice cream[46-48]. The subjects got the calories, but without the fun. Apparently it was a bit like eating a dry cracker. Participants ate 90 percent fewer calories from Oreo cookies, 60 percent fewer from M&M's, and 46 percent fewer from Snickers bars[48], demonstrating that there isn't enough incentive to eat as much without the feel-good hit.

Researchers at Rockefeller University found that regularly eating fatty foods can quickly reconfigure the body's hormonal system to want more fat. They also found that early exposure to fatty food could influence children's choices to seek a similar diet as adults.

Does this indicate these foods are addictive? While some individuals may meet the lax psychiatric definition for addiction, I am hesitant to take this seriously. It just illustrates that we have pleasure pathways in our brain which are designed to reinforce certain survival behaviors. Eating is one of them, sex another. Narcotics use this same brain pathway. In so doing, the narcotics usurp a brain pathway meant to reward us for eating or attempting to reproduce.

There are of course some other considerations that make use of the term "addiction" problematic. I just can't conjure up the same level of concern when I consider someone eating ice cream compared to their shooting heroin. Nor does taking a kid to a McDonald's drive-through elicit the same reaction as carting them along while you visit your drug dealer. I also doubt that many murders have been committed to support a Kentucky Fried Chicken habit.

Regardless of whether the term "addiction" is appropriate, a drive towards eating particular foods can be an extremely painful experience. Should you avoid this drug-like high that you might get from some foods, and "just say no" to chocolate? To the contrary, I think we should celebrate that food makes us feel good. Why not enjoy your biologic reward system?

For optimal health and well-being, I'd like to add a couple suggestions to go along with the dictum to enjoy foods. First, know that you have a lot of other biologic systems that also support you in getting the nutrition you need. Remember the discussion of negative allesthesia earlier – your taste buds toning down after initial exposure? Pay attention to this as well and try to get the maximum enjoyment from foods. This will support you in eating moderate amounts.

It also helps to have other tools in your arsenal that make you feel good. Is your sugar/fat habit causing you harm? Are there other things you can sometimes do that are more effective at giving you the comfort or the high you seek? Occasional food indulgences keep us happy and pose little concern. Moderation seems to be the key.

It may be helpful to remember that you can change your tastes and take back your power to enjoy foods. You will find that food can taste so much better than what you currently believe to be good and that there is a wide range of taste sensations beyond sugar and salt!

Not only can you change your taste buds, but studies show that repetitive consumption of high-sugar and high-fat foods actually leads to neurochemical changes in the brain in areas involved in appetite and reward[49-51]. You essentially re-wire your brain to adapt to your new diet, resulting in cravings for that new diet.

Earlier I mentioned an interesting line of research which demonstrates that there is a gradual shift in tastes as a child progresses towards adulthood. Children's taste buds are initially set to enjoy one taste: sweet. Over time, the preference for sweet decreases and enjoyment of other tastes increases.

However, interesting studies in rats have shown that rats on high-fat diets never show the adult pattern, but continue to have predominantly sweet tastes. Because of similarities in physiology between rats and humans, it is anticipated that humans react similarly, although these studies have not been conducted[52]. So if you were fed a high-fat diet as a child, your taste buds may not have matured to allow you to be fully sensitive to pleasures beyond fat and sweet.

The Taste Preference Makeover

A large part of your taste preferences is a result of your past experiences. Many cells that play a role in your perception of taste adapt to the foods you are accustomed to. Apply a little conscious effort to get out of your rut and you can change your tastes.

For example, do you want to lose your sweet tooth? Taste buds have about a 3 week life span. Try cutting sweets out for 3 weeks. Because the sweet taste buds are now less used, your gene activity will adjust and regenerate less of them. Sweets that you used to like may now seem overly sweet and unappealing. (Apples may be much more tempting after this experiment than ice cream!) The same process can also work if you cut back slowly; it will just take more time.

Want to enhance your sense of taste? Eat slowly, and allow the food to mix throughout your mouth. The longer you chew, the more taste cells get exposed; and as food becomes more liquid, additional molecules vaporize, taking it into the olfactory zone. The flavor intensifies and becomes more complex.

Also, maximize variety. Taste and smell, like all senses, react strongly to change and surprise, but stop responding if they keep getting the same stimulus. That's why wine-tasters wait about 30 seconds between sips, a strategy that also works with food.

Check out this experiment to take advantage of negative allesthesia. Get some good chocolate (or some other food that tastes particularly good to you), and take a bite. Savor that first bite, let it roll around your mouth before swallowing. Notice all the sensations. Then take another bite, same process. Then another. At some point you will notice that the chocolate stops tasting as good. If you become more attentive to the taste, you may find that it takes less to satisfy you; you are only interested when the chocolate tastes really good!

Action Tips…

Food is good stuff, and I hope that we can all learn to reclaim the joy of eating good-tasting food. However, you may find that the foods that are most pleasurable to you conflict with other values you have – for example, the drive to eat health-enhancing foods or "environmentally-sensitive" foods. What to do? I suggest a two-step process.

The first step is to figure out if the food is really as pleasurable to you as you think it is.

Are you really enjoying your food?

Don't underestimate the importance of tasty food. When you eat what you want, and allow yourself to truly experience the pleasure, you feel satisfaction and contentment, which allows you to comfortably stop eating.

Many people eat out of habit, without being conscious that they are making a choice and that choice has an impact. For example, you may love the Sunday family brunches and consistently overeat. Then you feel too tired and lazy afterwards to participate in the fun of throwing around a football. Once you start to make the connection that the food is not as pleasurable an hour after you have eaten, you may choose to moderate your intake. You do this because it makes you feel better, not because you are trying to restrict your calories and diet –a much more effective strategy in the long run.

Or perhaps you always eat rice, whether or not you like it, because it is a part of your family culture. As you make your underlying reasons explicit, you recognize that you are making a choice and that you have the option to choose differently.

Be more attentive to how the food tastes. Focus on noticing negative allesthesia (your taste sensitivity toning down after initial exposure), and choose quality, fully tasting and enjoying each bite, as opposed to prioritizing quantity. Demand pleasure from your food. In fact, make it a priority.

The next step I suggest is to change your taste. Wouldn't it be great if you craved broccoli and tofu?

How to fully taste and enjoy your food
- Before eating, take some time to let go of your day, so you can appreciate your meal.
  - Establish a ritual that will help you become more present and connected with others. (In my family, we all hold hands, close our eyes, and take a minute of silence before eating our dinner. My 7-year-old son then asks a question which we all answer: the typical question is "what made you happy today?")
- Eat when you're hungry and stop when you're comfortably full. (There are actual physical mechanisms that make food taste better when you are appropriately hungry.)
- Eat your meals in a pleasant environment.
- Surround yourself with people you like.
- Make sure there are appealing smells that don't detract from your food. (The kitchen might not be the best place for the kitty litter box!)
- Pay attention to eating.
  - Turn off the television.
  - Eat slowly.
- Make your food look appealing.
  - Think about colors when you create your meals, use garnishes.

How to change your tastes
- Part of your taste biology adapts to what it is presented with. Change to the diet you want, and be patient. For many aspects, your tastes will eventually catch up.

- Experiment with different food preparations.
    - Try new restaurants/different ethnic treats.
    - Try recipes from cookbooks.
        - There are more ways to cook carrots than steaming or boiling them!
    - Have cooking clubs with friends/potlucks.
    - Join food-related organizations that regularly host potlucks.
    - Use a variety of spices (don't just limit yourself to salt and pepper).
    - Hate vegetables? Look for sauces that remove the aspects you don't like and highlight more appealing flavors.
        - Example: lemon eliminates the bitterness PROP tasters sense in vegetables.
- Educate yourself about the implications of your food choices. What you learn may just change your tastes. For example, your produce may taste better when you buy it directly from the friendly neighborhood farmer and know the culture you are supporting. You may lose your taste for fast food as you learn about its social and environmental costs.

Be patient and persistent. Know that your tastes won't change immediately.
- Your taste buds may change relatively quickly, but it is hard to erase a lifetime of habits and associations.
- You may not like some foods the first time you try them, but repeated exposure may change your mind.
- You can learn to be creative in the kitchen and make delicious foods!

Get informed...

Check out *Fast Food Nation* by Eric Schlosser. A kids' version of this book is also available: *Chew on This* by Schlosser and Wilson, targeted to teenagers.

Transforming Animals into Food

We eat food everyday without giving it much thought, rarely considering how the food was grown or made. We buy our bacon cured or our hamburger pre-ground into patties, neatly wrapped in styrofoam and cellophane and bearing no resemblance to the pig or cow that it once was. It is difficult to understand the consequences of modern agriculture and food processing when we are so distanced from the source of our food.

I believe that people should know how their food gets to their plate. Education enables us to make informed choices and be responsible consumers. This chapter provides some details about how we raise and slaughter animals for our food, with a focus on animal welfare. (Future chapters will examine this issue from other perspectives, such as the food safety and ecological ramifications of our farming practices.)

Farm animals are sentient beings. Like humans and our animal pets, they are intelligent animals, capable of a full a range of feelings, including pain, fear, boredom and joy. As farms have become larger and more industrialized, we began to view animals as a commodity, treating them as units of production rather than living, breathing beings.

The result – factory farming of animals - is horrifying. Hundreds of thousands of animals confined in a small space with no access to sunlight or the outdoors, no space to turn around, systematic mutilation procedures such as the painful debeaking of birds, fire branding, tail docking and castration of cattle - performed without anaesthesia. Chickens crammed tightly into tiny cages too small to allow them to even spread their wings.

And these practices are entirely legal: agriculture is exempt from most animal welfare laws that apply to our pets and wildlife and there is no federal law that protects animals from cruelty on the farm. When the New York Times (7/20/2004) reported on sadistic practices at Pilgrim's Pride slaughter plant in West Virginia, where plant workers were videotaped "jumping up and down on live chickens, drop-kicking them like footballs, and slamming them into walls," the workers hadn't violated any federal laws.

The following are excerpts from a pamphlet prepared by Vegan Outreach (www.veganoutreach.org) called "Transforming Animals into Food," which helps to educate on factory farm conditions. Vegan Outreach has generously given me permission to reproduce them.

THE TRANSFORMATION OF ANIMALS INTO FOOD

Many people believe that animals raised for food must be treated well because sick or dead animals would be of no use to agribusiness. This is not true.

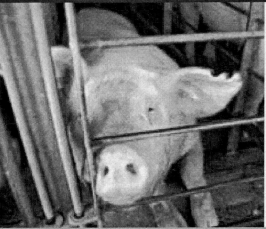

INDUSTRIALIZED CRUELTY: *FACTORY FARMING*

The competition to produce inexpensive meat, eggs, and dairy products has led animal agribusiness to treat animals as objects and commodities. The worldwide trend is to replace small family farms with "factory farms"—large warehouses where animals are confined in crowded cages or pens or in restrictive stalls.

"U.S. society is extremely naive about the nature of agricultural production.

"[I]f the public knew more about the way in which agricultural and animal production infringes on animal welfare, the outcry would be louder."

BERNARD E. ROLLIN, PhD
Farm Animal Welfare, Iowa State University Press, 1995

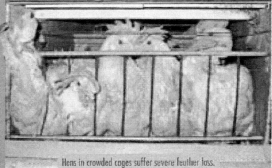

Hens in crowded cages suffer severe feather loss.

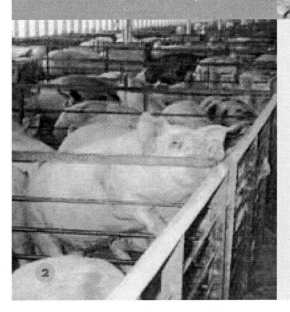

Bernard Rollin, PhD, explains that it is "more economically efficient to put a greater number of birds into each cage, accepting lower productivity per bird but greater productivity per cage... individual animals may 'produce', for example gain weight, in part because they are immobile, yet suffer because of the inability to move.... Chickens are cheap, cages are expensive."[1]

In an article recommending space be reduced from 8 to 6 square feet per pig, industry journal *National Hog Farmer* suggests that "Crowding pigs pays."[2]

2

Inside a broiler house.

Birds Virtually all U.S. birds raised for food are factory farmed.[3] Inside the densely populated buildings, where they are confined their entire lives, enormous amounts of waste accumulate. Manure fumes can cause eye and respiratory infections and other diseases.[4]

Egg-Laying Hens Packed in cages (typically less than half a square foot of floor space per bird),[5] hens can become immobilized and die of asphyxiation or dehydration. Decomposing corpses are found in cages with live birds.

Stress can make caged birds peck each other. To combat this, the ends of their beaks are cut off with hot blades, causing severe pain for weeks.[6] Some, unable to eat afterwards, starve.[1]

When her production declines, a U.S. hen is either slaughtered or "force molted"— deprived of food for days to shock her body into another laying cycle.[3]

1 Bernard E. Rollin, PhD, *Farm Animal Welfare* (Iowa State University Press, 1995).
2 11/15/93.
3 Peter Cheeke, PhD, textbook *Contemporary Issues in Animal Agriculture*, 2004.
4 *Diseases of Poultry*, 1997.
5 USDA APHIS VS, *Reference of 1999 Table Egg Layer Management in the U.S.*, 1/00.
6 *Appl Anim Behav Sci*, 1990;27:149–57.

"For modern animal agriculture, the less the consumer knows about what's happening before the meat hits the plate, the better.

"If true, is this an ethical situation?

"Should we be reluctant to let people know what really goes on, because we're not really proud of it and concerned that it might turn them to vegetarianism?"

PETER CHEEKE, PhD
Oregon State University Professor of Animal Agriculture
Contemporary Issues in Animal Agriculture, 2004 textbook

For more information on factory farming (including its impacts on the environment), and other reasons to become vegan, please see WhyVegan.org

3

Chick being debeaked.

Pigs In the September 1976 issue of the industry journal *Hog Farm Management*, John Byrnes advised: "Forget the pig is an animal. Treat him just like a machine in a factory."

Today's pig farmers have done just that. As Morley Safer related on *60 Minutes*: "This [the movie *Babe*] is the way Americans want to think of pigs. Real-life 'Babes' see no sun in their limited lives, with no hay to lie on, no mud to roll in.

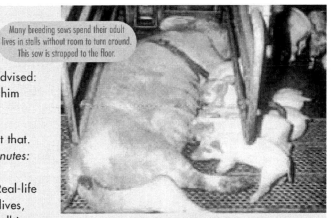

Many breeding sows spend their adult lives in stalls without room to turn around. This sow is strapped to the floor.

The sows live in tiny cages, so narrow they can't even turn around. They live over metal grates, and their waste is pushed through slats beneath them and flushed into huge pits."[7]

Dairy Cows From 1940 to 1999, average per-cow milk production rose from 2.3 to 8.9 tons per year;[8] some cows have surpassed 30 tons.[9] High milk production leads to udder ligament damage, mastitis, and lameness.[3,10]

It is unprofitable to keep cows alive once their milk production declines. They are usually killed at 5–6 years of age,[10] though their normal life span exceeds 20.

Dairy cows are rarely allowed to nurse their young.[10] Many male calves are slaughtered immediately, while others are raised for "special-fed veal"—kept in individual stalls and chained by the neck on a 2–3 foot tether for 18–20 weeks before being slaughtered.[11]

Cow with swollen udder on modern dairy farm in California.

"Mrs. DeBoer said she had never milked a cow by hand, and never expected to. In the factory that is her barn, the employees, almost entirely Latino, manage the machinery.

"'It's just a factory is what it is', she said. 'If the cows don't produce milk, they go to beef.'"

"Urban Sprawl Benefits Dairies in California", *The New York Times*, 10/22/99

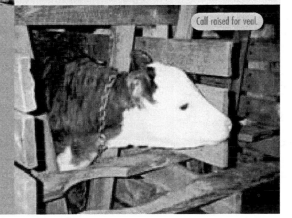

Calf raised for veal.

Transport Crammed together, animals must stand in their own excrement while exposed to extreme weather in open trucks, sometimes freezing to the trailer.[12] These conditions can result in "downers"—animals too sick or weak to walk, even when shocked with electric prods or beaten. Downers are dragged by chains to slaughter or to "dead piles" where they are left to die.[13]

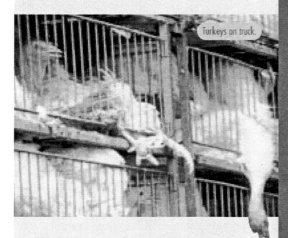

Turkeys on truck.

What about Fish? An Institute of Medical Ethics (U.K.) panel tentatively concluded that fish feel pain. Panel member Patrick Bateson wrote, "Few people have much fellow feeling for fish even though many fish are long-lived, have complicated nervous systems, and are capable of learning complicated tasks."[14]

Industrial fishing is seriously damaging ocean ecosystems.[15] Each year, in addition to countless fish, approximately 80,000 dolphins and thousands of other marine mammals are snagged in fishing nets worldwide. Most die.[16]

"Like this bull I had last year— this bull was one of the biggest bulls I've ever seen. It was at the very front of the trailer. And the spirit it had, he was just trying his hardest to get off the trailer. He had been prodded to death by three or four drivers...but his back legs, his hips have given out. And so basically they just keep prodding it. So it took about 45 minutes to get it from the front nose of the trailer to the back ramp....

"Then from there it was chained with its front legs, and it fell off the ramp, smashed onto the floor, which I don't know how many feet that would be but quite a racket...I just said, 'Why don't you shoot the damn thing? What's going on? What about this Code of Ethics?'

"This one guy said, 'I never shoot. Why would I shoot a cow that can come off and there's still good meat there?' When I first started, I talked to another trucker about downers. He said, 'You may as well not get upset. It's been going on for many years. It will go on for the rest of my life and your life. So just calm down about it. It happens. You'll get kind of bitter like I did. You just don't think about the animals. You just think that they aren't feeling or whatever.'"

interview with a Canadian livestock trucker from *A Cow at My Table*, 1998 documentary

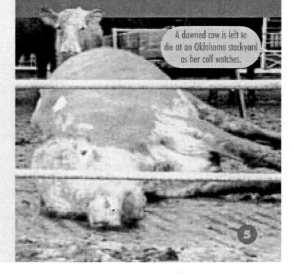

A downed cow is left to die at an Oklahoma stockyard as her calf watches.

7 "Pork Power," *60 Minutes*, 6/22/03.

8 USDA NASS, *Agricultural Statistics 2001*.

9 Associated Press, 9/20/96.

10 Textbook *Scientific Farm Animal Production*, 6th edition, 1998.

11 USDA, *Animal Welfare Issues Compendium*, 9/97.

12 USDA, *Survey of Stunning & Handling*, 1/7/97.

13 Video footage from *The Down Side of Livestock Marketing* (Farm Sanctuary, 1991).

14 *New Scientist*, 4/25/92.

15 "Overfishing Disrupts Entire Ecosystems," *Science*, 2/6/98.

16 *Science*, 5/14/99.

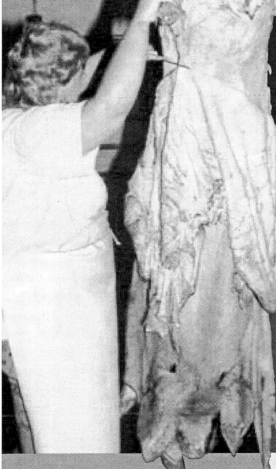

IF SLAUGHTERHOUSES HAD GLASS WALLS...

If they survive the farms and transport, the animals—whether factory-farmed or free-range— are slaughtered.

Federal law requires that mammals be stunned prior to slaughter (exempting kosher and halal). Common methods:

▶ Captive bolt stunning – A "pistol" is set against the animal's head and a metal rod is thrust into the brain. Shooting a struggling animal is difficult, and the rod often misses its mark.[17]

▶ Electric stunning – Current produces a grand mal seizure; then the throat is cut. According to industry consultant Temple Grandin, PhD, "Insufficient amperage can cause an animal to be paralyzed without losing sensibility."[12]

"It takes 25 minutes to turn a live steer into steak at the modern slaughter-house where Ramon Moreno works....

"The cattle were supposed to be dead before they got to Moreno. But too often they weren't.

"'They blink. They make noises', he said softly. 'The head moves, the eyes are wide and looking around'.

"Still Moreno would cut. On bad days, he says, dozens of animals reached his station clearly alive and conscious. Some would survive as far as the tail cutter, the belly ripper, the hide puller.

"'They die', said Moreno, 'piece by piece.'"

"Modern Meat: A Brutal Harvest"
The Washington Post, 4/10/01

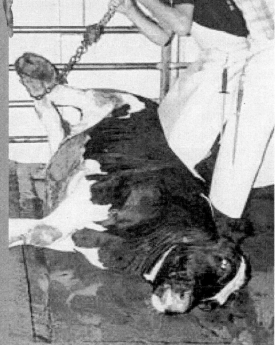

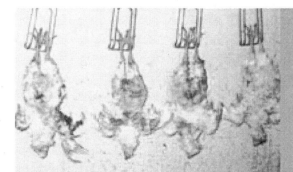

"In my opinion, if most urban meat eaters were to visit an industrial broiler house, to see how the birds are raised, and could see the birds being 'harvested' and then being 'processed' in a poultry processing plant, they would not be impressed and some, perhaps many of them would swear off eating chicken and perhaps all meat."

PETER CHEEKE, PhD
Contemporary Issues in Animal Agriculture, 2004 textbook

"Hogs, unlike cattle, are dunked in tanks of hot water after they are stunned to soften the hides for skinning. As a result, a botched slaughter condemns some hogs to being scalded and drowned. Secret videotape from an Iowa pork plant shows hogs squealing and kicking as they are being lowered into the water."[18]

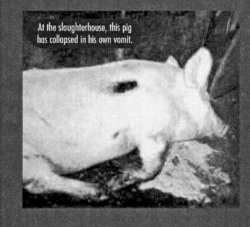

At the slaughterhouse, this pig has collapsed in his own vomit.

To induce paralysis in birds for ease of handling, electric stunning is normally used. However, it is not known whether stunning renders the birds unconscious;[1] the shock may be an "intensely painful experience."[19] Each year, large numbers of chickens, turkeys, ducks, and geese reach the scalding tanks alive and are either boiled to death or drowned.[20,21]

17 *Meat & Poultry*, 3/97.
18 "Modern Meat: A Brutal Harvest," *Washington Post*, 4/10/01.
19 "Humane Slaughter of Poultry: The Case Against the Use of Electrical Stunning Devices," *J Ag & Env Ethics*, 7/94.
20 USDA FSIS Animal Disposition Reporting System, 1998.
21 USDA FSIS, *Meat and Poultry Inspection Manual*, part 11.

"You have just dined, and however scrupulously the slaughterhouse is concealed in the graceful distance of miles, there is complicity."

RALPH WALDO EMERSON
"Fate," *The Conduct of Life*, 1860

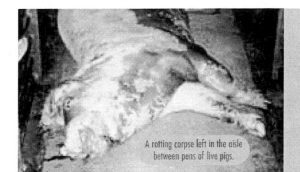

A rotting corpse left in the aisle between pens of live pigs.

Stories from
BEHIND THE WALLS

If you go behind the walls the industry erects to hide the truth, you will find the situation worse than you could have imagined.

Not Your Childhood Image by lauren Ornelas, VivaUSA.org

When I saw what life is really like for pigs on today's farms, I was left feeling physically sick for days. I suppose I knew they lived on concrete, indoors in factory farms. However, I was not prepared for the intensity of their confinement, and the awful reality of their boredom.

"Do we, as humans, having an ability to reason and to communicate abstract ideas verbally and in writing, and to form ethical and moral judgments using the accumulated knowledge of the ages, have the right to take the lives of other sentient organisms, particularly when we are not forced to do so by hunger or dietary need, but rather do so for the somewhat frivolous reason that we like the taste of meat?

"In essence, should we know better?"

PETER CHEEKE, PhD
Contemporary Issues in Animal Agriculture, 2004 textbook

In the gestation shed, I heard a constant clanging noise. It was the sows hitting their heads against their cage doors as if trying to escape. After a while, some would give up and lie down, while others again took up their futile action.

I saw the pens where pigs are fattened up for slaughter—essentially concrete cells, each holding about a dozen pigs. In one pen, there was a pig missing an ear. Another had a rupture the size of a grapefruit protruding from his stomach. A dead pig was constantly nudged and licked by others. The stench in these places is overwhelming.

Pig with stomach rupture.

At the larger farms I visited in North Carolina, there were thousands of pigs housed in sheds. Many were dead or dying—one actually died right in front of me as I videotaped. Dead pigs had been left in the pens with the living; other pigs had been tossed in the aisles— barely alive, unable to reach food or water.

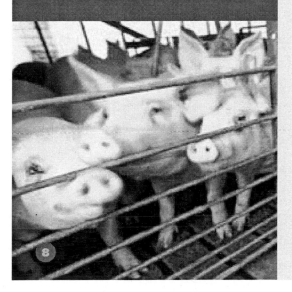

8

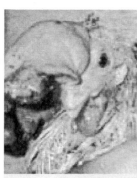

Lynn, just rescued from the manure pits, her comb caked with feces.

The Rescue from ISECruelty.com

On May 23, 2001, investigators openly rescued eight hens, in dire need of immediate veterinary care, from a factory farm in Cecilton, Maryland.

Jane, a hen found pinned by one wing in the wire bars of her cage, survived the amputation of her wing and enjoyed sunbathing, running through the grass, dust-bathing, jumping onto her perch at night, and eating her favorite treat—grapes. Jane was free from the exploitation of the egg industry for six months before succumbing to cancer.

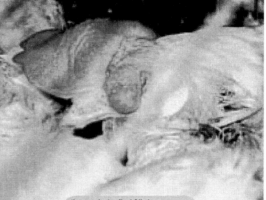

Christina had a fluid-filled cyst covering her eye when rescuers found her.

Above: Jane, immediately after rescue, waiting to be examined by a veterinarian before being taken to her new home. Right: Jane, just three months after rescue.

The hens, practically featherless and very despondent when rescued, were given a second chance at life. One year later, Jane's seven friends are alive and doing well—enjoying a virtual paradise compared to their former existence inside a factory farm. Unfortunately, approximately 280 million hens remain in U.S. battery cages.

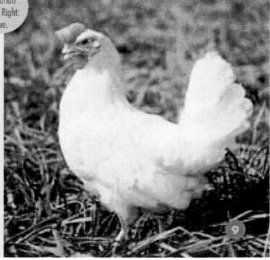

9

Widening the Circle

Male chicks, of no economic value to the egg industry, are found dead and dying in a dumpster behind a hatchery. Typically they are gassed[1] or ground up alive.[11] Other standard agricultural practices—often performed without anesthesia—include castration, tail docking, debeaking, dehorning, toe trimming, and branding.[11]

Entangled in the bars of her cage, a hen is left with no access to food or water.

"Historically, man has expanded the reach of his ethical calculations, as ignorance and want have receded, first beyond family and tribe, later beyond religion, race, and nation.

"To bring other species more fully into the range of these decisions may seem unthinkable to moderate opinion now. One day, decades or centuries hence, it may seem no more than 'civilized' behavior requires."

"What Humans Owe to Animals"
The Economist, 8/19/95

"True human goodness, in all its purity and freedom, can come to the fore only when its recipient has no power.

"Humanity's true moral test, its fundamental test (which lies deeply buried from view), consists of its attitude towards those who are at its mercy: animals.

"And in this respect humankind has suffered a fundamental debacle, a debacle so fundamental that all others stem from it."

MILAN KUNDERA
The Unbearable Lightness of Being, 1984

Crated calves live in their own excrement.

"Humans—who enslave, castrate, experiment on, and fillet other animals—have had an understandable penchant for pretending animals do not feel pain. A sharp distinction between humans and 'animals' is essential if we are to bend them to our will, make them work for us, wear them, eat them—without any disquieting tinges of guilt or regret.

Ducks and geese are force-fed to produce liver pâté.

"It is unseemly of us, who often behave so unfeelingly toward other animals, to contend that only humans can suffer. The behavior of other animals renders such pretensions specious. They are just too much like us."

**DR. CARL SAGAN &
DR. ANN DRUYAN**
Shadows of Forgotten Ancestors, 1992

10

Humans are omnivores, meaning that we have the ability to eat and obtain nutrients from a wide range of foods. We have evolved to have choice: we can survive with animal foods as part of our diets or as vegans, and a well-chosen diet in either of these categories can supply us with all of the nutrients we need.

After learning about how farm animals are raised and slaughtered, some people choose to become vegan and eliminate animal products from their diets entirely. Some vegans believe that we don't have a right to kill animals for food, while others assert that there is no way to continue eating animal products without being part of an inhumane system. (There are of course many other reasons people choose veganism.)

Becoming vegan is clearly one option, and the sections of the Vegan Outreach pamphlet that I chose not to include give more details on veganism. I encourage interested readers to view the full pamphlet available at the Vegan Outreach website.

Others choose to buy their animal foods from farmers who show more respect for the animals they raise. While most acknowledge that there is no pleasant way to kill an animal, there are ways to make the process less objectionable. For example, the U.K. Farm Animal Welfare Council proposes that animals should at least be protected from unnecessary suffering. They suggest that an animal's welfare be considered in terms of the following "5 Freedoms"[53]:

1) Freedom from hunger and thirst—by ready access to fresh water and a diet to maintain full health and vigour;
2) freedom from discomfort—by providing an appropriate environment including shelter and a comfortable resting area;
3) freedom from pain, injury, or disease—by prevention or rapid diagnosis and treatment;
4) freedom to express normal behaviour—by providing sufficient space, proper facilities, and company of the animal's own kind;
5) freedom from fear and distress—by ensuring conditions and treatment which avoid mental suffering.

Legal reforms would be necessary to ensure that the "5 Freedoms" are adopted (and enforced!).

The Humane Society of the United States suggests the "three Rs to humane eating:" refine, reduce and replace.

- "Refine" refers to recognizing that some practices are more cruel than others, and that you can use your consumer power to choose more humane options. For example:
  - ➢ You can pass on the foie gras, a product of particularly extreme cruelty. To make foie gras, ducks are confined to dark sheds and force fed enormous quantities of food through a metal pipe shoved down their throats. These ducks have difficulty walking, standing, and even breathing, but are prized for their fatty livers, considered to be a delicacy.
  - ➢ You can reconsider eating veal[d]. Veal calves are separated from their mothers within days of birth and crammed into individual stalls or crates, barely bigger than their own bodies. They are tethered by their necks to ensure minimal movement and deprived of certain essential nutrients, both of which result in more tender meat.
  - ➢ You can choose to support producers who are raising animals without intensive confinement.

---

[d] More humanely raised veal is available though it's hard to find. Look for "pink veal," which comes from calves raised in group pens or on pasture. They are fed a normal diet of grass, hay and milk.

With a little research you can learn more about the practices involved in producing your favorite foods and options for finding foods produced under less objectionable practices.

- "Reduce" refers to cutting back your consumption of animal-derived foods. In other words, the Humane Society suggests that we don't need to be pure - even a small reduction in the amount of animal foods we eat, particularly when amplified by many people making this choice, can make a difference.
- "Replace" reminds us that we can choose vegan alternatives.

Discussing these issues with your friends is another powerful way to amplify your statement. Of course, you can also get involved politically, supporting animal welfare organizations and sending a message to corporations and government that we can do better.

Fortunately, change is happening. Veganism is more commonly practiced. Many consumers are choosing more humane eating. And there are several campaign ballot measures and legislative bills under consideration which would improve various conditions. Free-range, humanely treated, and organically raised animals (free of hormones, routinely administered antibiotics, and genetic modification) are currently the fastest growing agricultural sector – and sales of "veggie meats" are also dramatically on the rise. You can join the growing movement of compassionate consumers.

Get informed...

- Check out *Fast Food Nation* by Eric Schlosser and *The Omnivore's Dilemma* by Michael Pollan.
- If you are interested in learning more about factory farming, check out:
  www.factoryfarms.org
  Vegan Outreach at www.veganoutreach.com
  Humane Society of the United States at www.hsus.org
  The Grace Factory Farm Organization, at www.factoryfarm.org
- View a short video clip called Meet Your Meat, which contains underground footage filmed at a slaughterhouse: www.peta.org or an animated video clip about factory farming at the Meatrix: http://www.bancruelfarms.org/meatrix/
- Here are some of the many activist organizations combating animal cruelty:
  Humane Society of the United States (www.hsus.org)
  Vegan Outreach (www.veganoutreach.org)
  People for the Ethical Treatment of Animals (www.peta.org)
  Fund for Animals (http://www.fund.org/Home/)
  Compassion Over Killing (http://www.cok.net/)
  Viva! USA (http://www.vivausa.org/)
  East Bay Animal Advocates (http://www.eastbayanimaladvocates.org)
  The Farm Animal Welfare Council (http://www.fawc.org.uk)
- Read about industry's perspective on animal cruelty or factory farming by checking out the website for the largest meat and poultry trade association, the American Meat Institute, at http://www.meatami.org, or another trade organization for the meat industry, the National Cattlemen's Beef Association (http://www.beef.org/).

Energy and Metabolism

Energy is the fuel our body runs on. Just as a car needs gas energy to power its movement, our body needs energy to operate.

Metabolism is a common term that gets bandied about to describe our use of energy. Most of us think of metabolism as calorie burning, in other words, getting rid of energy from our bodies. We say that those folks who use energy very quickly have a fast metabolism. Conversely, those folks who seem to pack on pounds even though they don't eat much are considered to have a slow metabolism.

For scientists, metabolism is a more general term used to refer to all the chemical reactions that occur within your body. It includes the chemical reactions in which you create larger molecules from simpler ones (anabolism), or break a larger compound down into smaller units (catabolism). For example, when you eat fat, your digestive tract breaks dietary fat's large molecules into smaller molecules that your body can absorb, and tissue cells further "catabolize" these smaller molecules to release their energy. Over-eat fat, and anabolic reactions take the small molecules that were absorbed (after the fat was digested) and link them up into molecules called triglycerides. Those are the molecules that plump up your hips and thighs, in the form of body fat.

Calories are your friend

Energy is measured in **calories**. Calories have a bad reputation in our modern industrialized world. We try to avoid them, and we willingly pay extra for food that's billed as having maximum taste and minimum calories. What we're really doing is paying extra for fuel that's been watered down to half of its original potency. You get less energy to run on. So why do we feel so self-righteous about paying top dollar to be duped?

Re-framing the bad guy

To get a grip on weight and good health, you need to reframe the role that the calorie has taken on. Open your mind to calories as essential sources of fuel required to survive, as opposed to villains who pack on pounds. (In other sections of the book, I hope to also open your mind so that you don't view body fat as a negative either.)

Counting Calories

It's interesting to note that for all the attention that's been paid to the calorie over the years, we never got it right. A calorie is actually a very small measure of energy, and its generic use is technically incorrect. The correct term is "**kilocalorie**," which refers to 1,000 calories. Kilocalories are abbreviated as kcals and often referred to as "k-cals."

Technically speaking, a calorie is the amount of heat flow required to raise the temperature of 1 gram of water 1 degree Celsius. In practical terms, think of a calorie as just a measure of energy, whether it's used to describe the energy in food or the energy that powers movement. For example, if you could harness food energy and put it to work, there is sufficient energy in 5 pounds of spaghetti to brew a pot of coffee. Or you could light a 60 watt light bulb for 90 minutes with a piece of pie.

When I was in graduate school, I burned a peanut to try to understand more about the energy it contained. I put the peanut in a loop of wire, and placed it under a test tube that contained 10 grams of water, and then lit it on fire. As the peanut burned, the water in the test tube started boil. When the peanut had finally burned in its entirety, the water in the test tube was reduced to 8 grams. Why did this occur? Energy was stored in the chemical bonds that held the peanut together, and the burning released this energy, converting the chemical energy into heat energy. The heat then raised the temperature of the water, causing some of it to evaporate.

Every time you eat, you engage in a similar process. Digestion is nothing more than a series of chemical reactions: you start with a large piece of food and progressively break it down into smaller and smaller pieces. Many of those small pieces then get absorbed into your body, and further broken down. In the process, you release the energy that is stored in the chemical bonds. Your body captures some of this energy, and transforms it to a form it can store or use to maintain itself. Some of the energy cannot be captured and dissipates from your body in the form of heat.

Let's take this a step further and see how much energy was contained in that peanut.

The burning peanut first warmed 10 grams of water from a tap water temperature of 20 degrees to a boiling temperature of 100 degrees. In other words, there was an 80 degree temperature change for 10 grams of water, which means an 800 degree change for each gram of water, or 800 calories. Next, two grams of water boiled away. Scientists have calculated that it takes 540 calories to boil one gram of water, so it therefore took 1080 calories to boil those two grams. This means that the burning peanut delivered 800 + 1080 calories, or a total of 1880 calories to that test tube of water. That translates to 1.88 kilocalories (abbreviated kcals), which is how much energy I was able to capture from that peanut in my experiment.

That's the general process nutrition scientists use to determine the amount of energy in food; they just use more technical equipment so they can keep the energy better contained. The equipment, called a bomb calorimeter, is a metal container surrounded by a water bath. The food sample is dried and made into a powder, and placed in the calorimeter. The calorimeter is then pumped full of oxygen at high pressure, and the food is ignited. There is a quick energy release - much like a bomb - the food is completely burned, and the energy is transferred to the metal and water, raising the water temperature and revealing the number of calories of energy that was contained in the food. The experiment I described earlier measured 1.88 kcals in a peanut. However, a great deal of the energy was lost in the air. This energy would not be lost in a calorimeter, and if we burned our peanut inside the calorimeter, we would find that a peanut actually contains about 6 kcals of energy.

"Eating Energy"

You have just one way to get energy into your body – and that's through eating. The food on your plate is described as "potential energy." Every time you eat, your body captures energy and turns it into something it can use or store. The energy your body doesn't use or store slips away in the form of heat.

Your body "burns" energy, not with flames, but with controlled chemical reactions that release the energy slowly. But the food releases the same amount of energy when it is broken down in the body as when it is burned.

For example, when you digest a banana, your body breaks the energy bonds that hold the food molecules together and captures the energy. A medium banana packs about 100 kilocalories of potential energy. If you digest and fully metabolize the banana, you capture much of that energy, which you can use as fuel. Whatever energy you don't use, you store. The laws of nature dictate that energy can never just disappear – you either use it, transform it into heat - or store it.

There is nothing magical about the amount of energy contained in foods. Only the macronutrients (and alcohol) provide energy in foods. The energy-producing nutrients always have the same calorie content. **Carbohydrates and protein always contain 4 kilocalories per gram, and fat always contains 9 kilocalories per gram**, so you can calculate the amount of energy provided by a nutrient by multiplying the kilocalories in a gram by the number of grams in the product. (Alcohol contains 7 kilocalories per gram.) You can then calculate the total amount of energy in a food by adding up the energy from each of the macronutrients. Other compounds in food (such as water, vitamins, minerals, or phytochemicals) don't contain usable energy, so they aren't considered when calculating the energy content of foods. We'll practice this in the "Food Label" section.

So, if you compare the same weight of foods, protein and carbohydrate contain less than half the energy that fat contains. Water is a filler that adds weight and bulk to foods, but no calories. That's why high-fat, dense foods are high in calories (like peanuts), while low-fat, water-packed foods (like celery) are lower in calories. Peanuts are 48% fat, 26% protein, 20% carbohydrate and 6% water. For comparison, celery is low in calories: it contains no fat, 1% protein, 5% carbohydrate, and 94% water.

There is a vast difference in calorie content between the peanut and a stick of celery because of the higher fat content and lower water content in peanuts. You get 550 calories in 100 grams of peanuts, compared to only 15 calories in the same weight of celery. This contradicts the myth that carbohydrates are fattening. They contain no more calories than protein, and both carbohydrates and protein contain less than half of the calories found in the same weight of fat.

Energy Balance/Imbalance

You have to do something with energy

Energy cannot be created or destroyed – it can only be converted from one form into another. This is an immutable fact, and one of the most important laws of nature. It is called the law of conservation of energy or the First Law of Thermodynamics.

When you eat food, its energy changes forms in one of these ways:
- Gets used for work – such as dancing, walking, thinking, fidgeting, breathing, etc.
- Flows from your body in the form of heat
- Packs away into storage.

In other words, when energy intake equals energy use, body energy stays the same (and so will weight, except for fluctuations due to water). Tip the balance, and you lose or gain energy. Take in more energy than you use, and you'll store the extra, leading to energy (and weight) gain. Spend more energy than you take in, and you have to use some of the energy stored on your body, resulting in energy loss (weight loss).

We can express the above in a simple mathematical formula, called the **energy balance equation**:

$$\text{Body Energy Change} =$$
$$\text{Amount of Energy Consumed} - \text{Amount of Energy Spent}$$

Or to use other words:
$$\text{Body Energy Change} = \text{Energy In} - \text{Energy Out}$$

Let's take a look at both sides of the energy balance equation.

Gaining Energy (Energy in)

Every time you eat, your body captures energy and turns it into something it can use or store. You have just one way to get energy into your body – and that's through eating.

Using energy (Energy out)

How we use energy (calories) is a little more confusing. There are three major components:
- resting metabolism

Copyright © Linda Bacon 2008.

- thermic effect of activity
- thermic effect of food.

Resting Metabolism

Every second you are alive, your bone marrow is making 2.5 million red blood cells to keep your body supplied with oxygen and nutrients and to tote away your cellular waste. Your brain is processing information through its trillion nerve cells, each connected to a hundred thousand others, helping to ensure that your heart beats and your lungs expand and contract.

No wonder we need a lot of energy to keep these complex processes cranking. Most of your energy goes to maintain these unseen functions. The rate that you use energy for these vital functions is called your **basal metabolic rate** (BMR).

Because it is so difficult to measure the energy consumed for basal metabolism (survival functions) alone, scientists frequently use a more expansive term, **resting metabolism**, which includes all of the energy consumed when one is in a resting state (e.g., lying down, fairly still). Resting metabolism is typically the largest component of energy use, accounting for about 60-70% of the average person's daily energy use.

That madly whirring brain of yours is the most energy-hungry of all organs. Even at rest, your brain is using about 20% of your body's energy, 10 times the rate of the rest of the body! (This is what makes the brain so vulnerable; cut off its energy supply for just 10 minutes and you get permanent brain damage.)

Each person has a characteristic resting metabolic rate. You use energy at a different rate than anyone else, even when you are doing nothing. The largest determinant of your resting metabolic rate is the amount of muscle tissue you have. That's because muscle is very active and requires a lot of energy to sustain. A large muscular man has a higher resting metabolism than a small woman. Fat tissue, on the other hand, is relatively inert and requires very little energy to sustain – which means it doesn't contribute much to your resting metabolism.

Many factors other than size figure in to resting metabolism; some of them are genetic and immutable. You may have been born with the ability to burn a lot of energy quickly and effortlessly, while others have a "sluggish metabolism" and don't use energy at a very fast rate.

For some people, that pumpkin pie will go right to the storage depots on their hips. Others use energy at such a fast rate that they'll burn it off before it settles on their body.

Wasting energy

What if you could just burn off extra energy from your body without doing anything? It is possible, and in fact the average person wastes about 7% of their energy every day. Scientists call this "adaptive thermogenesis." A protein called uncoupling protein (UCP) made in your fat tissue is the handy helper. (This protein essentially uncouples the burning of fat from energy production, meaning that when you burn fat, you create heat, but no usable energy.)

Some people make more UCP than others, and the amount you make plays a large role in your body size. If your gene for making UCP is very active, you have a faster metabolism and less body fat than most other people[54].

As you can imagine, scientists have examined UCP extensively in their efforts to find a magical weight loss technique. They've studied mice and found that ones bred with a specific UCP gene, human UCP-3, ate more than control mice, but were thinner, even though their activity levels were the same. One study showed that UCP-3 mice had only half as much body fat even though they ate as much as 50% more than normal mice[55].

Naturally, scientists are hard at work trying to figure out what activates the genes that create UCP. The answer to this question could help find a way to trigger this gene in people for whom it is suppressed, and rev up their sluggish metabolism.

One way to activate the gene that directs your body to make UCP is overeating. When some people overeat, their body compensates by making more UCP, thus burning off the excess calories. They can eat major quantities of food, without gaining weight. On the other side of the fence are those who make less UCP, and are more likely to gain body fat when they overeat.

Thermic effect of activity: moving to burn calories

Activity is the second highest calorie burner for most people. This category includes intentional exercise, such as running or jumping, as well as any activity your body performs beyond your resting metabolism. Technically called "thermic effect of activity," or TEA, it includes the fuel for unconscious activities (such as transmitting nerve messages as you read this page) and conscious movements (such as writing).

TEA accounts for about 30 percent of the average person's daily energy use (although of course it varies tremendously). If you're a young woman training to run a marathon, you may expend more energy on activity than you do supporting your basal metabolism. But if you're a sedentary older man, it may take only 15 percent of your energy to fuel your daily activity.

NEAT, an acronym used for non-exercise activity thermogenesis, is a part of TEA, and refers to the energy associated with unconscious behaviors such as maintaining your posture, fidgeting, crossing and uncrossing your legs, or just generally being restless.

The energy you use in NEAT matters a great deal in your weight[56]. If you're a constant fidgeter, this ongoing energy-burning can really add up and have a dramatic effect.

In one study designed to find out what happens to excess energy, scientists overfed participants 1,000 kilocalories a day for eight weeks[57]. As it turned out, only an average of 34 percent of the extra calories were stored as body fat. Surprisingly, two-thirds of the increase in energy use was on increased NEAT. Overeating simply pumped up their unconscious activity levels to "waste" the excess energy. Those participants who couldn't turn their NEAT switches on as readily stored more as body fat. Weight gain in the 16 participants varied from 2 to 16 pounds. Clearly, NEAT activity counts - and varies quite a bit between individuals.

But I don't advise you start pumping your legs or tapping your fingers as a route to weight loss. It's unlikely that you can consciously manipulate your NEAT to a great degree; you are either a fidgeter or not, and you are unlikely to change this for enough time to really matter.

Thermic effect of food: eating to burn calories

The thermic effect of food (TEF) refers to the energy it takes to metabolize the food you eat. This includes energy used for digestion, absorption, transport of nutrients, and storage or use. Your TEF is typically about 10 percent of the energy you use in a day.

Some foods need a higher TEF than others, and yes, this means that you can boost your TEF through your food choices. Protein stimulates your metabolism a little more than carbohydrates, and both of these stimulate your metabolism far more than fat, resulting in extra calories burned[58, 59].

Also, you need a lot of energy to convert carbohydrates and protein into fat and store it in your fat cells, so even if you overeat carbohydrates and protein, you're not going to be storing as much as you would if you overate high-fat foods. And the same amount of calories consumed in one meal results in a smaller TEF compared to spreading those calories out over several meals. So grazing - eating smaller, more frequent meals – also results in a higher TEF.

You will also have a higher TEF if you are efficient at storing carbohydrate energy and using fat as an energy source.

Going a long way on minimal fuel

The human body is remarkably efficient at using energy. It doesn't take much food energy to power us.

Suppose you wanted to run a marathon (26.2 miles). Depending on your conditioning and several other factors, you would burn about 100 calories per mile, or a total of 2,600 calories to fuel the run. A car, on the other hand, may be able to travel those 26 miles on a gallon of gasoline, which contains about 31,000 calories.

Think about it: a car needs twelve times as much energy! Viewed in another way, if you could drink gasoline instead of ice cream as a calorie source, you could run more than 300 miles to the gallon.

Too bad we can't build a car that's as fuel efficient as your body. We would celebrate that. But not too many of us appreciate this feature in our bodies – this level of efficiency is one of the main reasons you gain weight so easily.

Your personal metabolism: check it out?

Curious about how much energy you burn in a day? This can be calculated with a fair degree of precision by using high-tech lab equipment that measures the amounts of certain gases you exchange with the environment, but it's impossible to come up with an accurate number through mathematical formulas because of the high degree of variation among people. I suggest you ignore all the formulas (though one is provided in the Appendix if you're really curious). Knowing how many calories you burn in a day won't help you in regulating your weight anyway.

The average person consumes one million or more calories per year, yet weight changes very little in most people. What this tells us is that energy balance is regulated with a precision of greater than 99.5 percent[60]. This clearly far exceeds what you can consciously monitor. So why try? You won't be losing out when you give up on calorie counting. You're equipped with a much more effective system for healthy weight regulation.

Losing/Gaining Weight

You don't need to be a scientist to understand the basic theory behind weight loss and weight gain. The law of thermodynamics appears fairly straightforward. Weight loss is the result of simple math: eat fewer calories than you use. Diet and/or exercise plans based on this idea work well for short-term weight loss. On the other hand, whenever your body has excess calories, it converts them to fat, saving them for a rainy day and causing your weight to inch up.

The common weight loss prescription to eat less and/or exercise more seems logical enough. Does it work? Unfortunately not!

You're going to have to hold off until the weight regulation section for an explanation of why this fails, but for now, the short response is because you're not in control of the energy balance equation. Attempts you make to manipulate the equation may be met by compensatory changes that are beyond your control. You've got a fairly complicated built-in weight regulation system for weight control that can undermine your efforts. (For example, suppose you cut your calories. In response, your body could slow your basal metabolism, resulting in fewer calories burned.)

The news that your body can undermine your efforts at weight control is actually good, because it also demonstrates that your body is enormously successful at manipulating your weight. You don't have to take charge. Your body is perfectly capable of helping you maintain a healthy weight, if you let it do its job. (Details follow in the weight regulation section.)

Food Labels: How to Read Between the Lines

Food labels are an important tool to help assess the nutrient content of foods (although we will see that they do not provide us with all the information we need). Manufacturers manipulate labels to present their products in the best possible light. Our task is to learn how to read the label – and to read between the lines - so we get the important information we need, but don't get duped by trick labeling. In this section we'll cover some important introductory points to know about reading labels. Stay tuned to learn about food labels in much more depth throughout the book.

Units of Measure

The first surprise you get hit with is that most nutrients are measured in grams, not a unit familiar to many native-born Americans – unless you buy or sell cocaine. Those with ties to Europe or Asia are more likely to be familiar with the metric units used on labels, as opposed to the more clumsy units more commonly used in the United States. If it helps to visualize the conversion, a teaspoon is equal to about 5 grams.

Product Names

Be wary of product names: they are designed to sell products, not convey accurate information about the ingredients. Many "cheese crackers" don't contain any cheese, "Sunkist Fruit Gems" don't contain any fruit, the "blueberries" in Trader Joe's blueberry granola are actually made out of propylene glycol (antifreeze for RVs...), and Kraft's Guacamole Dip contains less than 2 percent avocado (hydrogenated oils and food coloring are much cheaper than avocado).

Serving Size

The best place to start when looking at a nutrition label is to figure out how much food was analyzed. At the top of the label under Nutrition Facts, you'll see the serving size and the number of servings in the package. The rest of the nutrition information on the label is based on one serving. If a serving size for a box of macaroni and cheese is "2," that means that if you eat the whole box of macaroni and cheese, you're eating two servings, not one, so you'll have to multiply all of the information on the facts panel by two to get accurate nutrition information.

The serving size rarely represents the amount that I actually eat, and this is an important way we get duped by the manufacturers. That 100 calories you glanced at on the label of a 20 ounce soda becomes 250 when you gulp down the whole bottle. And does anyone actually eat only half of a snack size bag of potato chips?

Calories

Next, the label lists the energy content, telling you how many total calories are in a serving of the product (but remember that they really mean kilocalories).

By itself this number means little, and most Americans would be far better off being less calorie conscious than we are. There are much more accurate and appropriate ways to monitor how much energy goes into your body, and we'll be learning about these later in the book, particularly in the carbohydrates and weight regulation sections.

Nonetheless, there is some handy information to be gleaned from knowing how much energy is in a product, and the following guides you in **calculating the amount of energy from the macronutrients:**

Find the number of grams of each of the macronutrients (protein, fat and carbohydrate) in the product. This information is provided on a food label.

Multiply the number of grams of the macronutrient by the amount of energy that is contained in one gram of that nutrient.

Facts to know:

- Carbohydrate (including all types, such as sugar, fiber and "other" carbohydrate) and protein both have 4 kcals in one gram.
- Fat (all types) has 9 kcals in one gram.

Example: A label from Grandma's Mac'n Cheese gives us the following information:

Nutrition Facts	
Serving Size 4.5 oz (126 g.)	
Servings Per Container: 2	
	Amount Per Serving
Calories	407
Total Fat	15 grams
Total Carbohydrate	50 grams
Dietary Fiber	0 grams
Sugars	30 grams
Other Carbohydrate	20 grams
Protein	18 grams

1) Determine how much energy is contained in each of the nutrients.

    Answer: Fat   15 g x 9 kcal/g = 135 kcals

                      Carbohydrate 50 g x 4 kcal/g = 200 kcals

                      Protein   18 g x 4 kcal/g = 72 kcals

Remember that the information on a food label applies to one serving, and the amount in a serving is defined on the label. If you have more or less than one serving, you need to adjust your answer. For example, if you eat two servings, you get twice as much energy from that nutrient. (In 2 servings, for example, there is 2 x 135 kcals of energy from fat, which equals 270 kcals.)

Another helpful hint: "Other carbohydrate" refers to starches.

Since protein, carbohydrate and fat are the only nutrients that contain energy, you can add up the energy from each of them to get the total energy in the product. Because of rounding off error, this may not be exactly equivalent to the total calories listed, but it should be close. Another possible explanation for an inconsistency is that some food items include the dietary fiber in the calculation of total calories, while others don't.

2) Calculate the percentage each of the energy nutrients contributes to the total:

First, why is this step even important? We previously calculated the amount of energy from each nutrient. Is this a high-fat product? A high-carbohydrate product? Sometimes it's difficult to tell from the numbers alone. A percentage helps us to better compare the amount of energy that each nutrient contributes to the total energy.

Divide the amount of energy that you get from each nutrient by the total energy in the product. This gives you the fraction the nutrient contributes. Then multiply by 100 to turn the fraction into a percentage.

    Example: (from above Mac n' cheese info)

    Fat   (135 kcals/407 kcals) x 100 = 33 percent

Carbohydrate (200 kcals/407 kcals) x 100 = 49 percent
Protein   (72 kcals/407 kcals) x 100 = 18 percent

Percent DV (Percent Daily Value)

Percent daily values tell you how much of something, whether it's fat, sugar or vitamin A, one serving will give you compared to how much the government estimates an adult would need for the entire day. It is intended to help you gauge the percentage of a nutrient requirement met by one serving of the product. Some percent daily values - like those given for the macronutrients - are based on the assumption that you require a 2,000 calorie a day diet (an average that is meaningless for most individuals), while others - like the micronutrients - stay the same no matter how many calories the government recommends you ingest.

The government recommendations aren't always based on accurate science, and I don't recommend strict attention to this information. For the micronutrients, a common rule of thumb used by nutritionists is that if it ranks at less than 5 percent, the product is a poor source of that nutrient; if the percent DV is between 10 percent and 20 percent it's a good source, and when the percent DV is over 20 percent, the product is high in that nutrient.

The percent DV is perhaps more helpful in comparison shopping. For example, if you're concerned about excess sodium, you can look at two foods and choose the food with the lower percent DV. And here's a key point to note: we just practiced calculating the percent of energy that each nutrient contributes to the total energy. This is not what the percent DV refers to! You have to calculate that information yourself.

Ingredients

The ingredients are listed beneath the Nutrition Facts panel. They are always listed in descending order of weight. If sugar is listed as the first ingredient, for example, that should give you an easy clue that you are looking at a high sugar product. But not every food is as it seems, and be wary of getting duped by clever marketing. Sometimes manufacturers use different types of sugar (like cane sugar, honey, high fructose corn syrup). Each type might be in small quantity so they aren't listed early in the ingredients, but if you sum them all up, sugar is in high quantity!

And you could get fooled in the opposite direction. Sometimes manufacturers pad the ingredients list with wholesome-sounding ingredients, but in such small quantity as to make them meaningless. Flaxseed is nutritious stuff, but when its the last ingredient in your cereal there's probably not enough to have a health impact. "Label padding" is a common tool used by junk food manufacturers who want to capitalize on the health food bandwagon without actually making nutritious products.

Another trick is to hide ingredients under different names. "Yeast extract" sounds innocuous, doesn't it? Those who try to avoid MSG (monosodium glutamate) may not realize that MSG lurks inside.

And of course, manufacturers aren't required to document the contaminants, so you'll never see an ingredients list which identifies the pesticides, heavy metals, perchlorate (the primary ingredient in rocket fuel and explosives), and other chemical compounds that lurk.

Vitamins and Minerals

Note that manufacturers are only required to list the percent DV of certain vitamins and minerals, so just because something isn't listed, doesn't mean it's not in the product. We'll discuss whether the percent DV is meaningful when we get to the vitamins and minerals section.

Advertising and Nutritional Claims

I suggest you ignore any advertising and nutritional claims made by manufacturers. There are many ways manufacturers can manipulate health claims. You can't trust that if a food manufacturer tells you, for example, that a product is 95 percent fat-free, that it really gets less than 5 percent of its calories from fat. Likewise, be wary if they tell you the product improves memory, relieves stress, or supports your immune system.

What – you believed in truth in labeling? Did I pique your curiosity about how they can get away with false claims? Here's a common example of how you get duped. You buy low-fat milk which advertises that it is 2 percent fat. What they don't tell you is that milk – like many foods and drinks – is high in water content, and they calculated the percentage of fat by weight. In fact, had they calculated the percentage by calories – a more appropriate measure – they would have to report that its fat content is actually 35 percent. But I suppose that might not sell as well.

Even the lesser water content in meat allows manufacturers to exploit this easy loophole in "truthful" labeling. A "95% fat-free" sandwich ham means that fat makes up just 5 percent of the ham's weight. It has nothing to do with the information most people are seeking - the measurement of calories that come from fat. Sandwich ham actually gets from 40 to 60 percent of its calories from fat, making it a high-fat product despite the low-fat declaration (legally) made by the manufacturer.

Manufacturers also have the right to make "structure/function" claims, meaning that they can describe how a food (or supplement) affects the body structure or its function – regardless of whether evidence exists to back it up. The law says that it can't be misleading, but as there are no specific rules defining this, the manufacturers get to interpret it themselves. They could probably back up a claim with one study that they conducted in-house, even if a dozen others show otherwise. (On the other hand, manufacturers can't make a "disease" claim without approval from the Food and Drug Administration (FDA). The silly result is that they get to legally claim that a product "helps maintain normal cholesterol levels" without government approval, but to claim that it "lowers cholesterol" requires approval.)

Bottom line: don't trust manufacturer claims!

Certifications

Many food producers use specialty certifications to attract consumers, and it's a challenge to read a food label and know what to trust. The most meaningful label is one that is certified to be "USDA Organic." To be labeled organic, a food must meet strict standards. The food cannot be grown with synthetic fertilizers, chemicals, sewage sludge, and cannot be genetically modified or irradiated. Organic meat and poultry must come from animals fed organic feed, and they cannot be treated with hormones or antibiotics. The animals must have access to the outdoors (although this doesn't necessarily mean that they go outdoors). (Note: "organic" as applied to seafood, on the other hand, is a meaningless term defined by the seller.)

For more details on certifications, see the Appendix page entitled "Guide to Sustainable Food Label Terminology."

What products contain labels?

Food labels are required on almost all foods, except those that don't provide many nutrients such as coffee, alcohol and spices. Although some restaurants provide information about the food they serve, they aren't required to have labels. While it is recommended that sellers provide nutritional information on produce, meat, poultry and seafood, it is strictly voluntary.

Get informed…

Want more information about reading between the lines of a food label? Check out the *Unofficial Guide to Smart Nutrition* by Ross Hume Hall. Chapter 7 gives some good tips.

Want comprehensive nutrition facts (including amount of macronutrients and micronutrients), beyond what you see on a label? Look up foods in the U.S. Department of Agriculture's nutrient database: http://www.nal.usda.gov/fnic/foodcomp/search/.

Scientific Reductionism

There are profound limitations inherent to any discussion or research about nutrition. Foods in their original form contain a mix of different nutrients. A simple soybean contains hundreds of bioactive compounds, including sugars, starch, fiber, mono-unsaturated fatty acids, poly-unsaturated fatty acids, protein, magnesium, potassium, phosphorous, calcium, manganese, Vitamin C, isoflavones, and possibly pesticides, genes that were modified through biotechnology, ... and that soybean is typically eaten in the context of several other foods in a meal, which are eaten in the context of numerous other foods over the course of a day. Yet when we study and report on nutrition, we focus on specific nutrients or foods, and lose the larger context of foods or nutrients that accompany them, in addition to losing the larger context of other lifestyle habits that affect their metabolism and our health, such as exercise, stress, or our attitudes towards food.

There's a name for this: scientific reductionism.

It is inevitable that if you take any nutrient or food out of context, you are sure to generate findings that are confusing, contradictory, and difficult to interpret. Let me give you three examples that help illustrate this point.

Extensive research indicates that a high-fiber diet will lower your risk for many diseases. But how much of that benefit can be attributed to the fiber itself, to the fact that fiber-rich foods tend to be nutrient-dense in general, or to the fact that people with high-fiber diets may have other health-enhancing habits, is not entirely controllable in research and often hard to discern. Consume the fiber out of context (through taking fiber supplements, for example) and its benefits considerably diminish – and sometimes disappear.

Next, consider the calcium debate. Calcium is the primary component of bones. Though your bones are hard and seem static, they are not; their calcium is constantly dissolving and being replaced. To maintain strong bones as an adult, you need to absorb enough calcium to balance calcium loss.

Some nutrients will help your body absorb or retain calcium, such as magnesium and Vitamin D. Others, such as protein, phosphorous and sodium, promote calcium excretion. Because of this, that a food contains calcium tells you little about its ability to maintain your bone strength. Furthermore, non-dietary factors, such as how active you are and whether you smoke cigarettes or consume alcohol, will also play a role in calcium absorption and excretion.

Osteoporosis, a disease of bone strength, is a huge problem in the United States, affecting over 50 percent of Caucasian women. Calcium is consumed in significantly lower quantity (less than half the calcium recommended to Americans) in several countries where osteoporosis is almost non-existent. Clearly, calcium consumption is not the principle issue in bone strength: in fact, the jury is out: that our diets are high in dairy, a significant source of calcium, may actually play a role in our vulnerability to *decreased* bone strength.

As another example, extensive research demonstrates a correlation between diets high in saturated fat and increased risk for numerous diseases. It makes sense that saturated fat plays a causative role, as we can trace some of the physiological mechanisms through which this occurs. For example, saturated fat is used as the starting material for cholesterol synthesis, and the cholesterol could contribute to build-up of atherosclerotic plaque, which in turn increases risk for heart attack or stroke.

However, diets high in saturated fat are also likely to be high in animal foods, which may also indicate excessive consumption of cholesterol, protein, oxidants and pesticides, and a low intake of fiber and beneficial micronutrients. To what degree we can implicate the saturated fat itself in disease risk is unclear, as many of these other factors increase risk for the same diseases.

And is there a threshold below which saturated fat ceases to be problematic? Dietary saturated fats are often used as an energy source. If we are not taking in excessive energy, dietary saturated fat just may be burned off, not causing any detriment. Its metabolism is affected by the quantity of total fat

– and energy - in your diet – and the failure to consider other energy sources could explain why many research studies don't show the same correlation between saturated fat and disease risk.

As much as we'd like to simplify the rules, "eat this" or "avoid that" just doesn't work. Nutrients - and even foods - have little meaning when viewed in isolation. You are better off paying attention to your overall dietary habits than getting bogged down in the details, and there will always be limitations to expressing nutrition in terms of the details.

Food marketers work hard to convince you that their products will dramatically improve your health. They won't. The choice of any one food or nutrient at a given time will have little impact on your overall health; it's what you habitually consume that's important – and the context that the foods are consumed in.

So I want to encourage you to hold this in mind as you read the remainder of this book. To help you understand nutrition, the next chapters will be reducing nutrition to its constituents. But by itself, each chapter is woefully inadequate. Interpretation needs to take place in the larger context.

Organizing this book was a challenge given the complicated interactions between the different constituents. Throughout my discussion of the nutrients and food categories, I loosely chose to focus on their metabolism and impact on personal health. Issues of food safety, ecology and sustainability, and biotechnology are addressed later, in separate chapters devoted to these topics. This means that you are going to have to skip around a bit to get the full picture of the ramifications of a particular food choice. But the good news is that all of the information in this book brings you back to the same place, as it turns out that the recommendations to nurture a healthy body also support a healthy planet, and there are some simple dietary patterns that get you there. The final chapter, called *Reclaiming the Joy in Eating*, will help you come back to seeing the holistic picture.

Digestion and Absorption

After an apple falls from a tree, it slowly starts to degrade. Return to the site a few months or years later, and the apple will have disappeared without a trace. That is because every raw food contains the perfect mix of enzymes to digest itself (break down) completely. (An enzyme is a molecule that helps to build or break molecules apart.) All food, regardless of whether it is plant or animal, eventually decomposes and returns to the earth from which it came.

When we cook or process the food, we destroy some of these natural food enzymes. (They start to degrade at about 106 degrees, and are almost completely degraded by the time the heat reaches 118 degrees.) The naturally high acidity in our stomach also degrades some of the enzymes not otherwise destroyed in cooking.

Fortunately, our body makes its own enzymes, some of which can replace those which are naturally found in food, and others which speed the process along or activate otherwise dormant enzymes in food. We don't have to wait the years it may take for some foods to naturally decompose in order to get its energy and nutrients!

How do you get large complex foodstuffs into our body and then into a form that you can later use? The action unfolds before the food even enters your mouth: when you see, smell, or even think about food, you trigger nerve responses that control your digestive tract.

When the food enters your mouth, digestion begins. **Digestion** refers to the process of turning the food you eat into smaller units, while **absorption** refers to the movement of those small units from your digestive tract into your circulatory system.

Your digestive tract is essentially a long hollow tube that starts with your mouth, travels through your esophagus, stomach, and intestines, and out your anus. (I do mean "long:" if you could spread your digestive tract out end to end, it would be about 30 feet.)

Since the digestive system is continuous from the mouth to anus, scientists consider digestion to be an "out-of-body experience." Once the food is completely digested and broken down into small by-products, these breakdown products are then absorbed, meaning that they cross the wall of your gastrointestinal tract and enter your body. Anything that can't be absorbed never enters your body: it continues through your digestive tract to your anus and is excreted.

The organs the food passes through are called **digestive organs**, and include your mouth, esophagus, stomach, small intestine and large intestine; the earlier part of your large intestine is called the colon and the end is called the rectum. Your anus is the opening at the very end of your digestive tract. "**Accessory digestive organs**," including your salivary glands, liver, gallbladder and pancreas, help along the way, releasing enzymes and chemicals that support the digestive process.

There are two different aspects to the digestive process: chemical and physical. As their names suggest, **chemical digestion** refers to chemical breakdown of food (including enzymes, acids, bile, etc.), while **physical digestion** – also known as mechanical digestion – refers to the physical breakdown of food, such as your teeth chomping down or muscles contracting to break up and propel food along.

The Action Begins

Digestion begins long before you take that first bite. The sight, smell, and even the thought of food get your digestive juices rolling and the muscles churning, preparing for the incoming action. Your mouth waters, releasing juices and enzymes ready to soften the food and start its journey. Your stomach starts to contract to be ready to receive the food, your pancreas starts to secrete chemicals that will break down the food. Be sure to be attentive to your food so you can get these important pre-digestive steps rolling.

Smell something you don't like? Or perhaps the food being served looks a bit like excrement? You experience a "rejection reaction:" your throat tightens and your muscles contract, preparing to push out the offending food (vomit).

But let's assume the food looks good. You take a bite. Your teeth grind the food into smaller, more manageable pieces, breaking any fibrous packaging on the outside so you can get at the nutrients inside. Your salivary glands inject saliva into your mouth, which moistens your food, making it more malleable, and contains amylase enzyme, which digests some of the starches into the sugars they're composed of.

When you are relaxed, your salivary glands produce watery saliva that contains a lot of digestive enzymes. When you are stressed, on the other hand, it's thicker and contains fewer enzymes. Also interesting, chewing stimulates the parotid glands to release certain hormones which contribute to a strengthened immune system.

The combination of chewing and saliva production is designed to put less stress on the rest of your body's digestion process. All kinds of additional things go wrong when you eat while stressed: you release less stomach acid, there's less blood flow to the stomach, and the muscle contraction which would ordinarily push food through the digestive tract gets slowed. So be kind to your gut and eat under peaceful conditions.

Try this experiment to actually feel starch digestion happening: put a plain, unsalted cracker in your mouth and let it slowly dissolve. You'll notice a sudden sweetness after a few minutes: that's because the amylases broke the starch into sugar, and you then taste the sweetness of the released sugar.

Food stays in the mouth for such a short time that only a small percentage of the starch typically gets broken down in your mouth – and starches don't usually taste nearly as sweet as foods that are already in the form of sugar.

Let's continue through the digestive tract. The moistened food is pushed by your tongue to the back of your mouth, and then slides into your esophagus. Muscle contractions, called **peristalsis**, rhythmically push it along, supported by gravity. The food then passes through a valve called your esophageal sphincter, and into your stomach. The stomach has three main jobs: storing the food you've eaten, breaking it down into a liquidy mixture, and slowly emptying that mixture into the small intestine.

Glands in your stomach release some chemicals, including a blend of enzymes, hydrochloric acid, and mucus. The mucus coats the inside of your stomach wall, protecting it from potential damage from the acid. The acid inactivates the amylases, stopping their action in the digestion of starch. It also denatures the protein chains, which means that it straightens them, making the chemical bonds in the middle of the protein chain more accessible to digestive enzymes. To a minor extent, the acid may also break some carbohydrate bonds. The enzymes get to work breaking down the protein and fat. Strong peristaltic muscle contractions make your stomach work like a food processor, blending its contents into a soupy mix called chyme. Gastric juices also help to kill some of the bacteria in your food that could cause you harm.

Although some digestion has taken place already, it is relatively minor compared to the action in the small intestine, the next organ in the route. "Small" intestine is poorly named, as your small intestine is actually pretty big: perhaps about 20 feet long if you were to straighten its tight coils. Amazing that you have so much stuff jammed inside you, isn't it?

Your food may spend as long as 4 hours in the small intestine and will become a very thin, watery mixture. The small intestine gets help from three accessory organs: your pancreas, liver and gallbladder. The pancreas secretes a host of helpful substances, including alkaline compounds that make the chyme less acidic, amylase enzyme that breaks down carbohydrates, proteases to break down the proteins, and lipases to break down the fats. Some enzymes are also generated by the intestine itself. Additionally, fat in the small intestine signals the gallbladder, which squirts bile into the small intestine. Bile is a greenish fluid that is made in the liver and stored in the gallbladder; it "emulsifies" fats, meaning that it breaks up the fat globules. This increases the surface area of the fats that are exposed to the digestive juices, allowing lipases, which are enzymes secreted from the pancreas, to digest the fat.

While this chemical digestion is happening, peristaltic contractions continue to propel the food along. By this point, just about all the digestion that can occur has. Now you're ready for the next step: absorption, which refers to actually getting the nutrients into your body.

The lining of your small intestine is covered in folds, which has projections called villi sticking out. The villi are covered in projections that are smaller still, called microvilli. These tiny projections increase the surface area of the small intestine by a factor of 600. Each villus and microvillus is specialized to accept a specific nutrient – and when that nutrient finds the projection specialized to receive it, it attaches and can then cross over your intestinal wall and into your circulation.

Stuff that can't be absorbed travels on to your large intestine. The first part of your large intestine is called your colon, and its job is to absorb water from this mixture and squeeze the remaining stuff into a solid bundle called feces. (For those who prefer simplicity here, feces is the technical term for "poop.") Feces contain all the indigestible portions of the foods you eat, along with the intestinal cells that sloughed off during this process, and lots and lots of bacteria. (In fact, about 50 percent of your feces is bacteria[61].)

Bacteria are so numerous in your body that they outnumber all the cells in your body, probably by as much as a factor of ten. (Think about that: most of the cells in the human body aren't human!) Before you start to panic about all those bacteria hanging out in your body, its time to reframe your ideas about bacteria. Most of the bacteria that live inside you are good guys, helping to take care of you. Bacteria in your intestines help to keep your intestines clean by feeding on harmful bacteria, poisons and other nasty substances, and foods you would not otherwise be able to digest. They also produce some vitamins and help to regulate gut and immune function, and play many other roles, many of which aren't well understood.

Like you, bacteria need to eat, so you should be sure to feed them well. Their favorite food? Fiber! In the carbohydrates section, we'll talk more about why lots of fiber is a great thing for your digestive tract (and for many other reasons), though you absorb very little.

The colon leads to the rectum, and the end of the rectum is called the anus, which is controlled by a powerful muscle called a sphincter. When feces arrive in the rectum, nerves that are responsive to stretch send a message to the nerve centers in the spinal cord, and these send a message to the sphincter muscles, making them relax to open the anus. If it is inconvenient for us to have our bowels open, the brain sends a message to prevent the "open anus" message being sent. We are not aware of this until the rectum becomes very full, when we have to make a conscious effort to keep the anus closed. When we allow the anus to open, the muscles in the wall of the large bowel and rectum contract to push the feces out.

Wondering if there's a typical pattern to bowel movements, or whether it's healthier to be "regular?" The answer is no – being regular is probably just a sign that you're boring! The timing and quantity of bowel movements is a product of the types and quantity of food you have eaten and when you eat them. Probably the largest contributor is fiber – the more you eat, the more you poop. (That's because most fiber is indigestible, and therefore becomes a large part of your feces.)

And here's some other important advice: be sure to choose food you like. It turns out that people actually absorb more nutrients from meals that appeal to them than from meals they find less appetizing. In one interesting study[62], researchers fed a traditional Thai meal of rice and vegetables spiked with chili paste, fish sauce, and coconut cream to two groups of women, one Swedish and one

Thai. The Thai women, who presumably liked the meal better than the Swedish women, absorbed 50 percent more iron from the same food than the Swedish women. And when the meal was blended together and turned to an unfamiliar and unpalatable paste, the Thai women's absorption of iron from the meal decreased by 70 percent!

So choking down the plate of steamed broccoli (if you hate steamed broccoli) is not likely to do you as much good as you think. Enjoying your food is an important nutritional practice!

Here's a little cheat sheet that summarizes the main actions in the different organs.

DIGESTIVE ORGAN	ACTION(S)
Mouth	Chewing Saliva moistens, contains enzymes
Esophagus	Muscles propel
Stomach	Muscles mix Chemicals denature and digest Mucus protects
Small Intestine	Muscles propel Chemicals digest
Large Intestine	Temporarily stores Undigested foods exit body

ACCESSORY DIGESTIVE ORGAN	ACTION(S)
Salivary Glands	Secrete saliva and enzymes (amylase, lipase) into mouth
Pancreas	Secretes alkaline substances, and enzymes (amylase, protease, lipases) into small intestine
Liver	Makes bile
Gallbladder	Stores bile, sends to small intestine

And the various digestive secretions:

SECRETION	ORGAN		DIGESTIVE ACTION(S)
	Origin	Site of Action	
HCl acid	Stomach	Stomach	Denatures proteins
Bile	Liver/Gallbladder	Small Intestine	Emulsifies fats
Amylase	Salivary Glands Pancreas	Mouth Small Intestine	Digests carbohydrates
Pepsin	Stomach	Stomach	Digests proteins
Protease	Pancreas	Stomach	Digests proteins
Lipase		Mouth Small Intestine	Digests fats

Digestive Disorders: When digestion goes awry

That was a quick rundown of normal, healthy digestion, but I'm sure we all know from personal experience that things don't always go smoothly. Now let's discuss what could happen when things go wrong.

Halitosis (Bad Breath)

There are two main forms of halitosis: physiologic halitosis describes when it occurs in otherwise healthy people, and pathologic halitosis is the name used when it occurs as a by-product of disease.

The root causes of pathologic halitosis include sinusitis (infected or inflamed sinuses), gum disease (gingivitis, periodontitis), an absccssed tooth, food impaction, kidney failure, liver failure, bowel obstruction, diabetes or an uncommon metabolic condition called trimethylaminuria (otherwise known as fish odor syndrome).

Physiologic halitosis is related to the food or drinks you consume, tobacco, or perhaps to unclean dentures or bacteria in your mouth or other parts of your digestive tract. The most commonly recognized food culprits are onions or garlic, but there's an even more common cause of offensive odor: the sulfur compounds that are released when certain proteins are digested. Those sulfur compounds are part of the amino acids methionine and cysteine which are found in highest quantities in animal-derived foods.

<u>Tackling bad breath</u>

Be sure to discuss your concerns with your dentist and/or physician to determine if there is a pathologic root that needs to be addressed. Solve the root problem and the halitosis should disappear.

To minimize physiologic halitosis, I have two suggestions. The first is to observe good hygiene. Brush and floss regularly, and use a tongue scraper to get at those bacteria that congregate on your tongue. And be sure to get regular professional cleanings by a dentist or hygienist.

But good oral hygiene won't do the trick alone. Foods are broken down in the intestine, and then the sulfurous gasses are absorbed into the bloodstream, where they circulate to the lungs and eventually out through your breath. So dietary change is also helpful: minimize obvious culprits like garlic and onions as well as foods high in sulfur (particularly animal-derived foods such as red meat, poultry, fish, shellfish, cheese...). Also, be sure to stay well-hydrated: a dry mouth encourages bacterial proliferation.

And of course - in case you need another reason - quit smoking!

Hiccups

Your diaphragm is a muscle in your chest, just below your lungs. When it contracts, your lungs expand and you inhale; when it loosens, your lungs contract and you exhale. With hiccups, your diaphragm muscle jerks, resulting in you sucking in air quickly. That causes the epiglottis to quickly snap shut, making the "hic" sound. Scientists aren't really sure what causes this process, but sometimes eating or drinking too quickly seems to start it. Some suspect that a gas gets lodged on the wall of your gastrointestinal tract and the irritation causes the repetitive contractions.

A silly fact: according to the Guinness Book of World Records, the longest recorded bout of hiccuping was over 69 years. Some guy actually began hiccuping in 1922, and continuing hiccuping every 1-1/2 seconds until 1990. He died only a year later.

There are thousands of suggested cures for hiccups, but most of the methods that are successful are based on increasing carbon dioxide levels in the blood. Breathing in deeply and holding your breath may work, for example. Or try breathing into a paper bag so that you fill it with exhaled carbon dioxide, and then inhaling that carbon dioxide.

If someone surprises you or scares you, most of the time the hiccups will disappear. Of course, to be surprised you have to be unaware of what is about to happen. I've never quite understood how to get someone to startle me without being aware that they are going to!

Eructation (Burping)

Eructation is such a fancy word that you may be surprised to learn that it simply refers to the act of burping. Both eructation and flatulence (farting) are caused by escaping gases, but they're different gases and of course at different ends of your body.

Every time you drink or gobble down food, you swallow gas, particularly when you eat or drink quickly. Other behaviors that can cause you to swallow extra air include chewing gum, drinking carbonated beverages, sucking on hard candies, drinking through a straw, talking while you eat, and cigarette smoking. (Did you need another reason to quit smoking?) All of those practices result in more saliva which has to be swallowed – and every time you swallow saliva, you swallow air.

Of course your body (and its resident bacteria) makes some gas as well. Those gases have to go somewhere! You probably pass the equivalent of about a pint – or maybe even as much as a gallon - of gases every day. Burps result when excess gas is forced out the stomach, back up your esophagus and out your mouth. The remaining gas travels through the intestines and eventually out the other exit, resulting in flatulence.

Overeating tends to lead to burping. This is because the stomach normally contains air, and when you overeat the stomach attempts to relieve the distention by expelling the stomach air upwards. (You don't have any control over this reflex.)

And yes, there are some foods that may make you more likely to burp: onions, tomatoes and mint, for example, relax the muscles at the lower end of your throat, allowing air from the stomach to escape through burps.

Flatulence (Gas)

The scientific term for gas is "flatulence." The major source of gas is the normal breakdown of undigested carbohydrates by bacteria in your colon (called "fermentation"). Gas is often a good sign, indicating that we are keeping our intestinal bacteria well-fed, which enables them to perform important functions in maintaining our health.

Given that so many people are lactose-intolerant, the number one source of farts in the United States is dairy products. (Michael Greger jokes that perhaps that's how the saying "cutting the cheese" evolved[63].) Greger checked the medical literature and found that the two most flatulent patients - who produced loud farts every ten minutes around the clock - were both lactose intolerant and were cured once they stopped eating dairy products. Yet another interesting tidbit Greger reports is a farting record in the Guinness Book of World Records – one lucky man got his claim to fame by drinking a glass of milk and then farting 70 times in four hours.

The second leading cause of gas is beans ("bean bombers" as I've heard them called), which contain two poorly digested sugars, raffinose and stachyose. Because beans are so nutritious, however, I don't recommend limiting them. Instead, I suggest that you experiment with ways to keep them in your diet. Lentils, split peas and canned beans produce less gas, so you may want to try them. Products made from soybeans, such as tempeh, miso, tofu, and soymilk, usually don't cause gas. A helpful tip if you cook your own: soak your dried beans and throw out the soaking water.

Other common raffinose-containing foods that are notorious for producing gas include cabbage, cauliflower, brussels sprouts, broccoli, and asparagus.

Other indigestible sugars include sugar alcohols, such as sorbitol and xylitol, which are frequently contained in sugar-free candies, or a newer one, erythritol, more commonly sold in packages for use as a drink sweetener. The fructose in high fructose corn syrup that sweetens many drinks and candies may also contribute to gas. Bread can also do you in; there is a sugar in wheat that the body can have a hard time digesting. In Old German, the word "pumpernickel" actually means "goblin that breaks wind"![63])

Starch also contributes to gas formation: potatoes, corn, noodles, and wheat are among the culprits. Soluble fiber (found in oat bran, peas and other legumes, beans, and most fruit) additionally can cause gas formation.

Constipation can also cause gas. Normally, most intestinal gas is expelled out the anus in small amounts that we aren't aware of. However, when we're constipated the gas becomes trapped behind the feces, and then suddenly emerges as a noticeable amount. Also, when we're constipated the food residues stay in our intestines longer and have more time to ferment and give off gas.

Anxiety seems to make gas worse, for two reasons: 1) when we're anxious we swallow more air; and 2) our intestines become more active due to increased hormones and, as a result, expel gas more forcefully.

And yes, some of us are just biologically designed to be stinkier, which results from our particular composition of intestinal bacteria. Some bacteria make more methane (odorless), while others help hydrogen to combine with sulfur to make hydrogen sulfide, the stinky stuff. Also, the more sulfur-rich your diet, the more your gas will stink. Foods such as cauliflower, eggs and meat are notorious for producing smelly gas, whereas beans may produce copious amounts of gas, but it's not particularly redolent.

Vegetarians are more likely to produce gas than carnivores because of their higher fiber intake. However, if they're fortunate enough to not have the stinky type, they may be more likely to get away with it socially because their sphincters tend to be a little looser. The sound of releasing gas is produced by vibrations of the anal opening and depends on the velocity of expulsion of the gas and the tightness of the sphincter muscles of the anus. While omnivores may produce less, they're likely to be louder given their tighter sphincters.

Any time you increase your fiber, you will probably see an increase in gas. Increase your fiber slowly and within a couple weeks your body should adapt.

Also, there is a commercial product called Beano that contains enzymes which break up those difficult to digest bean sugars. It comes in liquid form that can be added to foods after cooking, or tablets that can be chewed before or with your meal. Other companies make similar products.

In terms of what you can take once you have gas, Pepto Bismol and generic equivalents can bind to the sulfur in your digestive tract and eliminate odors. While this may help in the short term, it's not recommended that you take it for more than a few days at a time; you can actually get bismuth toxicity.

If you're feeling desperate, you can actually buy an activated charcoal-lined cushion you can sit on to absorb the smell. They used to call it the "Toot Trapper" but later tried to go for a more serious image and changed the name to the Flatulence Filter[63]. Another company sells it under the even more innocuous sounding name, Flat-D Chair Filter.

And if you're embarrassed about stinking up the bathroom, lighting a match makes the smell disappear quickly.

Wondering if those stories of lighting farts on fire are true? They may well be. The methane and hydrogen that are components of gas are both flammable. An informal survey by a now non-existent website (Fartcloud), revealed that about a quarter of the people who ignited their farts got burned doing it, so it's not a party game I recommend.

You can also try peppermint, which can aid digestion; it helps to relax smooth muscles, and minimizes cramping or bloating. Also, exercise helps your body absorb gas. If you are in a lot of pain, keep in mind that gas rises, so if you kneel down, put your head down and your butt in the air, things may start to move. (This helpful tip is also attributed to Michael Greger[63].)

The take-home message is that intestinal gas is often normal and healthy. Tolerance and slow dietary changes are the best way to handle it.

Choking

To understand what happens when you choke, let's start with a little anatomy lesson. The esophagus is like a stretchy pipe that's about 10 inches long, and its role is to move food from your mouth into your stomach. It runs parallel to your windpipe, also known as your trachea, which is the conduit for air to travel between your mouth and lungs. When you swallow food or liquids, a special flap called the epiglottis flops down over the opening of your windpipe to make sure the food enters the esophagus and not the windpipe.

When you eat or drink too fast, or you're talking while eating, your epiglottis might not be properly covering your trachea, and the food goes down the wrong tube. The typical response is to cough involuntarily, which helps to dislodge the food. Of course, you might not be so lucky. Then you hope that a nearby good Samaritan is trained in the Heimlich maneuver. They'll wrap their arms around you and sharply push up and against your diaphragm to help you expel the offending food.

Lactose Intolerance

Lactose is a type of carbohydrate found in milk products. You need a particular enzyme, called lactase, to break down lactose into the glucose and galactose that its made of, and these sugars can then be absorbed by the body. Almost all infants have very high lactase activity, as you would expect since they have a high intake of milk. The sweet taste of the sugar encourages them to nurse. Lactase activity starts to drop off after you're around two years old, and many people lose this ability as they age; in fact, only about 30 percent of adults make enough lactase to digest lactose efficiently. We call this lactose intolerance.

Without sufficient lactase, your body can't properly digest lactose-containing food. This means that if you eat lactose-containing foods, the lactose stays in your intestines and gets attacked by the bacteria. This leads to gas and to small molecules that attract water into the intestine, causing cramps, bloating, and diarrhea.

If you are lactose-intolerant, your body will usually start acting up within 2 hours of eating or drinking lactose-containing foods. Not everyone reacts in the same way - or within the same amount of time - because some people can handle more lactose than others can.

Lactose intolerance can start suddenly - even if you've never had trouble with dairy products or other foods containing lactose. You'll do a better job diagnosing it than a doctor because the best way to diagnose it is by experimenting: if you eat lactose-containing foods you experience the symptoms. (Your physician can also measure hydrogen gas in your breath to give some indication.) Sometimes people have a minor degree of lactase activity and can do fine with processed milk products like ice cream and yogurt – but experience symptoms with the more concentrated blast of lactose that comes in milk.

For most people, lactose intolerance is genetic. It's less common among descendants of people who consumed milk from domesticated animals during prehistoric times than among people whose early ancestors did not drink milk. Studies show its prevalence to include greater than 80 percent of Southeast Asians; 80 percent of Native Americans; 75 percent of African Americans; 70 percent of Mediterranean peoples; 60 percent of Intuits; 50 percent of Hispanics; and 20 percent of Caucasians. (Seems a bit racist that our nutrition recommendations push dairy so heavily, given the high prevalence among non-Caucasians, isn't it?)

People can also develop lactose intolerance for other reasons. Sometimes another illness may keep the intestine from producing enough lactase. For example, people with inflammatory bowel disease, such as Crohn's disease, or other long-term problems that affect the intestines, are often lactose intolerant. Certain medications can also cause people to develop lactose intolerance, as can some infections – but these types of lactose intolerance are usually temporary.

What to do if you have lactose intolerance? Two choices: either you can avoid lactose-containing products, or you can purchase lactase enzyme at a pharmacy (over-the-counter) and take some when you eat lactose-containing foods. Commercially-produced lactase is harmless – no different than the lactase that humans naturally produce. You can also buy some products, like milks, that have been fortified with lactase. The commercial lactase enzyme works well for most people, but not all. Avoidance won't set you up for nutritional deficiencies: despite the hype conjured by the dairy industry; there's nothing in dairy products that you can't easily get elsewhere.

Heartburn (Dyspepsia)

Earlier we learned that your stomach secretes acid, and that it has a mucus lining which protects your stomach lining from the burning effects of the acid. Suppose you over-fill your stomach quickly, and most of the food just isn't in a form that allows it to travel on to the small intestine. With nowhere to go, it heads back where it came from, pushing against the esophageal sphincter as it floods into the esophagus. But the problem is that the food is now mixed with acid, and your sphincter and esophagus don't have the mucus protection that the stomach does. Ouch! That's what the burning sensation is all about – the burning feeling usually travels from your chest up to your neck and throat. (Contrary to what the name implies, the heart itself is not involved.) You might also get a sour or bitter taste in your mouth.

You can do permanent damage to your sphincter and esophagus if heartburn persists (see section on GERD), so best to use heartburn as a learning experience and change your habits.

Heartburn can also result from a hiatal hernia (see section on hernias later in this chapter).

How to avoid heartburn? The key is to avoid over-filling your stomach. Eating smaller meals is the most helpful advice – and slowing down may also do the trick.

Below are some other culprits. Note that not everyone is sensitive, so you will need to do some experimenting.

- High-fat diets[64-66]: Meals that are lower in fat may go down easier, since fat floats on top of the watery digestive juices and stays in your stomach longer.
- Coffee [67-70]: Coffee weakens sphincter functioning[67]. The effects of decaf are somewhat milder, but still exist[68, 69]. Both also generate large amounts of stomach acid[70], which exacerbates the problem.
- Cigarette smoking[71]: As if you need another reason to quit?
- Alcohol[72]: Alcoholic beverages irritate the stomach lining and increase acid production. Wine and beer are more problematic than hard liquor[73].
- Onions[74]: Can't imagine life without onions? Don't worry: cooking destroys most of the substances associated with indigestion.
- Green peppers, cucumbers, radishes (when consumed raw).
- Chocolate[75-77]: you don't know how sorry I am to deliver this news!
- Fruit juices[78]: Citrus juices, like grapefruit and orange juice, and tomato juice, can cause heartburn by irritating the lining of the esophagus and the stomach[78]. (Surprisingly, their acid doesn't contribute – research shows neutralized orange juice has the same effect[79].) Whole fruit doesn't cause the same problems – some of the protective substances found in the whole fruit may be damaged in the process of juicing.

The worse thing you can do is lie down after eating – you want gravity to help the food along, not work against you. Stress reduction is also helpful.

If you get heartburn, there are plenty of over-the-counter medications available, and while most can provide temporary relief, none are recommended. Best to avoid heartburn in the first place. For example, antacids neutralize the acid for a little while, but eventually trigger your stomach to make more acid. Also, some ingredients can interfere with absorption of nutrients. (Common antacids include Rolaids, Tums, Mylanta, and Maalox.) Acid reducers and acid controllers reduce the stomach's ability to produce acid so much that digesting food becomes harder. They may also cause indigestion and diarrhea. (These include Pepcid AC, Tagamet HB, and Zantac 75.)

Gastro-esophageal reflux disease (GERD)

When people regularly get heartburn, it is called gastro-esophageal reflux disease, or GERD. (The official diagnosis usually comes when someone experiences recurring, significant heartburn two or more times a week.)

Over time, the reflux of stomach acid damages the tissue lining the esophagus, causing inflammation and pain. Untreated GERD can lead to permanent damage of the esophagus and sometimes even cancer.

Food Allergies

Normally, your immune system protects you from germs. It does this by making antibodies that help you fight off bacteria, viruses, and other micro-organisms. But if you have a food allergy, your immune system mistakenly treats something in a certain food as if it's dangerous to you and creates antibodies to attack it. Allergies are caused by proteins and the most common foods that cause allergies include peanuts and other nuts, seafood (especially shrimp), eggs, soy and wheat, and to a lesser degree, milk.

Antibodies cause mast cells (a type of immune system cell) to release chemicals into the bloodstream, one of which is histamine. The histamine then causes symptoms that affect a person's eyes, nose, throat, respiratory system, skin, and digestive system. The reaction could be mild or severe, and could happen right away or a few hours after the eating the allergen. The first signs of an allergic reaction could be a runny nose, an itchy skin rash such as hives, or a tingling feeling in the tongue or lips. Other signs include tightness in the throat, wheezing, cough, nausea, vomiting, stomach pain and diarrhea. In a serious case, an allergy can cause anaphylaxis; in addition to the previously-mentioned symptoms, anaphylaxis may include a drop in blood pressure, narrowing of the breathing tubes, and swelling of the tongue.

People who may be susceptible to an anaphylactic reaction should be prepared for an emergency, as these symptoms could result in death without appropriate care.

Many kids outgrow allergies to milk and eggs as they age. But severe allergies to foods like peanuts and some types of seafood often last a lifetime.

Sometimes it's easy to figure out that you have a food allergy, particularly if you get overt symptoms soon after eating something. But sometimes you have to do a little detective work to figure out which is the offending food.

Most allergies are believed to be hereditary. Some people are born with allergies, whereas others develop them over time.

Ulcers

An ulcer is a sore, which means it's an open wound. The ulcers that form in the stomach or the upper part of the small intestine are called peptic ulcers. Peptic ulcers are very common - almost one in every 10 people in the U.S. will get an ulcer at some time during their lives.

We used to believe that stress, spicy foods, and alcohol caused most ulcers. Now we know that most peptic ulcers are caused by a particular bacterial infection in the stomach and upper intestine, although sometimes they may be caused by certain medications, or by smoking. The bacteria that causes most ulcers is called Helicobacter pylori (or H. pylori, for short). Experts believe that 90 percent of the people who have ulcers are infected with H. pylori.

Strangely enough, however, most people (80 percent?) infected with H. pylori never develop an ulcer. No one is completely sure why, but experts think that part of the reason depends on the individual person - for example, people who develop ulcers may already have a problem with the lining of their stomachs. It is also believed that some people may naturally secrete more stomach acid than others - and it doesn't matter what stresses they're exposed to or what they eat. Peptic ulcers may have something to do with the combination of H. pylori infection and the level of acid in the stomach.

Sometimes ulcers can also occur when people take nonsteroidal anti-inflammatory drugs (NSAIDs), like aspirin or ibuprofen, in high daily doses over a long period of time. Smoking is also associated with peptic ulcers as the nicotine in cigarettes causes the stomach to produce more acid. Drinking a lot of alcohol can also increase a person's risk of ulcers because alcohol can wear down the lining of the stomach and intestines.

In certain circumstances stress can help cause ulcers. But this usually only happens in situations of illness involving severe emotional or physical stress - such as when someone is so sick that he or she cannot eat for a long period of time. They are then susceptible to an ulcer because of uncontrolled increased acid production in the stomach. If their body's ability to heal is severely challenged because of a weakened immune system, they are at greater risk.

Stomach pain is the most common symptom; it usually feels like sharp aches between your chest and belly button. This pain often comes a few hours after eating or when your stomach is empty.

Untreated ulcers grow larger and can lead to other problems, so best to recognize it early and get help.

The best advice in ulcer prevention is to observe good hygiene to minimize the risk of becoming infected with the bacteria. The bacteria appear to be spread through fecal contact. Flies may also be a vector for spreading the bacteria.

Hiatal Hernia

A hernia occurs when an organ slips through the muscle wall that holds the organ in place. A hiatal hernia refers to the upper part of the stomach pushing through an opening in the diaphragm and up into the chest. What would cause this? There are several possibilities, including tight clothing, an abdominal injury, sudden physical exertion such as weightlifting, or most commonly – frequent constipation. Straining to defecate actually causes the stomach to be pushed into the chest cavity, weakening the diaphragm muscle.

The diaphragm helps the sphincter between the esophagus and the stomach keep acid from coming up into the esophagus. When a hiatal hernia is present, it is easier for the acid to come up. In this way, a hiatal hernia can cause reflux (heartburn).

Gallstones/Gallbladder Disease

Bile is a substance made in the liver, then stored in the gallbladder until the body needs to digest fat. When fats arrive in your intestine, they signal your gallbladder, which contracts and pushes the bile into a duct that carries it to the small intestine.

Bile contains water, cholesterol, fats, bile salts, and bilirubin. Bile salts break up fat, and bilirubin gives bile and stool a brownish color. If the liquid bile contains too much cholesterol, bile salts, or bilirubin, it can harden into stones. Gallstones can be as small as a grain of sand or as large as a golf ball. They can block the normal flow of bile if they lodge in any of the ducts that carry bile from the liver to the small intestine.

Cholesterol build-up is the most likely cause of gallstones, and fiber is the key to prevention. A diet low in saturated and trans fat will also serve to reduce cholesterol production.

Ironically, losing weight, particularly if it's quick, can also trigger the development of gallstones. When you lose weight, stored cholesterol is released from body fat and concentrated into bile. (This is a common side effect of quick weight loss programs.)

If a duct becomes blocked by a gallstone, we call it a gallbladder attack. It feels quite painful, with the pain radiating from the gallbladder to the right shoulder. A gallbladder attack can last anywhere from fifteen minutes to six hours, often at times unrelated to meals. Nausea and vomiting may also occur. When the blockage is prolonged, inflammation and possible bacterial infection can also develop.

Gallstones are diagnosed through a relatively safe and painless ultrasound examination (sound waves are directed to the abdomen to pinpoint stones).

Dietary change is always recommended as a first strategy for dealing with gallstones (increased fiber, decreased saturated and trans fat). Regular exercise is also beneficial; researchers theorize that it works its effects through helping to normalize blood glucose and insulin levels, which may contribute to gallstones. Sometimes stones won't cause any discomfort if these recommendations are followed.

Other treatment possibilities include oral dissolution or mechanical extraction. Even if these treatment methods are initially successful, gallstones are likely to return in the absence of changing diet or exercise habits.

Surgical removal of the gallbladder, called cholecystectomy, is the more aggressive treatment. Some contend that doctors are too quick to recommend cholecystectomy and that patients should consider their options carefully before jumping to this step. Without a gallbladder to control the timing of bile delivery, bile drips into the small intestine even in the absence of food. When concentrated like this, the bile acids can irritate the intestinal lining, often causing diarrhea and making the individual at slightly higher risk for intestinal cancer. To reduce these risks, individuals who have their gallbladders removed should choose their foods wisely, and follow a high-fiber, low-fat diet.

Fatty Liver Disease (Steatohepatitis)

The liver is the largest internal organ, and it works hard, breaking down dietary carbohydrates, proteins and fats, and regulating cholesterol and triglycerides in the blood. It's also the primary site for detoxifying and clearing toxins. Abuse your body with toxic substances - the most well known being alcohol - and your liver takes a beating.

Sometimes fats accumulate in your liver, which is usually discovered when routine blood tests reveal elevated liver enzymes.

The secret to reversing liver disease is to stop abusing alcohol, if that's the cause, or decrease fat consumption, the other main underlying factor of a fatty liver. The liver has an astonishing capacity to recover when treated well.

Liver abnormalities may also be due to infections or medications. For example, hepatitis (inflammation of the liver) is usually the result of a viral infection, though it can also be caused by chemical toxins or medications. When its viral, we classify it with letters: hepatitis A, B or C.

Hepatitis is spread through bodily fluids. Hepatitis A is usually spread through food or water, while hepatitis B and C are almost always associated with drug use, transfusions or sexual contact. Immunization does a pretty effective job of minimizing risk for hepatitis A and B.

Oftentimes, an infection can be chronic. Currently available medications (interferon, ribavirin) are only about 40 percent effective at eliminating chronic infection and are quite costly ($10,000). Some herbal remedies are showing promise although they haven't been extensively tested.

Difficulties with Elimination

If the muscles in the colon don't work at the right speed for proper digestion or if the coordination with muscles is somehow hampered, the contents of the colon are not able to move along smoothly. When this happens, you can get abdominal cramps, bloating, diarrhea or constipation. Let's take a look at what happens when your stools are too loose (diarrhea) and too compact (constipation), and other disorders related to these two.

Diarrhea

Diarrhea refers to loose, watery stools. It usually results from some kind of irritation to the intestinal lining, which causes increased peristalsis. The intestinal contents move too quickly, and the colon doesn't have a chance to remove enough fluid.

Diarrhea is a common problem, and one that usually lasts only a day or two and goes away without any special treatment. However, prolonged diarrhea can be a sign of other problems.

A few of the more common causes of diarrhea are bacteria (common culprits include Campylobacter, Salmonella, Shigella, and Escherichia coli), viruses (such as rotavirus, Norwalk virus, cytomegalovirus, herpes simplex virus, and viral hepatitis), food intolerances (like lactose intolerance), parasites (such Giardia lamblia, Entamoeba histolytica, and Cryptosporidium), reaction to medications (such as antibiotics, blood pressure medications, and antacids containing magnesium), intestinal diseases (such as inflammatory bowel disease or celiac disease), bowel disorders (such as irritable bowel syndrome), or emotional stress.

If you get diarrhea, try eating foods with soluble fiber. Oats, barley, flaxseed, and the soft parts of fruits, vegetables, dried beans and peas, are examples of soluble fiber. Soluble fiber soaks up water in the digestive tract, making stool firmer and slower to pass. Make sure to get plenty of fluids to replace those you are losing. The dehydration that follows diarrhea is a common cause of death among malnourished people.

Irritable Bowel Syndrome

Irritable bowel syndrome, or IBS, affects the bowel, which is another name for the large intestine. The word syndrome refers to a cluster of symptoms, and the symptoms typical of IBS include cramps, bloating, gas, diarrhea, and constipation. (Most people have either diarrhea or constipation, but some people have both.)

With IBS, the nerves and muscles in the large intestine are hyper-sensitive. The muscles may contract too much after you eat, and these contractions can cause cramping and diarrhea. Or the nerves can be overly sensitive to the normal stretching of the bowel that may occur as a result of gas, causing cramping or pain.

Contrary to popular belief, emotional stress is unlikely to cause a person to develop IBS, although it can trigger symptoms in someone who already has IBS. In fact, the bowel can overreact to all sorts of things, including food and exercise.

Foods that tend to cause symptoms include milk products, chocolate, alcohol, caffeine, carbonated drinks, and fatty foods. Simply eating a large meal may trigger symptoms. Women with IBS often have more symptoms during their menstrual periods.

Fiber reduces IBS symptoms. Helpful pharmaceutical treatments are available, but over-the-counter peppermint oil also proves to be effective, without the side effects[80]. (Recommended dosage is 1-2 enteric-coated peppermint oil capsules three times a day for 2 to 4 weeks.)

Constipation

By world standards, America is a constipated culture! This is because of the low fiber content to our diets that is a result of our meat-centered focus, particularly when compared to the fiber rich plant-based diets of many traditional cultures.

Constipation refers to dry, hard stools that may be painful to pass. It occurs when waste remains in your colon for too long so that too much water is absorbed.

The first key to preventing constipation is: when you gotta go, go! If you don't respond to the need to defecate, you give your colon more time to absorb water, making your stool drier and more difficult to pass. Next, be sure to get plenty of fiber and fluids. Insoluble fiber is particularly valuable, and can be found in flaxseed, whole grains, vegetables, and the peels of fruit. It acts as a natural laxative that speeds the passage of foods through the stomach. It also gives stool its bulk and helps it move quickly through the gastrointestinal tract. Regular exercise will also make the muscles of your digestive tract stronger.

Hemorrhoids and diverticulosis may result from persistent constipation. Both disorders are much more common in industrialized countries, where diets are low in fiber. Diverticulosis first appeared in the U.S. in 1900, which is about the same time that processed foods were introduced. (Processed grains are typically stripped of the fiber that was present in the whole grain, so food processing marked a sharp transition to a lower-fiber diet.)

Hemorrhoids

Wondering why Napolean is always pictured side-saddle? The discomfort of hemorrhoids!

We all have small veins at the end of our rectum that allow circulation of blood. Straining to eliminate stool (especially when you're constipated) causes these veins to temporarily swell. Repeated straining causes them to remain swollen – and this is when you start to call them hemorrhoids.

You know you have hemorrhoids if you have pain and/or itching of your anus; you may also see some blood in your stool if any veins burst.

Hemorrhoids are very common. In fact, about half of the population have hemorrhoids by age 50. Pregnant women are particularly susceptible due to the pressure exerted by the fetus in the abdomen, as well as hormonal changes, which cause the hemorrhoidal vessels to enlarge. These vessels are also placed under severe pressure during childbirth. For most women, however, hemorrhoids caused by pregnancy are a temporary problem.

Over-the-counter creams and suppositories are usually pretty helpful at alleviating the symptoms. Fiber, fluids and regular exercise are the long-term helpers.

Diverticulosis

Diverticulosis refers to the presence of weak areas or tiny pouches in the colon wall. The pouches, called diverticula, look like small thumbs or tiny balloons poking out of the side of the colon. Sometimes one or more of these pouches becomes inflamed or infected, a condition called diverticulitis.

Abdominal pain is the main symptom, and you should have this pain checked out by a physician. Fiber and fluids are the best dietary guidelines.

How Well Do You Treat Your Digestive Tract?

Put a check mark in the box before the questions that you respond "yes" to.

- [ ] Do you eat a low-fiber diet - one lacking fruits, vegetables, whole grains, and beans (legumes)?
- [ ] Are you physically active less than 30 minutes a day?
- [ ] Do you seldom drink water or low calorie beverages?
- [ ] Do you suffer from constipation and/or diarrhea?
- [ ] Do you feel abdominal pain, bloating, or gas after consuming some dairy products?
- [ ] Does eating certain foods routinely give you discomfort?
- [ ] Do you have digestive tract problems such as ulcers, hemorrhoids, diverticulosis, constipation or lactose intolerance?
- [ ] Do you have a family history of digestive problems?
- [ ] Do you often get hiccups?
- [ ] Do you lie down after eating?
- [ ] Do you wear tight clothes, such as jeans?
- [ ] Do you smoke?
- [ ] Do you take antacids, acid reducers, or acid controllers?

Any "yes" responses suggest that you may want to change your habits to reduce your risk for digestive disorders.

Action Tips...

Which of these are changes that would be helpful for your digestion?

- [ ] Eat slowly.
- [ ] Sit and relax while you eat.
- [ ] Don't lie down after eating.
- [ ] Avoid overeating.
- [ ] Avoid foods/drinks that cause problems.
- [ ] Exercise regularly.
- [ ] Quit smoking.
- [ ] Drink plenty of fluids.
- [ ] Get plenty of fiber.
- [ ] Avoid antacids.

☐ Know your family medical history and watch for symptoms.

Carbohydrates: Not all that Complex

Should you eat a high-carbohydrate diet? Or low-carbohydrate? The constant media debate obscures a simple truth: carbohydrates aren't all good or all bad. Some kinds promote good health and its to your advantage to load up. Others may be less beneficial, but are harmless in moderation and may add an enjoyable kick to your diet.

"Carbo" refers to carbon (C) and "hydrate" refers to water (H_20), and, as the name implies, they are built from carbon and water. In a process called photosynthesis[a], plants, using sunlight as a catalyst, absorb carbon dioxide from the atmosphere and combine it with water they get from the soil to form a ring which is called a sugar molecule; all carbohydrates are merely a chain of one or more sugars bonded together. (The more technical name for a sugar is a saccharide.) It's more than a figure of speech to say that plants create food out of thin air!

With the exception of lactose, a type of sugar that is contained in milk, all carbohydrates come from plants. Concentrated sources of carbohydrates include fruits, vegetables, grains and beans.

Carbohydrates that contain a single sugar are called monosaccharides, those that contain two sugars bonded together are called disaccharides, and those that contain between three and ten sugars are called oligosaccharides. Longer chains, called polysaccharides, can contain hundreds or thousands of sugar rings. You may have heard of some of the technical names of the more common monosaccharides: glucose, fructose and galactose; or the common disaccharides: sucrose, lactose, and maltose.

Carbohydrates come in two forms, simple and complex, which are distinguished by the number of sugar rings that are bonded together. Mono and disaccharides are simple carbohydrates, while oligosaccharides and polysaccharides are complex carbohydrates. Dieticians typically teach us to distinguish between these types of carbohydrates, explaining that complex carbohydrates get put to good use by the body, while simple carbohydrates are less valuable to your health and should be minimized in your diet. We will see that this is often meaningless. Sugar is not synonymous with "white death," and the complex carbohydrate found in most breads acts fairly similar in your body to the sugar that sweetens your soda. There are more important ways to distinguish the effect of carbohydrates on your health, which will be discussed in this section.

Complex carbohydrates are further divided into two categories, starches and fibers, which are distinguished by the type of bond that holds the sugars together. The human body contains enzymes that can break starch bonds during digestion. However, we do not have enzymes that can break the bonds in fiber. As a result, we can't digest it – which is a good thing, as we'll see shortly.

To store energy, plants chain sugar molecules together to form starch. When the plant needs energy, the bonds holding the glucose molecules together are broken, and the energy that was holding the bonds together is released. Starch is a better way to store energy than glucose because it can be stored in large amounts without taking up as much space as individual glucose molecules.

There are two principle types of plant starches, amylose and amylopectin, both of which are composed of glucose molecules. Amylose consists of a long straight chain of glucose rings, while the glucose chains in amylopectin have many side branches.

---

[a] This is part of an interesting process called the carbon cycle, a testimony to our interconnection with nature. Animals eat the plants and use the carbon to build their own tissues. Other animals may then eat that animal and use the carbon for their own needs. These animals (including humans, of course) return carbon dioxide into the air when they breathe, and also when they die, since the carbon is returned to the soil during decomposition. Carbon atoms in soil may then be used in a new plant or in a microorganism. The same carbon atom can move through many organisms and be recycled for millennia.

Carbohydrates in the body

Carbohydrates get used in a variety of ways by your body, but the most important role of sugar and starch is as an energy source. All cells use carbohydrates for energy, and some cells in your brain, nervous system and blood can *only* use carbohydrates efficiently for energy. Other cells can use protein and fat to supplement the carbohydrate energy, but they need carbohydrate to burn these other fuels efficiently.

Carbohydrate is also important in providing structure to certain cells, but the body is fully able to synthesize these carbohydrates from non-carbohydrate sources, making dietary carbohydrate almost completely available for energy.

Fiber is particularly valuable for good health, in large part because you can't digest it. It acts like a pipe cleaner as it travels through your digestive system, pulling harmful substances out of your digestive tract and your circulatory system, slowing the digestion and absorption of other nutrients, and strengthening your digestive tract along the way. Inadequate levels of fiber are associated with many diseases, including appendicitis, atherosclerosis, colon cancer, constipation, diabetes, diverticulosis, and hemorrhoids, while increased consumption provides many health benefits[81].

There are five primary ways that fiber is helpful:

- Although we can't digest fiber, our intestines are filled with bacteria that can. These bacteria help keep us healthy by manufacturing vitamins for us, aiding in digestion and immune function, and removing toxins from our body. When we eat fiber, we keep these microbes healthy and well-fed so they can do their important work.
- Fiber gives you a feeling of fullness because it absorbs water. It also delays the emptying of your stomach so that you feel fuller longer. For these reasons, it is helpful with diabetes and insulin resistance. (We'll learn more about these later.)
- Because it absorbs water, fiber increases the bulk in your intestinal tract. This stimulates the muscles, keeping them toned. The toned muscles can then better move food through the digestive tract, which minimizes your risk for digestive disorders.
- Fiber helps to sweep cholesterol out of your body (both dietary cholesterol and the cholesterol that is synthesized by your liver), lowering your risk for cardiovascular disease.
- Fiber grabs on to toxins and helps pull them out of your digestive tract, possibly lowering your cancer risk.

If you're switching to a higher fiber diet, you may have an increase in gas; you may be able to reduce this effect by making changes slowly, giving your body time to adjust along the way.

Can you get too much fiber? Consuming large amounts in a short time can result in intestinal gas and discomfort. If your fiber comes from dietary sources, you are unlikely to overdo it.

An extremely high fiber diet may result in mineral deficiency, as fiber binds to some minerals, lessening their absorption. This effect is minimal, however, and since high fiber foods are rich in minerals, they more than compensate for any losses. Fiber supplements are more likely to create mineral deficiencies if your diet is otherwise mineral-poor.

Be sure to drink plenty of fluids when consuming fiber so that you don't clog up your digestive tract. (Fiber "holds" water; in fact, insoluble fiber can swell to about 20 times its size in the presence of adequate water!)

Digestion, Absorption and Processing

The digestive system handles all sugar and starch in much the same way, clipping the bonds between the sugar rings and reducing them to single sugar units (monosaccharides). Monosaccharides are the only carbohydrates that are small enough to be absorbed through the intestinal lining and get into your bloodstream. Once in the bloodstream, they travel to your liver. Your body can only use carbohydrate energy in one form - glucose, also called "blood sugar" - so your liver converts any monosaccharide that is not already in the form of glucose into glucose. The liver can then release the glucose into the bloodstream so that it is available for delivery to individual cells that need it for energy, or convert the glucose into its storage form.

After carbohydrates are digested, absorbed and processed by the liver, they become indistinguishable. That the types of sugar affect our metabolism differently is in part the result of a difference in the speed of digestion and absorption and the processing time required by the liver.

Compared to the other nutrients, the digestion, absorption and processing of carbohydrate is rapid; glucose levels in your bloodstream increase fairly quickly after a carbohydrate-containing meal, although this elevation is only temporary, and your glucose levels return to normal within 2-3 hours.

The exception is fiber. Our body doesn't have the digestive enzymes to break the bonds holding the sugar molecules together in fiber, and so it passes through the body undigested.

Glycemic Index/Load

How fast a particular carbohydrate food (other than fiber) turns into glucose and raises your blood glucose (also known as blood sugar) is one of the more important determinants of its effect on your health. This idea is expressed numerically as the glycemic index (GI). The quicker a food raises your blood glucose levels, the higher its glycemic index.

This section will help you to understand the glycemic effects of foods, and will be followed up with a discussion of how glycemia affects your health.

There are four major issues to consider when forecasting a food's glycemic effect (which is just a fancy way of referring to how quickly the the glucose will get into your bloodstream).

Size. For the most part, the smaller a carbohydrate, the quicker it gets digested and absorbed. Many simple sugars, for example, don't even need to be digested as they are already in a form that your body can absorb. For this reason, you can use the simple rule of thumb that simple carbohydrates are likely to have a high glycemic index.

With complex carbohydrates, the more bonds that need to get broken, the longer time will be required to break these bonds, so an oligosaccharide composed of three or four sugar units will be digested much more akin to a simple sugar than to a polysaccharide chain composed of thousands of sugars. Many "sports bars" utilize short chain oligosaccharides as sweeteners, and their label will boast that they are high in complex carbohydrates. Though the label is technically accurate, the effect of those sports bars on your body may be similar to a candy bar sweetened with simple sugar.

Composition. Another issue that affects how quickly carbohydrates get into the bloodstream relates to the composition of the sugars. Glucose requires no processing by the liver, and when it is contained in foods it gets into the bloodstream quickly. (Table sugar, for example, contains 50 percent glucose.) An apple, on the other hand, contains 100 percent fructose, and no glucose. Since the fructose has to be converted to glucose, it takes a little longer to get into your bloodstream.

Even more important is the type of starch. Amylopectin has many branches, while amylose is a straight chain. The amylopectin branches offer more surfaces for enzymes to work on, and is consequently digested much more quickly. (The type of starch found in the white rice used in traditional Chinese and Japanese cooking is composed of amylopectin, which raises your blood glucose levels quickly, meaning that it results in a high glycemic index. This accounts for why many people describe feeling hungry soon after eating Chinese meals. White basmati rice used in Indian cooking, on the other hand, is composed of amylose, which takes longer to digest.)

The *physical nature* of the carbohydrate. The small particle size of flours results in quicker breakdown compared to the whole form of the wheat. The yeast in bread further has an effect of expanding the surface area, giving digestive enzymes more room to work. These both result in quickening the rise in blood glucose and a higher glycemic index.

Amount of *fiber* or other nutrients that may slow digestion/absorption. Fiber can't be digested, and as it travels through your digestive system, it binds to other carbohydrates, thus slowing their digestion and absorption and lowering their glycemic index. This is another reason why the sugar from the apple will be released more slowly than that contained in table sugar: some of the starch is encased in a fibrous coating. The presence of protein and fat in a meal will also slow the digestion of carbohydrates. Mono-unsaturated fats (which we'll read about later) lower the GI of foods they are eaten with by increasing secretion of a hormone (glucagon-like-peptide-1) which delays stomach emptying.

Because of these factors (and others), all carbohydrates are far from equal nutritionally, and there is much disparity in the effects they will have on your body. For example, if you drink soda (which has a high glycemic index), your blood glucose levels will rise at a rate of 30 kcals/min, whereas brown basmati rice will raise your blood glucose levels about 2 kcals/min. You ordinarily use energy at a rate of less than 2 kcal/min. When you down a Pepsi, you flood your body with much more energy than you can use, triggering your body to store the excess energy. The basmati rice, on the other hand, gets into your bloodstream at a much slower pace, more commensurate with your needs.

Dieticians often recommend avoiding simple sugars and maximizing complex carbohydrates for their purported glycemic effects. However, this simplistic advice may mislead you, as some complex carbohydrates have a higher GI than some simple carbohydrates. For example, many starchy foods, like baked potatoes and white bread, result in an even higher GI than table sugar[82].

To consume a diet with a lower glycemic index (and we'll discuss the value of this shortly), choose carbohydrates that are low in sugar and high in fiber. Also, minimize your intake of refined carbohydrates such as white bread; these enter the bloodstream almost as quickly as simple sugars. (A more in-depth discussion of refined grains follows later in this chapter.)

A certain amount of nutritional knowledge is necessary to implement a low-GI diet, and foods should not be selected only for the GI. For example, the GI is not significant for foods which are low in energy and in which the ratio of other nutritious compounds, like minerals, vitamins, and phytochemicals is high. That is where glycemic load (GL) comes in. The GL measures the glycemic index times the total amount of carbohydrate, and provides a better measure of low energy foods. The glycemic index value for carrots is much higher than potatoes, but because the amount of carbohydrate in carrots is minimal (7 grams in a serving) compared to potatoes (37 grams), the glycemic load is low, and there is no reason to minimize carrots in a healthful diet.

Learning more about the glycemic load of foods you commonly eat will help you have a better understanding of their impact on your health. But before we move to our discussion of glycemia and health, I want to encourage you to keep a healthy perspective about this concept. The glycemic load of foods is not always straightforward and foods don't always work as anticipated. The research is rife with conflicting values for the same foods. But the concept of glycemic load does alert you to the value of eating unprocessed foods that are high in fiber. It also alerts you to the undesirable effects of eating large quantities, or of eating processed foods, particularly those that are high in added sugars.

Understanding Blood Glucose Regulation

After carbohydrate digestion and absorption, glucose is in your bloodstream and available as a potential energy source for your body cells. However, only a limited amount of glucose can comfortably "fit" in the bloodstream (the equivalent of about 80 kcals worth!), and excess can do damage. After meals, our body takes excess glucose and stores it. During the periods when we are not eating, it then releases it from storage to help fuel us.

Let's add a little more detail to help you understand glucose storage and its subsequent release.

Carbohydrate Storage and Release

To obtain energy from glucose, the body goes through a series of metabolic reactions, breaking the glucose into smaller and smaller molecules, until it is reduced to its waste products, carbon dioxide and water. This process is called glycolysis.

Excess glucose molecules get packaged together in a long chain called glycogen. Glycogen is a short-term energy reserve, stored in your muscles and liver. When your blood glucose levels get high, you trigger the release of a hormone (insulin) which helps get the glucose into the cells for conversion into glycogen. This process is called glycogenesis (the roots of this term help you to see that it refers to "generating glycogen"). (If glycogen storage is full, the excess glucose then gets converted to fatty acids and stored as fat.)

When your blood glucose level gets low, you trigger the release of other hormones (notably glucagon, epinephrine, and cortisol) that act on your liver to convert the glycogen into glucose and release it into the bloodstream. The breakdown of glycogen into glucose is called glycogenolysis ("lysis" means breaking down).

You typically have enough glycogen stored in your liver to provide the glucose to get you through about four hours between meals, or about twelve hours overnight when you are not using as much energy. This is equivalent to about 2 cups of cooked pasta or 3 candy bars. This is your total reserve capacity to keep the brain functioning properly! Eating sufficient carbohydrates allows you to replenish depleted glycogen stores.

The glycogen stored in your muscles is for use by muscle cells only, and can't be released into the general circulation to raise your blood glucose levels.

Exercise vigorously and you will run out of glycogen quickly. (Endurance athletes call this "bonking" or "hitting the wall" and describe it as a sudden drop in energy. One moment they feel fine, the next they can barely lift their leg. "Bonking" represents the lag time between when they run out of glycogen and when their body switches into alternative methods to replenish their blood glucose.)

You can see that we don't have a lot of glucose energy available in the bloodstream, particularly when you consider that an average man uses energy at the rate of approximately 2 kcal/min. In other words, the 80 kcals of blood glucose, if it were the only energy source, could only support him for about 40 minutes! For this reason, your body has evolved complex pathways to help preserve blood glucose, both through utilizing other fuels and releasing the glucose that is stored in your liver in the form of glycogen.

Metabolism: Glucose Homeostasis

The main function of glucose is to supply energy for the body. Because the brain, nervous system, and red blood cells depend almost exclusively on glucose as an energy source, it is essential that glucose be always available, and your body has many different mechanisms to ensure that the right level of glucose is flowing in the bloodstream. In fact, maintaining appropriate blood glucose levels is the most important function of metabolism: a mere 10 minutes of deprivation can result in a coma.

The foods you eat can play a dramatic role in your mood, in part because of their impact on blood glucose. Adequate blood glucose levels are important for a feeling of well-being. When your blood glucose levels become too high, you may feel sleepy; when they become too low, you feel weak and shaky. Only when blood glucose is at a normal level will you feel alert and energized.

Your endocrine system (hormones) plays the largest role in helping you to maintain blood glucose homeostasis. It tries to keep a constant supply of glucose for your cells by maintaining a constant glucose concentration in your blood - otherwise your cells would have more than enough glucose right after a meal, which would damage them, and starve between meals and overnight. So when you have an over-supply of glucose - for example, immediately following a meal - it gets corrected by sending the excess to the muscles and liver to be stored as glycogen, or if those storage sites are full, it gets converted to fat and stored. When blood glucose gets too low - for example, after an overnight fast - it is replenished by releasing the glucose from stored glycogen in the liver. If you run out of glycogen reserves, your body can make new glucose from your body proteins.

In order to understand how we maintain glucose homeostasis, let's learn about the hormones of metabolism.

Hormones of Glucose Metabolism

Hormones are chemical messengers that help to regulate our metabolism. The major metabolic hormones are insulin and glucagon, and the stress hormones, epinephrine and cortisol.

Insulin is the leader of the storage team, while glucagon is the leader of the breakdown team. Your body releases insulin when your blood glucose concentrations rise, and releases the other hormones, which are called the counter-regulatory hormones (glucagon, epinephrine and cortisol), when your blood glucose levels fall.

Lowering Blood Glucose

Insulin does its job of lowering blood glucose in large part by helping get glucose into cells that need it for energy or can store it as glycogen, and by inhibiting your body from making new glucose. It acts as a gatekeeper to get glucose into cells. Without insulin (or if the cells have difficulty responding to insulin), you can eats lots of food and actually be in a state of starvation because that glucose can't get out of the bloodstream and into the cells that need it for energy.

Insulin has other metabolic jobs. Not only does it lower blood glucose levels, but it also works to lower blood concentrations of the other energy-producing nutrients after a meal. For example, it stimulates fat cells to form fats from fatty acids that are in the bloodstream, and stimulates liver and muscle cells to make proteins from amino acids, thus reducing blood concentrations of fatty acids (the breakdown product of dietary fat) and amino acids (the breakdown product of dietary protein). If there is excess glucose that can't fit into glycogen storage, insulin activates enzymes that convert the glucose into fatty acids and promotes their storage in adipose (fat) tissue. It also inhibits lipolysis (fat breakdown), ensuring that more glucose is taken up.

There are several stimuli for the release of insulin. These include a rise in blood glucose and amino acids, such as would happen after the digestion and absorption of carbohydrate and protein. Insulin release is also stimulated by some "satiety hormones" that are generated by the digestive tract in response to the presence of food.

Raising Blood Glucose

The counter-regulatory hormones convert glycogen back into glucose, and can create new glucose from amino acids. Thus, these hormones cause blood glucose to rise again.

When you haven't eaten for a while and your blood glucose levels fall, you release the hormone glucagon. Glucagon has effects that oppose insulin: it stimulates the liver and muscle to break down stored glycogen and release the glucose into your bloodstream, and it also stimulates your liver and kidneys to make new glucose out of amino acid remnants from proteins on your body, a process called gluconeogenesis. (You can understand this term by breaking it apart: "gluco" refers to glucose; "neo" means new; and "genesis" refers to generating; in other words, gluconeogenesis refers to generating new glucose.)

Like insulin, the major factor regulating glucagon release is blood glucose concentration. Elevated blood glucose stimulates the release of insulin and inhibits the release of glucagon, while decreased blood glucose triggers the opposite. Thus, these hormones act synergistically to maintain blood glucose homeostasis. These two hormones also have opposing effects on fat metabolism.

A different mechanism increases blood glucose during times of stress, whether that stress is physical, such as exercise, or psychological. The stress hormones, epinephrine and cortisol, both increase blood levels of glucose. (Epinephrine is more commonly referred to as adrenaline in the general public.) Epinephrine is released quickly and its effects are immediate; cortisol release is slower, and its actions are slower and more long-term.

Growth hormone also can elevate the blood levels of glucose and fatty acids. Like the stress hormones, it is typically of little importance during normal metabolism. However, it becomes important in helping to maintain blood glucose during severe stress or starvation (or very low energy diets).

Glucose regulation in simple perspective

The following is a diagram of a sample day's worth of healthy blood glucose regulation.

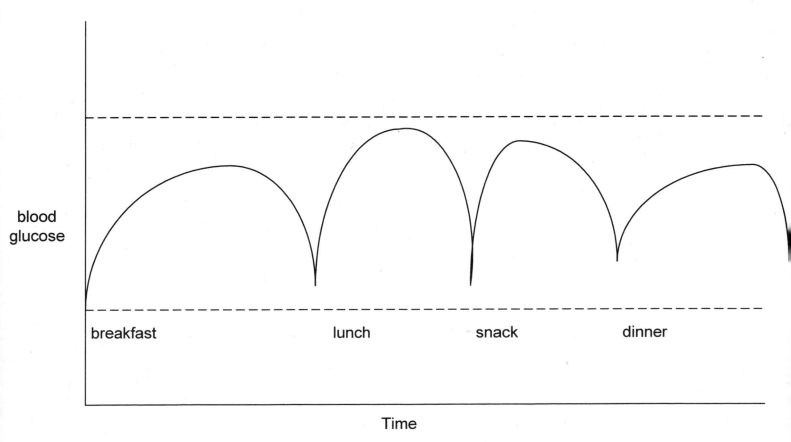

The dotted lines refer to the healthy upper and lower limits of blood glucose. This woman's blood glucose was low in the morning due to an overnight fast, during which her cells were using the glucose energy, thus removing it from the bloodstream. She ate breakfast and her blood glucose rose, then got lower again as she used her glucose following breakfast. She ate lunch, pumping up her glucose again, and continued this pattern with a snack and dinner. When her blood glucose got low and approached the lower limit, she felt hungry and ate. She stopped eating when she was full, keeping her blood glucose below the healthy upper limit.

Another way to eat healthfully is grazing - snacking frequently throughout the day - which keeps hunger and fullness levels steady.

The following example shows the flipside - undesirable blood glucose regulation:

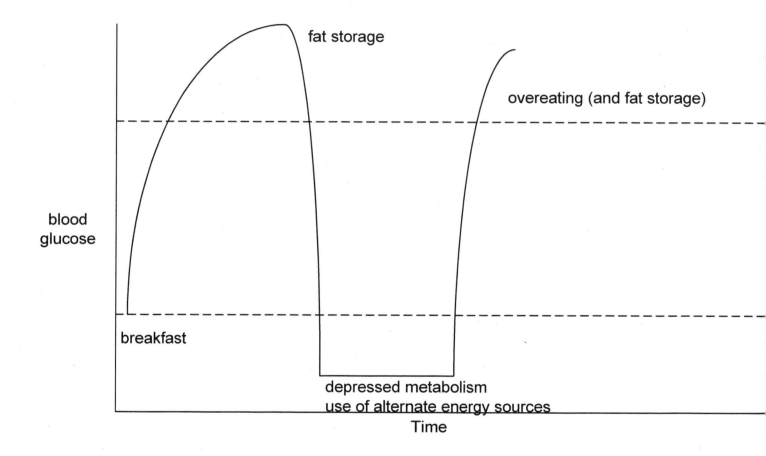

This person ate too much, spiking her blood glucose to an unhealthy level called transient hyperglycemia, or high blood sugar. You might feel "speedy" for a few minutes when your blood glucose gets this high, although not everyone experiences this.

When your brain senses high blood sugar, it signals "system overload!" This starts body reactions that bring your blood glucose down. Most important of these processes is the release of insulin, allowing energy-containing nutrients like glucose to get into cells. When insulin is released, the insulin binds to the cells, and the glucose enters. Your cells take up the glucose and use what they need.

Some cells, like muscle cells and liver cells, can make glycogen, and will pack away what they can't use. But when you exceed your modest storage capacity, you are out of luck.

Ah, but fat cells are much more accommodating. They can expand indefinitely to store extra energy. This means that the rest of the glucose gets converted into fat and your fat storage cells roll out the red carpet. Even a thin individual has probably 100 times as much energy stored as fat compared to glycogen.

High blood glucose *may* make your body over-compensate and release too much insulin. (Not everyone has this response – and there is much scientific debate as to whether its occurrence is overblown in the popular media. Genetic susceptibility and your past history define whether it occurs for you.) Too much glucose gets drawn out of your bloodstream (transient hypoglycemia). You feel the sugar crash: you're hungry, tired, irritable and anxious. You may also crave foods (sweets) that will ratchet your blood glucose levels quickly.

You may have eaten recently, but your body thinks it is starving because blood glucose is low and it can't access the pounds of fat that you've got socked away. This launches a refrigerator raid. Quick fix needed! The bottom line is this: over-eating and eating lots of carbohydrates that get into your bloodstream quickly may cause you to feel hungry and continue to crave them. These cravings can come anywhere from 20 minutes to 3 hours after eating.

Sugar cravings and the emotional lows are just a small part of the distress you undergo when your blood sugar gets too low. You may also experience a headache, which is a result of your brain not getting enough glucose. Another side effect is that your metabolism slows down to try to preserve the little blood glucose that you have. In other words, getting too hungry just causes you to use *less* calories! (Contrast this to eating, which actually speeds up your metabolism.)

Yet another side effect is that it triggers a second wave of hormones, including stress hormones, such as epinephrine and cortisol, in order to get your blood levels up. While these do work effectively to get your blood glucose levels up, it's at a cost to the body. One cost is an increased risk for heart attacks. Another cost is excess hunger, which continues even after eating.

Of course we can't forget the other side effect of low blood glucose levels: your body then has to scavenge for an alternative way to make glucose. The only way to make glucose is from the amino acids that are part of protein. You don't store protein on your body, and as all is in active use, your body in effect "cannibalizes" itself, compromising immune function and weakening your muscle.

What's a person with this experience to do?

This is where an understanding of glycemic load comes in handy: try to avoid the spike from a high glycemic load. Eat smaller amounts and foods that get into your bloodstream more slowly, and your blood glucose climbs more slowly and doesn't crest as high as it does with larger quantities and quickly digested carbohydrates. The glucose also falls more slowly, making it unlikely that you'll see your levels drop to the point of distress.

Try this and you can expect to experience noticeable changes in your cravings, your energy, and your emotional state. You may be shocked to discover that you feel better with less sugar, and that you no longer crave it.

Disorders of Blood Glucose Regulation

Now that you have learned how your body regulates blood glucose, let's look at what happens when something goes wrong with this system. The two most common disorders are insulin resistance and diabetes. Given how prevalent they are, odds are pretty good you know someone with one of these disorders – or you have one yourself.

We'll discuss each in general terms first, and then we'll focus in on more specific details.

Insulin Resistance

Millions of adults – perhaps one quarter of the U.S. population – have cells that are at least partially insulin resistant[83], although it is often undiagnosed. When a person has insulin resistance, many of their cells are resistant, meaning less sensitive, to the effects of insulin. When insulin gets released, it is limited in its ability to get glucose out of the bloodstream and into the cells.

The more common term for insulin resistance in the general public is "carbohydrate sensitivity." If the name doesn't ring a bell, the symptoms might: feeling hungry or tired after you eat and at other times that you shouldn't, mood swings, creeping blood pressure or cholesterol or weight.

<u>Diabetes</u>

Diabetes is a particularly malicious disease as it often goes unnoticed while it causes irreversible damage to many of the body's most vital systems. The fifth deadliest disease in the United States, diabetes affects 18.2 million people in this country and kills approximately 400,000 each year, according to the American Diabetes Association (ADA). In the eight years from 1990 to 1998, the incidence of diabetes increased 33 percent[84]. Particularly alarming is that one-third of people with diabetes aren't aware that they have it[85].

There are three major types of diabetes: type 1 diabetes, type 2 diabetes, and gestational diabetes. Previously, type 2 diabetes was referred to as "adult-onset diabetes" and type 1 diabetes was referred to as "juvenile-onset diabetes." However, because up to 45 percent of new diabetes cases in children are type 2 diabetes, the age-specific names have been dropped[86].

People who have **type 1 diabetes** don't make insulin or don't make sufficient insulin; they require insulin injections for survival. For this reason, it is also called insulin-dependent diabetes. It is an auto-immune disease in which the immune system attacks the insulin-secreting cells of the pancreas, typically in childhood. Type 1 diabetes accounts for approximately 5 to 10 percent of all diabetes cases.

Type 2 diabetes is characterized by insulin resistance, just a more severe form. The more common type of diabetes, it accounts for over 90 percent of all cases. Its incidence is on the rise, especially in the younger population, while at the same time, new government findings suggest that the rate of diabetes control is on the decline. Poor diabetes control is serious stuff: an estimated 90% of all patients with diabetes are not controlling it enough to prevent diabetes-related health risks, including blindness, amputation, kidney failure, heart attack, and stroke.

Some women get a temporary form of diabetes during pregnancy, called **gestational diabetes**, in which hormones that help the baby develop also partially block the action of insulin in the mother's body. Gestational diabetes typically occurs in late pregnancy, after the baby's body has been formed, and if the mother takes good care of her diabetes, the pregnancy can result in a healthy baby. However, poorly controlled or untreated diabetes can hurt both mother and baby.

Gestational diabetes usually goes away after the baby is delivered, although it may increase the mother's risk of developing type 2 diabetes later in life.

<u>Normal glucose metabolism versus insulin resistance/diabetes</u>

To understand insulin resistance and diabetes, let's first review normal metabolism. When a metabolically fit individual eats, they digest and absorb the food and their blood glucose rises. Glucose and other nutrients circulate through their bloodstream, triggering their pancreas to release insulin. Insulin then tells their cells to take up the glucose and other nutrients. Their cells are sensitive to insulin and can respond to its effects. The cells get the glucose energy they need; other nutrients are routed to storage.

People who have insulin resistance, type 2 diabetes, or gestational diabetes have a muted response to insulin, whereas people with type 1 diabetes can't produce sufficient insulin. Regardless of the type of metabolic disorder, the result is the same: insulin can't do its job properly. Glucose can't get into the cells that need it for energy, and the individual may feel as if he or she is starving, despite high blood glucose levels. (For this reason, diabetes is called "starvation in the midst of plenty.")

While type 1 diabetes has a sudden onset, insulin resistance is a progressive disease which can advance to become type 2 diabetes. When type 2 diabetes progresses, eventually the pancreas may become so tired that it loses its ability to produce enough insulin. That's why noticing and treating insulin resistance and type 2 diabetes in their early stages is helpful.

Here's the process for the progression of insulin resistance: because insulin can't have its full effect, its as if the cell "doors" are partially shut, and blood glucose levels remain high after a meal. (This is known as hyperglycemia.) That leaves the cells failing to get the energy they need, so they continue to send the "I'm hungry" message. That prompts the pancreas to release even more insulin and your appetite also increases to compensate. You eat more, causing increased hyperglycemia and the release of more insulin. This results in high levels of insulin in your bloodstream (called hyperinsulinemia). Your overwhelmed cells shut down to the effects of insulin even more, making you even more insulin-resistant.

Insulin resistance affects different cell types differently. Cells in your muscle and liver are more likely to develop insulin resistance, while fat cells are typically unaffected. The cells in your liver and muscles are most important for using and storing glucose, and it becomes difficult to get glucose into these cells to use for energy or storage. Because cells in fat tissue don't develop the same resistance, it is easy to pack fat into fat storage. In other words, there are plenty of energy nutrients in your bloodstream, and your liver and muscle cells are crying for this energy and unable to get it. With nowhere else to turn, the energy gets converted into fat, and the fat cells readily take it up for storage.

The result? You feel hungry and gain weight! In other words, weight gain is an early symptom of type 2 diabetes for some people, providing partial explanation for why type 2 diabetes is more common among heavier people. Research shows that high levels of insulin appear before weight gain in future diabetics[87, 88]. This means that the increase in obesity that we have seen in the last few decades may in part reflect increasing insulin resistance in our population. (However, keep in mind that people of all sizes get diabetes. Thinness does not protect you from diabetes.)

The relationship between type 2 diabetes and body fat appears to be self-perpetuating: the high levels of insulin characteristic of type 2 diabetes lead to weight gain, and high levels of visceral fat increase insulin resistance, worsening the type 2 diabetes.

The insulin myth

Because insulin helps you pack fat away, many people think insulin encourages weight gain. Popular weight loss diets demonize insulin and urge people to avoid foods that stimulate insulin release. However, those diets don't distinguish between normal insulin responses to meals and the chronic over-production of insulin that triggers insulin resistance.

In fact, insulin is one of the most important regulators of your weight regulation system – and is very effective at helping keep your weight down! One of the many effects of insulin production, for example, is triggering the release of leptin, which in turn helps to decrease your appetite and speed up your metabolism.

In moderate quantities, insulin is your friend – and avoidance of insulin is associated with weight gain[89]. Chronically over-produced, on the other hand, insulin can lead to insulin resistance and weight gain.

What causes insulin resistance and type 2 diabetes?

No one really knows. There is no doubt that genetic susceptibility plays a large role in their development, and that degree of susceptibility varies widely from individual to individual. Lifestyle habits – particularly those that play a role in insulin release and sensitivity - also influence their development – and can prevent or reverse them. Some people can get away with the lifestyle habits that encourage these disorders, whereas others are much more vulnerable to their effects.

Less well discussed (and understood) is the role of environmental pollution. Many pollutants are fat-soluble and stay in fat tissue for many years. Several studies have demonstrated an association of dioxin exposure[90, 91] or other organic pollutants[92, 93] and diabetes risk. This was most evident in an air force study of Vietnam veterans in which the servicemen who loaded the pesticide Agent Orange onto the planes had far higher rates of incident diabetes than the pilots. Also, after a chemical leak in a plant in Arkansas making Agent Orange, there were higher rates of insulin resistance and diabetes in people living nearby compared to a control population living 50 miles away. Other studies show that injection of dioxin into rats stimulates fat cells to secrete chemicals such as TNF-alpha, which are inducers of insulin resistance[94, 95]. Another study indicates striking dose-response relations (38-fold!) between serum concentrations of six selected pollutants and the prevalence of diabetes[96].

What causes Type 1 Diabetes?

To understand this question, let's start with a discussion of your immune system. Your immune system is designed to defend your body against foreign invaders, like bacteria or viruses. A substance that can produce an immune response is called an antigen.

To fight antigens, the immune system has a few tricks. Among them is the ability to create a protein, called an antibody, which can fit onto the antigen (like a lock fits a key) and destroy it.

The first time your immune system meets an invader, it needs to create the right defense. Once this is accomplished, it has a great memory. On initial exposure to streptococcus bacteria (the bacteria responsible for strep throat), for example, your immune cells struggle to create antibodies that can kill the bacteria. You might feel some nasty symptoms for a few days, such as a wicked sore throat or a high fever. However, the second time you encounter the strep virus you're prepared. The antibodies are more quickly created and mobilized and the fight is shorter and less difficult. You may not even feel sick.

Sometimes the foreign invaders that enter our body look a lot like our body cells. This is called molecular mimicry. In that case, the antibody that fits onto the invader may also fit onto your own cells. When this happens, the immune system could easily mistake one of your own cells for an invader and attack it. In other words, the body turns against some of its own cells. This is called an "auto-immune" response, where the word "auto" refers to your self. Your body becomes its own worst enemy.

So what does this have to do with nutrition? It so happens that the antigens that trick you into attacking your own cells may come from your food. Some proteins that you eat could slip through the digestive process without being fully broken down into the amino acids they are composed of and enter your bloodstream. They get treated by your immune system as invaders, and your immune system hustles to make an antibody that could destroy them.

Clearly, genetic susceptibility plays a large role in the development of type 1 diabetes. However, even though individuals may have genes that make them more susceptible, they will only get type 1 diabetes in response to certain lifestyle circumstances. (It has been observed that after one person with an identical twin gets type 1 diabetes, there is only a 13-33 percent chance that the other twin will develop it, making it clear that genetics alone is not responsible[18, 97-99].) There is an extraordinary amount of controversy over what those circumstances are for type 1 diabetes.

While there are many hypotheses about what triggers type 1 diabetes in genetically susceptible people, the strongest evidence suggests that it may be associated with cow's milk[18-20]. Cow's milk supplies several foreign proteins that mimic our own body proteins. Whether they contribute to development of type 1 diabetes, however, is one of the most contentious issues in nutrition today.

What's the evidence that cow's milk is involved? First, let's take a look at a study reported in the New England Journal of Medicine in 1992[19]. The researchers examined the blood of young children with and without type 1 diabetes, and measured the levels of antibodies formed against a milk protein called bovine serum albumin (BSA). If BSA antibodies were found, it meant that undigested milk proteins had entered the children's blood. Results were astonishing: there was no overlap in antibody levels of the healthy versus the diabetic children. All 142 of the diabetic children had higher antibody levels than the 79 "normal" children. Clearly, the type 1 diabetic children consumed more milk than the non-diabetic children, and the research raised the question of whether the BSA antibody played a causative role in the diabetes. Another study found that one hundred percent of diabetic children were positive for BSA antibodies compared to 1.9% for healthy controls[100].

An avalanche of studies have examined this relationship. The general theory that has arisen from the research works like this[a]: a genetically susceptible child drinks milk, perhaps weaned onto cow's milk too early. For whatever reason (perhaps a digestive disorder, for example), the cow's milk is not fully digested and protein fragments get absorbed into their body. The immune system destroys them. Unfortunately, some of those fragments look conspicuously like cells in the pancreas responsible for making insulin and the immune system destroys these as well.

In support of this theory, one study found that genetically susceptible children weaned too early onto cow's milk-based formula were 13.1 times more likely to develop type 1 diabetes than those who did not have the genes and were breast-fed for at least three months[101]. A similar study showed an 11.3 times greater risk[102]. While we would expect that genetically susceptible children would have a higher risk, this 11-13 times greater risk is very profound and cannot be explained by genes alone. (T. Colin Campbell puts this into perspective with the example that smokers have a 10 times greater risk of getting lung cancer compared to non-smokers[103].) Genes don't act in isolation but need an environmental trigger.

Providing further support that milk consumption may be that trigger is research documenting an almost perfect correlation between cow's milk consumption and type 1 diabetes in children under age 14; in other words, the greater the consumption of milk, the greater the incidence of type 1 diabetes[104]. On the extremes, for example, this research showed that type 1 diabetes is 36 times more common in Finland, where large amounts of cow's milk is consumed, compared to Japan, where little is consumed. Further research in Finland indicated that cow's milk consumption increased the risk of type 1 diabetes five- to six-fold[105].

Many other studies examining the relationship between cow's milk consumption and type 1 diabetes have been conducted or are underway. One recent scientific review evaluated ten human studies[106]. Five of the ten showed a statistically significant relationship – the greater the consumption of cow's milk, the greater the incidence of type 1 diabetes. The other five studies did not find a statistically significant relationship either way. There are many reasons why an experiment might lack a statistically significant relationship and these five studies – particularly in light of the five studies with positive findings – should not be interpreted to dismiss a relationship. For example, perhaps the study didn't include enough people, or the people were similar enough in their milk consumption so the little differences weren't enough to determine a relationship.

The point is that there is much evidence to suggest concern, even if it's not definitive. However, this issue has huge financial implications for the dairy industry, and is unlikely to receive fair scientific consideration nor reach the popular media anytime soon. Nonetheless, this data so impressed the American Academy of Pediatrics, that in 1994, families with known genetic susceptibility were "strongly encouraged" not to feed cow's milk to infants under two years of age[107].

Long-Term Risks of Diabetes

Hyperglycemia and hyperinsulinemia are insidious, resulting in many long-term complications[108], such as:

- cardiovascular disease;
- stroke;
- hypertension;

---

[a] For more information, see The China Study by T. Colin Campbell.

- blindness;
- kidney disease;
- nervous system disease;
- amputation;
- dental disease;
- pregnancy complications;
- and increased susceptibility to other illnesses.

Bottom line? Get help before it progresses.

Symptoms to Watch For

People with diabetes may have some or none of the following symptoms. Discuss your symptoms with a qualified health professional.

- Feeling hungry despite eating
- Frequent urination
- Excessive thirst
- Unusual weight change
- Increased fatigue
- Irritability
- Blurry vision
- Tingling or numbness in the hands or feet
- Very dry skin
- Sores that are slow to heal

Diagnosis

Blood tests are necessary in diagnosing insulin resistance and type 2 diabetes. The easiest test is to directly measure glucose levels in the blood after an overnight fast. In someone who has a normal metabolism, glucose levels should be low, given that they haven't eaten for a while and their cells removed some of the blood glucose (and stored glycogen) to fuel themselves through the night. With insulin resistance, on the other hand, the cells can't effectively remove the glucose from the blood and it remains elevated. (A value above 140 mg/dl on at least two occasions typically means a person has diabetes. Normal people have fasting glucose levels that generally run between 70-110 mg/dl.)

A more sophisticated test measures the body's ability to appropriately handle the excess glucose presented after consuming a glucose drink. The person being tested starts the test in a fasting state (having no food or drink except water for 10 to16 hours). Blood glucose is tested and then the person is given a glucose solution to drink. The person then has their blood tested again 30 minutes, 1 hour, 2 hours and 3 hours after drinking the glucose drink.

In a person without diabetes, the glucose levels in the blood rise following drinking the glucose drink, but then fall quickly back to normal (because insulin is produced in response to the glucose, and the insulin has a normal effect of lowering blood glucose). In a diabetic, glucose levels rise higher than normal after drinking the glucose drink and come down to normal levels much slower. This is because insulin is either not produced, as in type 1 diabetes, or it is produced but the cells of the body do not respond to it, as in type 2 diabetes.

Preventing/Reversing/Treating Insulin Resistance and Diabetes

Drugs are available to improve insulin sensitivity and deal with the symptoms of insulin resistance and type 2 diabetes, and may be necessary for some people. However, they don't treat the cause. Many people are critical that physicians are too quick to prescribe drugs for diabetes treatment when lifestyle changes can have better results - and without the harmful side effects.

Caught early enough, in many cases, the right lifestyle habits can prevent or reverse the problem[109-115] – and they are the same as those recommended for optimal health in general. An interesting epidemiological study assessed the effects of an improved dietary pattern (similar to that recommended here), increased activity and no smoking, and estimated that in the approximately 85,000 women in the study, 91 percent of the diabetes could have been prevented[116].

The key is to help your body by regulating your blood glucose levels through improved eating and activity habits. (Always remember that genetic susceptibility plays a large role in most diseases. Lifestyle changes will benefit some more than others.)

First, before you even look to dietary changes, become more active. Regular activity teaches your cells to become more sensitive to insulin.

The specifics of what type of activity is most helpful, however, may be different than what you've heard. If you believe that going to the gym or running around the block is a precondition for improved health, I've got some good news for you: it turns out that vacuuming the living room can be just as, or more, beneficial than conventional aerobic exercise for some people.

There is a new model for exercise that has emerged from the scientific research, called "active living." Active living refers to moving more and being more vital as part of your everyday life. It can involve taking the stairs instead of the elevator; raking the leaves yourself instead of recruiting a neighborhood child to do it; or parking at a distant spot at the movies instead of the closest one to the door.

You can get great health benefits from moving more in your life, without meeting those old-fashioned fitness recommendations. More importantly, moving can be pleasurable and light-hearted. It doesn't need to be penance, nor detract from your time for other pursuits.

Next, develop your ability to support your body in regulating your blood glucose through improved eating habits. The weight regulation section discusses the principles of intuitive eating, which helps you to figure out what, when and how much your body wants you to eat.

When considering nutrition, remember to keep perspective. What you eat will be less important than the previous two strategies – and it will be hard to make good nutritional choices if you don't first establish a comfortable relationship with food and your body.

Nonetheless, when you have diabetes, hunger and fullness aren't as effective at helping you to regulate your needs – unless they're combined with good nutritional choices. This is why: suppose you eat and get plenty of energy into your body. The rise in insulin may not effectively get the nutrients into your hungry cells (because of the insulin resistance), and your body might pump up the "I'm hungry" messages, despite the plethora of calories in your bloodstream. However, good nutritional choices can help circumvent this and make sure that your hunger drive is working effectively.

The trick is to consider strategies to lower your insulin output at a given time, such as eating smaller meals, increasing your fiber[117-119], and decreasing simple sugars and other high glycemic foods (such as refined grains). (The goal is not to avoid insulin-inducing foods, but to avoid those that *spike* your insulin. High GI foods need not be avoided, but consuming them in smaller quantities at any given time is beneficial.) Less widely publicized is the value of reducing animal proteins, which also stimulate a large insulin release[120], or increasing soy protein[121], which has been shown to reduce insulin production and insulin resistance[122]. Minimizing saturated[123-128] and trans fats is also valuable, as they can make your receptors less receptive to insulin. (However, increased incidence of diabetes was only found in one of three prospective studies that investigated the association between trans fat intake and diabetes[116, 129, 130].)

The conventional approach to diabetes, recommended by the American Diabetes Association, focuses on minimizing carbohydrates – the rationale being that any carbohydrate requires insulin production, which stresses the body. However, scientific research alerts us to the fallacies behind substituting protein or fat for carbohydrate. Some foods high in protein and fat raise insulin levels higher than carbohydrate, for example[120]. (Surprisingly, fish produces a bigger insulin release than popcorn[120]. And beef and cheese cause a bigger insulin release than pasta[120].) And some fats contribute to decreased insulin sensitivity. Additionally, reducing carbohydrate also results in reduced fiber, though fiber is very beneficial in reducing the rise in blood glucose and subsequent insulin production.

Many studies have actually shown an inverse relationship between the amount of carbohydrate consumed and the development of diabetes[131]. In fact, some groups of people who eat diets centered on high glycemic index carbohydrates, like white rice for Asians, and potatoes for Peruvians, have extremely low rates of diabetes[132, 133]. This may be because they consume their carbohydrates in conjunction with high-fiber foods (vegetables) that temper the insulin response.

The ADA also recommends careful monitoring of blood glucose with glucose meters. While this is generally good advice, be cautious about how you interpret the data. The number on the meter should not be your only consideration. For example, many diabetics choose high-fat diets in order to avoid a glycemic rush. It is true that fat slows the digestion and absorption of glucose and can help you to avoid the spike in blood glucose that may result from eating some high carbohydrate foods. However, this is just a short-term approach. As noted above, some fats can also result in increased insulin release or insulin resistance – facts which don't get instantly reflected on your glucose meter. And a low glycemic load doesn't necessarily equate to more wholesome nutrition.

For optimal health and well-being, you can't beat regular activity and a diet that is rich in vegetables, beans, and whole grains, and there is much research to support the benefits of a plant-based diet in preventing or reversing insulin resistance[109-111, 114, 115, 134-138]. Preliminary research finds that a whole foods, vegan diet is more beneficial than the more traditionally recommended American Diabetic Association diet, which encourages low-fat meats and dairy in addition to whole grains, beans and vegetables[115, 138]. The vegan diet, high in carbohydrate (80 percent of its energy), results in consuming less saturated fat, cholesterol and protein, and more fiber than the ADA diet.

One study showed that after 22 weeks on a vegan diet, 43 percent of the patients were able to reduce their diabetes medication, while many others showed marked improvements in glycemic control[115]. Patients in the control group (on an ADA diet) also improved, but to a lesser extent. Yet another study found that 13 of 17 patients on insulin and 21 of 23 patients on oral medications were able to stop their medications 26 days after following a near-vegetarian diet and exercise program[114].

Another study not only demonstrated similar improvements on a vegan diet, but also showed that most patients were able to maintain their gains 2 and 3 years later[111].

Participants in one study described the vegan diet as easier to follow than most because they did not measure portions or count calories[139]. Only three of the vegan dieters dropped out of the study (6 percent), compared to eight in the control group on the ADA diet (16 percent)[115]. Given the difficulties that people have in adhering to diets for diabetes, the high adherence to the vegan diet is particularly noteworthy.

Do you need to become a vegan to see benefits? No. But there has been little research to help tease out the "dose" response. An educated guess suggests that a shift in emphasis is what's really valuable: base your diet on unprocessed plant-based foods, and bring in other foods you enjoy as accompaniments.

It may also be helpful to limit your exposure to environmental toxins; one diet-related strategy is to choose organic foods whenever possible. (The chapter on Agriculture and Sustainability will help you to implement this.)

Weight Loss Myths

Notably absent from my list of suggestions - which is usually the first line of defense for the traditionally-minded diabetes "experts" - is weight loss. Let me explain why. I don't dispute that on a short-term basis, weight loss is very effective at improving control of blood glucose. However, it is difficult to determine whether this means that it is improving the diabetes - even skipping one meal will lower blood glucose, but this doesn't mean that the diabetes is being cured. A 1995 review of all of the controlled weight loss studies for type 2 diabetics showed that the initial improvements were followed by a deterioration back to starting values 6 to 18 months after treatment, even when the weight loss was maintained[140].

Surgical studies provide a way to determine the effects of weight loss without changing the lifestyle factors, such as nutrition or activity habits, which often accompany the weight loss. Gastric bypass surgery appears to reverse diabetes within days, before significant weight is lost, suggesting that it is not the weight loss that brings about the improvement, but probably some other factor (such as a change in hormone secretions from the gut).

Liposuction studies provide further support that it is not the weight itself that is problematic. For example, one study was specifically designed to examine the effects of weight loss through liposuction on people with insulin resistance. The researchers examined obese women (half of whom were diabetic) before and 10-12 weeks after an average of about 20 pounds of body fat was removed[141]. Despite the weight loss, their metabolic profile did not improve, including their fasting glucose and insulin levels or their insulin sensitivity.

So the jury is clearly out on how beneficial weight loss is for managing or reversing diabetes. (And incidentally, despite the media hype, the jury is also out on how beneficial it is in improving longevity, as we'll see in the weight regulation section.) But regardless of its value, the question is moot: as we will also learn in the weight regulation section, there are no methods that have been documented to be effective for accomplishing weight loss, and the pursuit of weight loss has been quite damaging (food and weight preoccupation, eating disorders, weight cycling and associated increased cardiovascular disease risk, etc.).

Moreover, the lifestyle changes that have been advocated here are very effective. Numerous research studies document that type 2 diabetes can be improved or reversed through changes in nutrition or activity habits, even when little or no weight is lost[142-146].

Of course, weight loss may be a side effect to healthy lifestyle changes, but this won't be true for everyone. Too many people make wonderful changes in their habits – improving their health – but then give up when they don't get the weight loss results they seek. So a change in emphasis is certainly valuable.

What are the recommendations for people with type 1 diabetes?

Those with type 1 diabetes will always need a source of insulin. However, the same recommendations apply for them, as these recommendations minimize the amount of insulin required, which can go a long way to warding off the complications that may result from the diabetes.

Metabolic Syndrome (Syndrome X)

Scientists have coined the terms "Metabolic Syndrome" or "Syndrome X" to describe how insulin resistance sets the stage for serious disease. The syndrome is characterized by additional traits: hyperglycemia, hyperinsulinemia, hypertension (high blood pressure), high triglycerides, low HDL, atherosclerosis, all of which are probably secondary to the insulin resistance.

Identifying carbohydrates on food labels

The carbohydrates section first tells you the total number of grams of carbohydrates. The total number isn't so important, but knowing the kind of carbohydrate is valuable, so keep reading.

Next it lists the grams of sugar and fiber. Sometimes it also lists "Other Carbohydrates" which refers to the amount of starch. If the "other carbohydrates" is missing, you can calculate the amount of starch by subtracting the sugar and fiber from the total carbohydrate. To get even more information about the impact of the starch, read the ingredients list to see if that starch has been processed. (A refined grain, for example, acts more like a simple sugar than a whole grain.)

But remember that knowing these numbers alone doesn't tell you much, and they need to be interpreted in context. And while food labels can provide you with a lot of valuable information to evaluate the nutritional punch, they are also inadequate. One notable deficiency is that a label doesn't give you all the details you need to determine the glycemic load, which is one of the largest distinguishing characteristics of how health-enhancing a carbohydrate is. The number of grams of each type of carbohydrate, combined with the information you can interpret about those carbohydrates from the ingredients list, can help you make a good guess, however. And of course, the most effective method will be to observe your own reaction to foods.

Taking Stock of your Carbohydrate Consumption

The glycemic rush...

How often do you...	Seldom or never	1 or 2 times per week	3 to 5 times per week	Almost daily	Several times a day
Drink soft drinks, fruit juices or sweetened drinks?					
Eat sweet snacks, such as cakes, pies, cookies and ice cream?					
Use canned or frozen fruits packed in heavy syrup or add sugar to cereal or other foods?					
Eat candy?					
Add sugar to coffee or tea?					
Use jam, jelly, or honey on bread or rolls?					
Eat refined breads, tortillas, or white rice?					
Eat low fiber or sweetened cereals?					
Overeat so you feel stuffed?					

The more often you choose the items listed above, the higher your diet is likely to be in foods that stimulate a quick increase in blood sugar (which is typically followed by an over-release of insulin and resultant low blood sugar). (The last item is not a food, but another way to stimulate an insulin surge.)

Check your diet for fiber...

To figure out how much fiber you consume in a day, write down the number of servings you eat in a typical day for each of the food categories below. Next, multiply by the factor shown (this number represents the average amount of fiber from a serving in that food group). Then add up the total amount of fiber consumed.

Food Group	Number of Servings		Amount (g)
Vegetables (½ c cooked; 1 c raw)	_____	x 2 g =	_____
Fruits (1 medium; ½ c cut; ¼ c dried)	_____	x 2 g =	_____
Dried beans, lentils, split peas (½ c cooked)	_____	x 6 g =	_____
Nuts, seeds (¼ c; 2 tbsp peanut butter)	_____	x 2 g =	_____
Whole grains (1 slice bread; ½ c rice, pasta; ½ bun, bagel, muffin)	_____	x 2 g =	
Refined grains (1 slice bread; ½ c rice, pasta; ½ bun, bagel, muffin)	_____	x 0.5 g =	
Fiber in your breakfast cereal(check label)	_____	x __ g =	_____
		Total	_____

Scoring

38+: Wow! According to U.S. government standards, this should keep anyone healthy. But getting significantly more may even be better!

38: If you are male, your fiber meets the recommended goal. If you are female, this is great, in excess of what is recommended.

25-37: You consume more fiber than the average American. If you are female, this is good news: your fiber meets the recommended amount (25). However, if you are male, this is still below recommended.

15-25: You consume more fiber than the average American (but not enough for optimal health).

10-15: Your intake is similar to the average American intake (but not enough for optimal health).

0-10: Uh oh!

Putting it All Together: Health Recommendations for Dietary Carbohydrate

The first half of the carbohydrate consumption scorecard dealt with consumption of carbohydrates that enter the bloodstream quickly and are typically low in nutrient density, while the second half helped to identify carbohydrates that get into the bloodstream slowly, and are typically high in nutrient density.

In moderation, foods in the first section (sugars and refined grains) are relatively harmless as part of an overall nutritious diet. However, when consumed in excess, they tend to squeeze more nutritious foods out of your diet and contribute to several nutrition-sensitive diseases and concerns. Fiber-rich foods, on the other hand, tend to be extremely high in overall nutrient density, and a high-carbohydrate diet which predominately consists of fiber-rich foods may prevent or cure many nutrition-sensitive diseases and contribute to better sustained energy throughout the day and increased mood stability.

Want to change to more health-enhancing carbohydrate consumption? Consider eating more fiber-rich foods, and cutting back on the foods or habits that induce a blood sugar surge, particularly the ones in the first section where you checked "3 to 5 times per week" or more. Note that this does not mean that you need to eliminate these foods. You can moderate your intake by choosing these foods less often and by eating smaller portions.

Body Language

What's the easiest way to move towards healthier patterns? Notice how foods affect you. If you pay careful attention to your moods, energy levels, and the feelings inside your body after you eat meals, you'll probably find that eating foods that help support more stable blood glucose just makes you feel better!

How do you know, from a felt sense, whether you are choosing the right quantity and type of carbohydrate? There are two key feelings to look for:

1) Your energy and mood should be fairly stable and consistent throughout the day, emotional events aside. If you find yourself crashing or irritable at times, that's possibly a sign of difficulty regulating your blood sugar. Perhaps you're not eating enough – or you overate in general or ate too high a glycemic load.

2) You should have comfortable bowel movements. Constipation, in particular, is often related to insufficient fiber.

Action Tips...

To optimize health, choose carbohydrates that are:
- high in fiber;
- high in nutrient density;
- with a low glycemic load.

To make low glycemic food choices, try these strategies:
- Switch from refined to whole grains. As far as your hormones and metabolism are concerned, there's not much difference between a bowl of unsweetened corn flakes (a refined starch), wheat bread (which is not the same as *whole* wheat bread) and table sugar. Breads, grains and cereals that aren't whole grain tend to have high glycemic indices; try tasty whole grain alternatives.
- Most pastas have modest glycemic indices, making whole grain pastas another winner.
- Bank on beans. They have a small glycemic effect, and their fiber lowers the glycemic index of other foods that accompany them.
- Eat plenty of whole fruits and vegetables.
- Eat mixed meals (a little protein or fat with your carbohydrates).
- Stick to small quantities when you consume simple sugars – or spread them out over time.
- Drink water, sparkling water, and herbal teas instead of sodas, juices and alcohol. Dilute juices with plain or sparkling water.
- We all have different metabolisms. Experiment with your diet. Try different amounts and types of carbohydrates, protein and fat in meals until you find combinations that give you mental focus, extended energy, and lack of hunger/cravings for the meal intervals you desire.

Get informed...

The low-carbohydrate food craze took over our country not long ago, but fortunately it finally seems to be going out of style! If you want some more information about low-carbohydrate diets, check out the website created by Dr. Michael Greger: http://www.atkinsfacts.org/ or his recent book, *Carbophobia: The Scary Truth Behind America's Low Carb Craze.*

If you want more details on the glycemic index of foods you eat, the most comprehensive list was published in the American Journal of Clinical Nutrition in July of 2002[147]. You can also find a searchable database maintained by the University of Sydney at http://www.glycemicindex.com/.

For more details on implementing the dietary recommendations for reversing or managing diabetes, check out any of the following. Note that they all advocate for a vegan diet. If you can get past the myths they promote about body weight and weight loss, you'll find valuable nutritional information.

Dr. John McDougall, at the McDougall Wellness Center, http://www.drmcdougall.com/

Physician's Committee for Responsible Medicine, at http://www.pcrm.org/

Dr. Dean Ornish, at the Preventive Medicine Research Institute, http://www.pmri.org/

Of course, if the traditional route is more your style, the American Diabetes Association is on-line at http://www.diabetes.org.

Fats: Here's the Skinny

Eat fat and die young? Fortunately, that old adage just isn't true: dietary fat and disease are not a package deal. We'll see in this section that the fear of dietary fat is simplistic and misinformed, and that one can live healthfully on a high-fat diet. The *type* of fat plays a larger role in health and longevity than the overall amount[148].

Let's start with the contradictory facts. The French eat more fat and suffer fewer heart attacks than Americans and the British. The Japanese eat less fat and suffer fewer heart attacks than Americans and the British. So what should you do, eat more or less?

Let's complicate the picture even more: The Italians drink more wine than Americans and the British, and suffer fewer heart attacks than the Americans and the British. Koreans, on the other hand, drink little red wine and suffer fewer heart attacks than the Americans and the British.

What's the moral of this story? Eat and drink what you like - it's speaking English as a country's first language that kills you! Kidding aside, the point I'd really like to make is that heart disease is a lot more complicated than how much fat you get in your diet - or the quantity of other nutrients for that matter. (And no, I can't claim credit for this joke – it's been circulating on the Internet, and I don't know the original source to credit.)

The Basics

Let's get started by examining the properties of fat. The more technical name for fat is "lipid," and it includes both fats and oils. Scientists don't consider oils (which, in contrast to fats, are liquid at room temperature) to be fats, but throughout this book we'll stick to general conventions and use the term "fat" to include both fats and oils.

The distinguishing feature of fats is that they are insoluble (don't dissolve) in water. Consider filling a bottle with oil and vinegar (which is water-based) and notice the separation that occurs. Sure, shaking the bottle will cause the oil to disperse, but the oil doesn't dissolve; that's why it separates out again when the bottle rests.

Plants often store their oils in seeds (nuts, sesame seeds, corn), occasionally in fruits (avocados, olives and coconuts) and rarely in quantity elsewhere. Animals are also rich sources; fat, which is jam-packed with energy compared to protein or carbohydrate, serves as a convenient and important energy reserve. Fat can also be commercially isolated from plant or animal sources, and gets into our diet in concentrated forms through butter, oil, margarine and shortening.

Like carbohydrates, all fats are composed of only three elements: carbon, hydrogen and oxygen.

Fats in the body

Although most of us think of fats as something to avoid, fats actually serve important roles in our body. As an example, about 50 percent of the dry weight of your brain is composed of lipids - and you'd be stupid without them. Since most cells are continually degrading and replacing lipids (like other compounds), there is continuous demand for them – and consuming the right type of fat is critical to good health and survival. Research documents that if a fetus or infant is deprived of sufficient fat, they are likely to have a lower than normal IQ (Intelligence Quotient) as an adult.

Avoidance of fat is not a good health strategy, although smart choices about the types of fat will work to your benefit.

Forms of fat

There are **three main families of fat: triglycerides, sterols** (cholesterol is the best known of these), and **phospholipids** (lecithin is an example of this).

Triglycerides make up 95 percent of the fat in our diet, and are also the primary type of fat that is found on our body. A triglyceride consists of backbone molecule, called glycerol, with three attached fatty acids.

The predominant role of the fatty acids (we'll discuss this term shortly) that are a part of triglycerides, particularly saturated fatty acids and mono-unsaturated fatty acids, is to **provide energy**; the triglycerides in food provide us with energy to power ourselves, and the triglycerides that are part of our fat tissue supply us with abundant energy reserves.

Poly-unsaturated fatty acids **serve important roles in our cell membranes** and as the **precursors to hormones**. They additionally help to **carry "fat-soluble" compounds**, like some vitamins, around in our body.

Fatty acids also provide **insulation, protect the body's vital organs**, and serve as a shock absorber. I guarantee you wouldn't want to sit on your butt if you didn't have a layer of fat to cushion you - nor would you want to be out on a cold day without your layer of fat insulation!

Phospholipids, another of the families of fats, help us in digestion, provide structure to cell membranes, and coat the outside of lipoproteins, which transport fats throughout the body. We'll learn about lipoproteins in more depth soon. One distinctive characteristic of phospholipids is their **ability to allow fat and water to mix**.

The best known of the third "fat" family, sterols, is *cholesterol*, which performs vital functions in our body – and that of other animals. (Cholesterol is not found in significant quantity in plants.) For example, cholesterol serves as the starting material to other important compounds, such as the sex hormones, Vitamin D, and bile (which, incidentally, is a phospholipid). Bile helps in the digestion of dietary fat, and the body can rid itself of excess cholesterol by adding it to the bile that is secreted during digestion. **Cholesterol's most important function, however, is the role it plays in cell membranes.**

Cell membranes are primarily composed of lipids, predominantly fatty acids which I will describe shortly. The unsaturated essential fatty acids make membranes more flexible, while the more saturated fatty acids make them more rigid. The flexibility of cell membranes varies day-to-day depending on the type of fatty acids in your diet. Cholesterol helps you to compensate for these daily variations and keep you within normal limits; it is added to stiffen membranes that are too fluid and removed to soften ones that are too stiff.

Since cholesterol is so helpful, why does it have such a bad reputation? It is also the major component of the plaque that narrows the arteries in a type of heart disease called atherosclerosis. In the right place, it's good stuff – it's when it gets dumped in the wrong places that it gets you into trouble.

Understanding Fatty Acids

The building block of triglycerides and phospholipids is a fatty acid, and a fatty acid is often attached to cholesterol as well. Fatty acids play a critical role in our health, so we will discuss them at length here.

Although there are many different types of fatty acids, all are basically a chain of carbon atoms that have attached hydrogen atoms, with a distinctive acid at the end of the chain. The carbon-carbon bonds in a fatty acid are more energetic than those in carbohydrates, which explains why lipids have more than twice the amount of energy than carbohydrates when the same weight is compared.

Fatty acids differ from one another in two ways: the number of carbons in the chain, and the degree of saturation. Most foods contain a mixture of different types of fatty acids, with differing numbers of carbons and differing degrees of saturation. The number of carbons in the chain is significant because it affects how "soluble" the fat is in water: short-chain fatty acids are somewhat soluble in water, which allows them to travel more easily in our watery blood. Longer chain fatty acids are less soluble, and need carriers to shuttle them around in our blood.

The degree of saturation is a more important distinction between fatty acids from the perspective of your health. Each atom has a characteristic number of bonds that it likes to form with other atoms. Carbon, for example, always has four bonds. With the exception of the acid on the end, two of the four bonds on each carbon in the fatty acid chain are to adjacent carbon atoms, leaving it with two bonds available for other atoms. If those two bonds are filled with hydrogen atoms, we say that the fatty acid is "saturated" with hydrogens. Saturated fats form straight chains which are very compact. Because they can stack together tightly, they are likely to be solid at room temperature. Butter and lard are examples of food fats that have high saturated fat content.

Sometimes adjacent carbons are attached by a double bond, leaving only one bond for a hydrogen atom; in this case, we say that the fatty acid is "unsaturated." A fatty acid that has one point of unsaturation is called mono-unsaturated, and one with two or more points of unsaturation is called poly-unsaturated. Unsaturated fats tend to be liquid at room temperature because the chain forms a kink at the point of unsaturation and they can't stack together as tightly as saturated fats. Olive oil and canola oil are examples of foods with high mono-unsaturated fat content, while corn oil and safflower oil are examples of food fats with high poly-unsaturated fat content.

The body is a good chemist and can make the cholesterol and phospholipids it needs, so it is unnecessary to get these in your diet. Vegetarians, for example, don't get significant dietary cholesterol and their bodies can make it in sufficient quantity. We can also synthesize most of the fatty acids we need, including all of the necessary saturated fats.

However, there are a few poly-unsaturated fatty acids that your body can't synthesize. We call these essential fatty acids. Nutritionists use the term "essential" to refer to compounds that you need to get from your diet. The two essential fatty acids are omega-3 fatty acids (the most common example of this is alpha-linolenic acid), and omega-6 fatty acids (the most common example is linoleic acid). We'll see later that modern food processing has gotten us into trouble, and diet alone is often insufficient in supplying the right type and ratio of essential fatty acids, leading to an increase in heart disease, among other maladies.

Now that you have a good understanding of lipids, let's briefly discuss their health implications.

The degree of saturation plays a particularly large role in your health. In moderation, saturated fats are used as part of cell membranes or for energy. However, most types of saturated fats can also be used by your body as the starting material in synthesizing cholesterol, and as a result, promote heart disease when consumed in excess. It is commonly agreed that saturated fats should not be eaten in excess for this reason. Saturated fats are found in high quantities in animal products, particularly red meat.

Nutritionists typically recommend that you replace saturated fats with poly-unsaturated fats, as these actually reduce LDL, a cholesterol carrier in your bloodstream (thus reducing risk for heart disease); we'll learn about this soon. However, the wisdom of this is questionable. While it is true that poly-unsaturated fats have this health-enhancing quality, they also lower your HDL (another cholesterol carrier, but this one is best in higher quantities as it reduces the cholesterol in your bloodstream), lead to an unhealthy ratio of essential fatty acids, and are more subject to oxidation. Whew, lots of new ideas there, huh! We'll save a discussion of HDL and LDL for later in this section, but let's tackle those other two concerns now

Essential fatty acids

As mentioned, there are two types of fatty acids that are essential to get in your diet: omega-3 fatty acids and omega-6 fatty acids. Omega-3s occur in only a few seeds and nuts (flax, hemp, pumpkin and walnuts) and fewer oils (canola and soy), and they are also found in dark leafy greens and seaweeds. Products made from soy (like tofu and soy milk) are particularly good sources.

Although other animals can't synthesize omega-3s either, they obtain them from eating foods containing them, and in turn also become a source of omega-3s for us when we eat them. Fish and egg yolks tend to be good sources, although new farming methods have resulted in a greatly decreased amount. Since salmon farmers don't typically provide sources of omega-3s to their farmed fish, for example, farmed salmon have a much lower omega-3 content compared to wild salmon; similarly, chickens confined to cages and fed standard feed will have a much lower omega-3 content compared to free range chickens that scratch and peck the ground for food. Most Americans are deficient in omega-3s, in large part due to our changing methods of food manufacturing.

Omega-6s are found in many seeds and nuts and the oil expressed from them, including all of the poly-unsaturated oils commonly sold (such as corn, safflower, sesame and sunflower). As a result, they are plentiful in the American diet, and most of us get well in excess of what we need.

Of more importance than the individual amounts of omega-3s and omega-6s is the ratio between the two. As the ratio of omega-6s to omega-3s rises, the efficiency of the omega-3s decline because both types compete for the same limited supply of enzymes. Since essential fatty acids serve a critical function in creating prostaglandins and prostocyclins, hormone-like compounds that play many roles, including regulating blood pressure and blood clotting, immune response, and inflammatory response, it is believed that a high omega-6/omega-3 ratio has played a crucial role in the declining health of Americans.

As an example, like most body control systems, these chemical messengers have ambivalent actions – some can increase and other decrease inflammation in your blood vessels or clotting of the blood. To maintain optimum health, these two functions must be balanced. If you are injured, the inflammatory response is critical to healing as it brings nutrients and immune cells to the injured area. Once healing is complete, the inflammatory response needs to stop, or cells could proliferate in the previously injured area, causing damage.

In general, prostaglandins that are derived from omega-6 fatty acids promote inflammation and blood clotting, while the prostocyclins derived from omega-3 fatty acids act in an opposite manner, as an anti-inflammatory and helping blood to flow.

As our diet – and the diet of the animals we eat – shifted from one based on green plants to one based on corn, the ratio of omega-6 to omega-3 that we obtain has gone from roughly 1:1 to more than 10:1. This may be the most damaging dietary change brought about by food processing and the industrialization of our food supply. There is mounting evidence that the high omega-6/omega-3 ratio common to the American diet has thrown off our balance, increasing our susceptibility to cancer, cardiovascular disease, and inflammatory and auto-immune disorders. It is more than possible that the epidemic of heart disease that we are now experiencing is not so much about excess of certain fats in our diet, but rather that we are now eating the wrong balance of fat, and are now deficient in the protection afforded by omega-3s.

More detail about essential fatty acids can be found in the Appendix.

Oxidation

Whether a poly-unsaturated fatty acid is in a food or your body, its points of unsaturation are like weak spots in the chain in that they are vulnerable to attack by free radicals. When an unsaturated food fat, like an oil, is oxidized, the result is rancidity. The more common ways that this occurs are from exposure to the oxygen in air, which builds over time, or when foods are brought to high temperatures, which often happens during commercial processing or cooking.

Trans Fatty Acids

I've given you sufficient reason to be cautious of the standard advice to replace saturated fats with poly-unsaturated fats in your diet (although I hope you'll remember that excessive saturated fats have much worse health implications). But now let me mention a specific type of poly-unsaturated fat that is dangerous, carrying an even higher risk than excessive saturated fats. These are called trans fatty acids.

Most fatty acids that occur naturally are called cis fatty acids. The term "cis" refers to the shape of the molecule that results from the way in which the hydrogens attach to the carbon. This particular shape is very important in helping to build our cell membranes and hormones.

Saturated fats are often more convenient for food manufacturers to use than unsaturated fats in that they are solid at room temperature, can withstand higher temperatures in cooking, and can last longer without going rancid (being oxidized). However, they are also more expensive to produce.

Years ago, manufacturers discovered a way to give unsaturated (cheaper) fats some of these "positive" characteristics of saturated fats. They did this by shooting hydrogen atoms with a high pressure gun onto a poly-unsaturated fat. The result is a fat that has a much longer shelf life, can withstand higher cooking temperature, and is solid at room temperature.

The added hydrogens make it look and act a lot like a saturated fat, but the hydrogens add in a slightly different conformation, and we call them "trans fatty acids" rather than cis fatty acids. Your body uses these trans fatty acids in the same way it would use a cis fatty acid, and the result is disastrous: defective membranes and hormones, resulting in increased risk for cancer and cardiovascular disease, among other illnesses[149].

Trans fatty acids, even in small quantities, are bad news. On a per-calorie-basis, they appear to increase the risk of cardiovascular disease more than any other macronutrient, even at low levels of consumption (1 percent of energy, which amounts to 2 grams for the average person)[149].

Digestion, Absorption and Processing

Dietary fat begins to appear in your bloodstream an hour or two after you eat. Fat levels peak after four to five hours, and are generally completely cleared by ten hours.

The different types of lipids face different fates in the digestion and absorption process. Digestion does little to change cholesterol and other sterols, for example, and they are poorly absorbed compared to triglycerides. Your body has mechanisms to protect you from getting too much cholesterol; surprisingly, the more cholesterol you consume in your diet, the less you absorb. Additionally, fiber binds to cholesterol in your digestive tract, providing another method of limiting the amount of cholesterol that will get absorbed (and also removing some of the excess cholesterol that was already contained in your body). On the other hand, the saturated fats that are found in many triglycerides in your diet, as well as trans fats, increase the amount of absorbed cholesterol.

There is a persistent myth that individuals who are concerned about high levels of cholesterol in their blood and its potential for causing heart disease should limit the amount of cholesterol in their diet. But this just isn't true: your body manufactures most of the cholesterol in your system and what food adds is relatively small. The research and physiologic mechanism convincingly demonstrate that dietary saturated fat contributes to high blood cholesterol levels to a much greater degree than dietary cholesterol. This is in part because the more cholesterol you have in your diet, the less gets absorbed. Also, your liver uses saturated and trans fat as a precursor for making cholesterol, and the more saturated and trans fats you get in your diet, the more cholesterol your liver makes. So the take home message for optimal health is to decrease dietary saturated and trans fat, and pay less attention to dietary cholesterol. (This is not to say that dietary cholesterol has no effect at all – just that it has a much lesser effect than is commonly believed.

Digestion breaks most other lipids (triglycerides and phospholipids) down into fatty acids, and some other small components (such as glycerol, monoglycerides, and in the case of phospholipids, a nitrogenous compound). For the purposes of understanding fuel, the fatty acids are the most important breakdown product.

Fatty acids arc very small and extremely mobile. It is very easy for them to pass through the walls of your bloodstream and cells. Because they are so mobile, they are sometimes called "free" fatty acids. Free fatty acids are important for two reasons: they can move into cells to be burned for energy, or they can enter a fat cell for storage. In other words, they can either provide fuel or make you fat.

After digestion, some smaller fatty acids get absorbed into the bloodstream and travel to the liver. However, because fat and water don't mix very well, most fatty acids can't travel freely in the watery blood. Instead, the fatty acids get re-formed into triglycerides in the intestinal cells, and then packaged into **lipoproteins**, which are molecules that can then transport them through the bloodstream.

All lipoproteins act as fat transport molecules. However, there are several different types, and they all serve different roles and have different effects on your health. The lipoprotein that gets formed in your intestinal cells immediately after digestion and absorption is called a chylomicron. **Chylomicrons** travel through your bloodstream, where there are enzymes called lipoprotein lipases (LPL) that cleave the fatty acid from the chylomicron, releasing the fatty acid so it can enter cells. Lipoprotein lipases are found in the walls of blood vessels, particularly those found in fat tissue, muscle tissue, and around the heart.

Chylomicrons do not last long in your bloodstream - only about 8 minutes - so any fatty acids from your diet that cannot be used or kept efficiently in the bloodstream, will get placed into storage quickly. The existence or absence of LPL determines whether or not a free fatty acid near a cell will be taken up into that cell, so you can see that LPL is a very important enzyme in determining your weight. If your fat cells make a lot of LPL, then you will store fat easily. If your muscle cells make a lot of LPL, then you will burn dietary fat easily.

Fatty Acid Storage and Transport

Although we only have a limited ability to store glucose (in the form of glycogen) and a complete inability to store amino acids (the breakdown product of protein), we have an almost endless capacity to store fatty acids on our body. Adipose is the scientific word for fat; fat cells are called adipose cells, depots of stored fat on your body are called adipose tissue, and we can refer to an individual's adiposity.

Fats are a great way for us to store energy, for two reasons. First, they contain a lot more energy in a comparable weight. (Remember that fats contain 9 kcals of energy per gram, whereas protein and carbohydrate contain 4 kcals/gram.) Second, because they don't need to be stored in water, they can be stored in a very compact manner. Protein and carbohydrate, on the other hand, need to be stored in about three to four times their weight in water. For these reasons, if energy stores were in the form of carbohydrate or protein, they would weigh about ten times as much as they are when stored in the form of fat. In other words, we would be extremely chubby if we stored excess nutrients in the form of carbohydrate or protein compared to fat, even if we couldn't literally call ourselves fat!

Adipose cells can also take up glucose and amino acids which have been absorbed after a meal, and convert them into fat molecules. Storing fat in a fat cell takes relatively little energy. In fact, if you have 100 extra fat kilocalories that need to get stored, it will only take about 2.5 calories to store it.

Converting glucose or amino acids into fat, on the other hand, takes a substantial amount of energy. If you have 100 extra kilocalories of either or both of these, it takes about 25-28 kilocalories to convert them into fat and put them into fat storage. In other words, if you over-eat 100 kilocalories of fat, 97.5 of those kilocalories will get stored; over-eat 100 kilocalories of carbohydrates and/or protein, and only 75 kilocalories get stored.

Given a choice, your fat cells will grab the fat and store it, rather then invest the extra energy in converting the other macronutrients. An excess of dietary carbohydrate causes you to shift the fuels you are using so that you reduce the use of fat and it makes a beeline for storage rather than being burned.

Lipoproteins

Earlier we mentioned that fat needs a transport vehicle to get around your body, called a lipoprotein. We discussed the chylomicron, which is the lipoprotein that transports newly digested fat. However, we get fat on our body not just from our diets, but as a result of synthesis by our liver. Our liver is like a fat factory, providing fat for all of our needs. Whenever there is excess glucose or amino acids, your liver uses these to make fat.

Let's now look at the lipoproteins that carry the fat from your liver. All lipoproteins are a mixture of lipid and protein, thus the name. They have an outer coating that is made out of a double layer of phospholipids. Fat and water ordinarily don't mix, but the phospholipid gives it the unique quality of allowing it to travel in the watery blood, while protecting the lipid inside. The lipid being carried inside includes both cholesterol and fatty acids (bound in triglycerides).

Protein is a lot denser than lipid, and if you keep this concept in mind you can understand the names and corresponding roles of each of the lipoproteins fairly easily. Picture punching a bodybuilder in the stomach, compared to punching a fat person. You could hurt your hand when you punch the bodybuilder because their stomach is so hard or dense. Muscle is comprised primarily of protein. However, when you punch the fat person, your hand would sink into the cushioning (non-dense) fat.

When the liver packages the fatty acid and cholesterol in the lipoprotein for transport to cells, there is a lot of fat compared to protein, so it is very low in density, and thus gets its name, **very low density lipoprotein (VLDL)**. The VLDL acts much like the chylomicron that is made by your intestinal cells, traveling around your bloodstream delivering fatty acids. As it travels, the enzyme lipoprotein lipase (LPL) plucks the fat off of the VLDL so it can enter cells to be used for energy or stored. After a while, there is less fat on the lipoprotein, although the protein content hasn't changed. It is no longer *very* low in density, now we just call it **"low density lipoprotein," or LDL**. LDL continues to travel through your bloodstream, delivering the fat to cells, although its job is to off-load more of the cholesterol (as opposed to the fatty acids that the VLDL was primarily delivering).

There is one more lipoprotein that also plays an important role in your health: **high density lipoprotein, or HDL**. As you would expect from the name, HDL contains a lot of protein and very little lipid. It is made in the liver, and travels through your bloodstream acting like a scavenger, picking up excess cholesterol and returning it to the liver for recycling or disposal.

Obtaining Energy from Fat

Lipid Storage and Release

To obtain energy from fat, the body goes through a series of metabolic reactions, breaking the fatty acid molecule into smaller and smaller components. This process is called lipolysis. Fat can't be converted to energy as quickly or as readily as glycogen can.

In order to get fat out of the adipocytes that store it, there is an enzyme that acts like lipoprotein lipase in reverse: it is called hormone-sensitive lipase (HSL), and it cleaves the fatty acids from the triglycerides in your adipose tissue and releases them into your bloodstream.

The complete breakdown of a fatty acid releases all of the energy that was contained in that fatty acid. We call this process fatty acid oxidation. Most, but not all, cells have the enzymes necessary to oxidize fatty acids. Muscle is particularly good at it and is very efficient at using fat as an energy source. Brain cells, certain other cells in your nervous system, and red blood cells, on the other hand, don't have all the enzymes necessary to completely oxidize the fatty acid, so they can't use fatty acid as an energy source.

In order to completely oxidize the fatty acid and release all of its energy, one of the metabolic reactions along the way requires a little bit of energy in the form of glucose. If you don't have sufficient glucose, then the fatty acid oxidation stops at this step. Instead of completely oxidizing the fatty acid and getting the waste products, carbon dioxide and water, you now have a molecule called a ketone or a ketone body, which still contains much of the original energy that was contained in the fatty acid. A ketone is merely a partial breakdown product of a fatty acid. When you run low on glucose, your liver produces ketones and releases them into the bloodstream.

Ketones can be used as an energy source by some tissues, such as the heart, muscle and kidney. Some cells in the brain (which ordinarily require glucose) can temporarily adapt to getting a portion of their energy from ketones, though your brain prefers to run on glucose. Excess ketones are excreted in the urine. However, if ketone production is high (or if there is insufficient hydration to excrete them), ketones can build up in the blood, a process called ketosis. Mild ketosis (such as might happen with a weight loss diet) causes symptoms including headache, dry mouth, bad breath, slowed metabolism, and reduced appetite. Ketones are acidic molecules and high ketone levels increase the acidity of the blood, called ketoacidosis. In diabetics, this can get particularly pronounced and result in coma or death.

Types of Fat Storage: Visceral vs. Subcutaneous Fat

How does your body distribute its fat? Are you "pear-shaped," with fat stored on your hips or thighs? Or "apple-shaped," holding your fat around your middle?

An apple shape is indicative of high levels of abdominal fat, also called visceral fat or visceral adipose tissue (VAT). This differs from subcutaneous fat, which is fat that lies just below the skin (so called "love handles"). VAT breaks down more readily than subcutaneous fat, releasing free fatty acids (FFA) into the bloodstream. Because it is in close proximity to the portal vein, which is the vein that feeds directly into the liver, it exposes the liver to high amounts of FFA, setting you up for a number of metabolic complications. High levels of FFA both increase the liver's production and output of glucose, and reduce the liver's capacity to clear insulin, leading to disorders such as insulin resistance and type 2 diabetes. Additionally, FFA stimulate the liver to produce VLDL, which increases risk of atherosclerosis (heart disease).

Using fatty acids as energy

As we've discussed, glucose is essential for your survival, and your body regulates your blood glucose levels tightly in order to ensure its ongoing availability. The key to understanding when you will use fatty acids as an energy source is remembering that your body's main goal is to maintain glucose homeostasis. If a tissue can use fatty acids, it will, in order to spare the available glucose. At rest, the energy your body needs is derived almost equally from fatty acids and carbohydrates, although there is quite a bit of individual variability.

Just about all cells in your body can use fatty acids as a valuable energy source, with the exception of your red blood cells and certain cells in your brain and nervous system. How much they use is in large part determined by how much is in your bloodstream, which in turn is largely dependent on the amount of lipoprotein lipase (LPL). So just because you have a lot of fat stored on your body doesn't mean that you will use it in high quantities as an energy source. You need to have LPL to help release it.

We all have a characteristic amount of LPL that we typically make, which was in part genetically determined and later altered by your lifestyle habits, predominantly the foods you eat and the amount and type of activity you get. The difference makes some of us "better butter burners" than others. (The amount of fat that gets used is also dependent on the amount of blood flow, so during times of exercise when the blood flow is greatly increased to your working muscles, there is much more fatty acid used.)

Atherosclerosis

Healthy arteries have flexible walls and a smooth lining that allows them to transport blood freely, much like a garden hose is a conduit for free-flowing water. The term "**atherosclerosis**" comes from the Greek words "athero" which means paste, and "sclerosis" which means hardness. When you have atherosclerosis, your internal "hose" gets rough and sticky, loses much of its flexibility, and gets a build-up of cholesterol-containing plaque on its walls. Plaque may build to such an extent that the blood vessel becomes narrowed, limiting blood flow. Particularly vulnerable are the arteries that supply blood to the heart (coronary) and the brain (cerebral).

The leading hypothesis about how atherosclerosis develops suggests that it begins with an insult or injury to the blood vessel. This could arise for a variety of reasons, including oxidative damage from free radicals (which are generated by smoking, breathing polluted air, eating oxidized fats, etc.), raised blood glucose, raised insulin, raised stress hormones, turbulent blood flow or high blood pressure, or a viral or bacterial infection. Heredity undoubtedly also plays a role.

The body's immune system responds to this insult or injury by initiating an inflammatory response. But sometimes things can go wrong with the inflammatory response. So wrong, in fact, that the body's response to injury is worse than the injury itself.

To understand inflammation, consider this experiment. Suppose you had a pile of dirt and you whacked it with a hammer. You would see the injury: there would be a dent in the dirt where it was contacted by the hammer. Now, whack your thumb instead of the dirt. After you stop swearing and jumping around, what do you see? You have a nasty bruise, and your thumb is hot, red, swollen, and throbbing with pain. There is a small trickle of blood on your thumb, indicating that you cut some small blood vessels. But it is a worthwhile learning experience, because now you can understand the inflammatory response.

Your body responded to the injury by trying to repair the damage. That heat, redness, and swelling are the result of your immune system sending over an arsenal of fix-it cells, chiefly white blood cells called macrophages. Your body had to repair those blood vessels and stop your blood from leaking out through the cut. Initially, you produced a blood clot, which is basically congealed blood that acts like a plug to seal the cut in the blood vessel. While this short-term fix is happening, your immune system got to work rebuilding the blood vessel for the long-term, stimulating neighboring cells to secrete substances like collagen and elastin, which span the cut and join the two sides together.

In a few days, the cut will be perfectly healed, and there will be no external manifestation that your skin or blood vessels were ever damaged. Pretty effective system, huh? Most of the time, this inflammatory response is quite successful at keeping you healthy and strong.

You don't need to whack yourself with a hammer to produce inflammation. You can get the same results from an infection. Think back to the last time you got infected with a cold virus. The swelling and pain you felt in your throat are part of the inflammatory response triggered by your immune system. The type of injury does not matter too much; when there is a problem your immune system kicks into gear, rushing to the site of insult. Inflammation is desirable, a sign that your body is hard at work trying to protect and repair you.

The examples of getting whacked with a hammer or being attacked by a cold virus describe acute difficulties. Most often, you know something is wrong since you feel the pain. However, sometimes the insult to your blood vessels is more gradual or more subtle, and you don't feel it. You may have chronic insult to your blood vessels, resulting in chronic inflammation, without knowing it.

Many things can contribute to chronic inflammation, such as the presence of certain bacteria or viruses, or a high stress lifestyle[150]. Chronic insult is not about giving your thumb a strong whack with the hammer – it's more like mild, steady taps with the hammer, that go on for minutes, hours, days – okay, years – at a time. Your thumb just doesn't stand a chance at recovering. Waves of immune cells rush to the scene of insult, keeping the inflammatory process going. It's like the biological equivalent of "friendly fire" in warfare.

Unfortunately, the cells and chemicals sent by the immune system can't always distinguish between the good guys and the bad guys, so they destroy not only the infecting or problematic cells, but healthy tissues as well. In addition, your immune system is working hard at repairing tissue, even if it's not needed. This leads to dense scar tissue replacing normal cells.

A vicious cycle has begun. As healthy tissues get damaged by the immune system, the body increases the inflammatory response.

So let's get back to atherosclerosis. So far we've talked about an insult to the blood vessel walls and the body's inflammatory response. Now let's talk about some other stuff traveling around in your bloodstream. You always have some free cholesterol and LDL (which contains cholesterol) traveling around in your bloodstream. Both compounds are very vulnerable to oxidation. Suppose LDL, for example, runs into a free radical bouncing around in your bloodstream and gets oxidized. In response, the white blood cells (macrophages) in the artery walls rush to the scene and attempt to remove the oxidized LDL by attacking and "eating" them. Unfortunately, after ingesting the LDL, they can't get rid of the cholesterol portion, and become engorged and swollen. The swollen cells, called foam cells, accumulate, producing plaque. Threads of cholesterol-containing plaque are called fatty streaks.

Fatty streaks start when you're young; they've been found during autopsies on the hearts of children as young as ten years of age. As the plaque grows over time, engorged foam cells burst and die, releasing their fat. This fat is often called soft cholesterol, and the soft cholesterol binds together inside the plaque.

We used to believe the mechanism behind a heart attack to be simple: clumps of plaque, building up on the coronary arteries, making the channel narrow. Eventually a clot gets stuck, choking off flow. The degree of blockage could be determined by angiograms, during which doctors inject dye into your heart arteries, and then aim an x-ray camera. They look for spots where the blood flow slows to a trickle, which highlights the areas of atherosclerotic blockage.

But this simple explanation is not a common occurrence: in fact, some scientists speculate that they are only to blame for about 15 percent of all heart attacks. So figuring out your degree of atherosclerotic blockage is not going to be the most effective predictor of your vulnerability for heart attack.

Instead, it seems the smaller stuff, called "vulnerable plaque," which can't always even be viewed by imaging equipment, may be more lethal. Because plaque doesn't usually bulge outwards into the bloodstream, but instead protrudes into the wall of the artery, an angiogram might look normal. That's why the first sign of a heart attack may be the heart attack itself.

That soft cholesterol I mentioned is a part of vulnerable plaque. It's called vulnerable because of its tendency to easily burst. And it could burst long before it gets big enough to protrude into the artery and cause angina. (Angina is the discomfort or chest pain or discomfort that results from inadequate blood flow to the heart muscle. The pain may also occur in the shoulders, arms, neck, jaw, or back, or feel like indigestion.) So you look and feel healthy up until the moment you drop dead. In fact, the most common time for a heart attack to occur is around 9:00 a.m. That's because the hormonal surge necessary to get you going in the morning can be enough to break vulnerable plaque. You don't need to get wildly physical.

When pieces of plaque break off (rupture) from the inside wall of large arteries, the plaque flows into smaller arteries, narrowing their passageway. Insufficient blood flow in the arteries that travel to the heart damages the heart. Complete blockage results in a heart attack, and complete blockage in blood flow in arteries that travel to the brain results in a stroke.

As you can see, the process of atherosclerosis involves many complicated factors. It is not simply a matter of high blood cholesterol levels. The dietary influences are wide-reaching, including the excesses of dietary lipids that result in increased blood cholesterol, namely saturated and trans fats, and to a lesser degree, cholesterol. Non-lipid dietary related factors also contribute to the increase in blood cholesterol, such as high glycemic index carbohydrates and animal proteins. (The contribution of animal proteins doesn't receive much discussion; nonetheless, there is a significant amount of research to support that it plays a large role in raising blood cholesterol levels – and that plant proteins can reduce blood cholesterol – even when other associated nutrients, such as saturated fat, are controlled for[151-157].)

However, increased cholesterol production is only one part of the story: also important are the lipoproteins that transport cholesterol. Since LDL is a vulnerable molecule and subject to oxidation, high levels of LDL will result in a greater likelihood of cholesterol being released and attaching to the artery walls. High levels of HDL will allow an individual to clear cholesterol from the arteries, regardless of what they eat.

Furthermore, while cholesterol can damage the artery walls, whether it does depends on other factors, not all of which are completely understood. But some kind of damage must occur to the artery walls in order for the cholesterol to deposit there, and this damage is in large part the result of oxidative stress. High levels of oxidants and low levels of antioxidants contribute to this.

Since poly-unsaturated fatty acids are more vulnerable to oxidation, excess poly-unsaturated fatty acids in the diet make oxidation more likely. And cholesterol is another easily oxidized molecule, implicating animal foods, including baked products made with eggs and butter. The damage that occurs from the high heats that deep fried foods are subject to, also results in highly oxidized foods. Another contributor to atherosclerosis is an inflammatory response related to an excess of omega-6 fatty acids relative to omega-3 fatty acids.

Less commonly discussed is the strong association between animal proteins and atherosclerosis[156, 158-160], which some research shows to be even stronger than the association of saturated fat and cholesterol to atherosclerosis[156, 158, 160].

High fiber intake, on the other hand, appears to quite protective. You can't get enough of that good stuff! (Well, actually you can – but as long as you make changes gradually and the changes come from foods as opposed to supplements, you should be okay.)

Fear of fat

Food fat has gotten a bad rap. I'm sure this is partly because its energy density threatens the values of our puritanical/weight-loss obsessed culture. Also, certain types of fat contribute to increased disease risk, and it's an easier message to vilify all fats as opposed to recommending moderation of certain types of fats.

But there is no reason to be scared of fat. Fat can enhance the flavor of many foods, and enjoying and feeling satisfied by your food can play an important role in supporting healthy moderation and healthy weight regulation. Try cutting an onion in half, sautéing half in oil, and boiling the other half in water. You'll notice a huge taste difference: the oil helps to carry some of the onion's flavor compounds to your taste buds.

The fat also helps your body to absorb certain nutrients. For example, one research study compared research participants eating a fat-free salad to another group whose salad had the addition of half an avocado (which is rich in mono-unsaturated fats)[161]. The avocado-eaters absorbed about ten times the carotenoids from the salad's greens than did the fat-free eaters. And adding avocado to salsa more than quadrupled the amount of absorbed lycopene, a phytochemical that can lower your risk for cardiovascular disease and some types of cancer. Another study compared people eating salads with fat-free dressing to those eating salads with traditional dressing and found similar results[162].

If you're successful in eating a very low-fat diet, you'll eventually feel the distress in your body: weakness, irritability, tiredness, brittle nails, increased susceptibility to infection, constipation and other digestive problems, joint pains, psoriasis, and (strangely) weight gain, in addition to a host of other problems. And you sure won't be any fun to be around.

So be sure to eat some fat… it's good for you. It's the fear of fat that does more damage.

Identifying fats on food labels

The fats section lists the total number of grams, as well as the number of grams of saturated fat and trans fat. Trans fat labeling can be deceptive, as manufacturers of foods that contain less than 0.5 grams of trans fats are allowed to list them as zero on the label. For these foods, inspect the ingredients list for the words "partially hydrogenated" to determine if trans fats are present. (Fully hydrogenated oils are typically listed as "hydrogenated" and don't contain trans fats. But beware: if a package simply lists "hydrogenated oil" without expressly stating whether it is partially or fully hydrogenated, it may contain trans fats. Sometimes the terms "hydrogenated" and "partially hydrogenated" are used interchangeably. Only when the package clearly states that it contains fully hydrogenated oil, can you rest assured that it is free of trans fats.)

Sometimes manufacturers will also list the number of grams of mono and poly-unsaturated fats, although they are not required to do this unless they make specific health claims.

Food Sources of the Different Fats

There are five types of food fat, all of which affect your risk for cardiovascular disease. Foods are generally a mixture of several different types of fat, although we usually identify them by the type of fat that predominates. (For example, although we refer to olive oil as a mono-unsaturated fat, it also contains small amounts of poly-unsaturated fat and saturated fat.)

Before you read the recommendations, however, heed this warning: it is always important to hold individual nutritional recommendations in context. One study, for example, showed that only 4 percent of the French consumed a diet that met the U.S. recommendations for saturated fat (<10% of total energy)[38], yet cardiovascular disease occurs at much lower rates in France compared to the United States[163]. (This phenomenon is called the "French paradox.")

Cholesterol: amount **in your diet** doesn't have a large impact on the amount **in your blood**. (Be sure to understand this: the amount of cholesterol in your blood is much more closely linked to dietary saturated fat than it is to dietary cholesterol.)

Food sources: animal products.
Food label fact finding: amount listed.

Saturated fat: not a killer, but in excess tends to lead to build up of blood cholesterol. No need to avoid entirely, but Americans in general get too much. The government recommendation is to get less than 10 percent of your total energy from saturated fat. (For people with established heart disease, the recommendation is less than 7 percent of total energy.)
Food sources: animal products (but not seafood).
Food label fact finding: amount listed

Mono-unsaturated fat: protects against heart disease.
Food sources: olive oil, canola oil, most nuts.
Food label fact finding: not required to be listed.

Poly-unsaturated fat: there are different types that have differing impact on your body and can either promote cardiovascular disease or help to prevent it.
Food sources: vegetable oils.
Food label fact finding: not required to be listed.

Food processing techniques often result in oxidation when plant products are converted to vegetables oils, turning them into highly reactive free radicals. (Processing also diminishes their vitamin and antioxidant content.) If you use added oils, buy those that have been processed using less damaging methods, such as cold-pressed or expeller-pressed. To minimize oxidation, store them in the refrigerator or at least away from the heat of your stove, and keep them in closed, opaque containers.
Some poly-unsaturated fats are essential. **Essential Fatty Acids** become part of body structures, and are needed to make hormone-like substances in your body. Two main types (**omega-3 fats and omega-6 fats**) are needed in appropriate balance. Changing food manufacturing methods have resulted in most Americans getting too many omega-6s relative to omega-3s, which results in increased risk for cardiovascular disease as well as many other diseases. Most Americans would benefit from decreasing omega-6s and increasing omega-3s.
Food sources of omega-6 fats: vegetable oils.
Food sources of omega-3 fats: fish, flaxseed, walnuts, soy products, beans.
(See Appendix for more specific details.)

Trans Fats (also called hydrogenated fats): predominately result from hydrogenation, which is a form of commercial processing of fats. No amount of trans fats is healthy for you – consumption may result in all of the negative health impacts of excess saturated fats, and worse.
Food sources: found in most processed foods (most margarines, shortenings, baked goods, crackers, commercial frying fats used for French fries, popcorn, egg rolls, donuts...)
Food label fact finding: the amount is required to be listed. If the amount listed is zero, double-check by scanning the ingredients list for the words "partially hydrogenated" as they may still be present in small quantity. If the food doesn't have a food label, assume that all deep fried foods – and indeed, most processed foods that contain fat - contain trans fats.

Food Source Summary

Saturated	PUFA (Poly-Unsaturated)	MUFA (Mono-Unsaturated)	Omega-3	Trans Fats
Butter Lard Meat Poultry Dairy products	Most vegetable oils	Olive oil Canola oil Avocados Nuts (most)	Fish Flaxseed Hemp Walnuts Soy products	Most processed and deep-fried foods

Action Tips...

- A fat-free diet is not a healthy diet! It is much more important to consider the *types* of dietary fat, as opposed to the absolute amount.
- Minimize trans fat (found in processed foods).
- Moderate your intake of saturated fat (predominately found in animal products).
- Replace saturated and trans with mono-unsaturated fats (e.g., olive oil, canola oil, avocados, most nuts).
- Reduce poly-unsaturated fats (most vegetable oils) – except omega-3s.
- Get more omega-3 fatty acids (e.g., fish, flaxseed, walnuts, soy products).
- Other nutrition tips that will enhance a healthy heart include eating foods with plenty of antioxidants (whole plant foods!) and a low glycemic load. And don't forget to keep active and lower your stress! Maintaining close friendships will also tremendously reduce your risk for cardiovascular disease.

And keep a healthy perspective. Elimination of saturated fats is not necessary; moderation will be more beneficial. And a far bigger dietary concern is the nutrients we're not getting. Sure, the fats in food affect your health, but they do so within a larger context. Hike up the good stuff, and you'll probably spontaneously reduce the less helpful foods.

Proteins

The word "protein" comes from the Greek word "protos," meaning "of prime importance." Proteins play an integral role in every living cell.

To make protein, plants combine simple sugars with nitrogen from the air or soil to make amino acids. The name "amino" means "nitrogen-containing." A protein is a chain of amino acids, and each protein is distinguished by different types and order of amino acids. Only twenty kinds of amino acids combine to make all the thousands of kinds of protein in your body. (It's the same concept as how only 26 letters combine to form all of the words in this book.)

Your body can make about 11 of the amino acids itself, given fragments derived from dietary carbohydrates or fat, and nitrogen from dietary protein. However, approximately 9 of the amino acids are called "essential amino acids" as your body can't make them (at all or at least in sufficient quantity) and they must be supplied by your diet. Because your body cannot store amino acids (or nitrogen) in the way that it can store carbohydrates and fat, your body will become compromised quickly without them.

Food Sources

Most people associate dietary protein with animal foods, such as meat, poultry, fish or dairy products. However, most plant foods also provide protein, including beans, grains, nuts, seeds, and vegetables – and sometimes are even more concentrated sources of protein than animal products. For example, when the same number of kilocalories are compared (which is how nutrient-density is defined), broccoli actually has more protein than steak! (Steak has 5.4 grams of protein per 100 kilocalories, compared to the 11.2 grams – almost twice as much – found in broccoli.) Even lettuce far surpasses steak in terms of protein nutrient density. The confusion in understanding the protein content of foods arises because of the different ways that we use to compare them, which is a highly political issue.

When people are typically presented with a comparison of broccoli and steak, for example, the comparison is either a serving of each or an equal weight of each, and in those cases, steak has a higher protein content. Many scientists suggest that this is an inadequate comparison (that has been promoted by the industries – predominantly meat and dairy - that appear rich in protein when viewed in this way).

Since people usually eat foods until their calorie requirements are satisfied, it is suggested that we switch to focusing on which foods are more nutrient-dense with regard to protein, instead of maintaining a focus on which has more protein per weight. (Acquisition of energy is arguably the main physiologic drive for eating, although modulated by other factors; the body is quick to send off hunger signals if there is insufficient food energy.)

The main point is that, contrary to popular wisdom, plant products can provide a substantial amount of protein – and in fact some are even more protein-dense than animal sources. As we will see, it is not necessary to consume the more traditionally known protein sources, such as meat, poultry, fish or dairy products – or even beans or nuts - in order to get sufficient protein.

Protein in the body

Proteins play more varied roles in the body than carbohydrates or fat. In their structural role, they form the basis of your muscles, hair, nails, and collagen, which is the connective tissue that holds your body together. They also play regulatory roles, particularly as enzymes. Enzymes are the work-horses of our bodies and help to make chemical reactions happen. For example, enzymes digest the foods you eat, help your heart muscle to contract, and help your body to send nerve messages. Receptors form another important category of protein in our body. They act to carry information within and between cells. For example, the hormone insulin binds to specialized insulin receptors. When it does this, it causes the cell conformation to change, so that glucose can enter the cell. If insulin can't bind to the receptor, glucose cannot get into the cell easily, and your cell may not be able to get the energy that it needs. Other examples of proteins in your body include antibodies, hormones, transport molecules, and oxygen carriers.

Like dietary proteins, body proteins are composed of chains of amino acids. In order to make a specific protein, your body needs all of the amino acids that it is composed of. Since body cells can't store amino acids, all of the essential amino acids must come from your diet. Your body can synthesize the non-essential amino acids from the atoms contained in dietary carbohydrate, protein, or fat, as long as there is sufficient nitrogen available from protein.

Although your body prefers to use carbohydrate and fat sources for energy, it can also use amino acids either for energy or to make glucose which can then be used as energy. If you take in more protein than your body needs to make its necessary body proteins, the excess amino acids will get burned for energy or turned into glucose, if either of these are needed. If not, the excess will get converted to carbohydrate (if glucose/glycogen levels are low) or fat, and stored in these forms (and the excess nitrogen will get excreted).

Digestion, absorption and processing

Proteins from foods don't directly become body proteins. Proteins are crushed and moistened in the mouth, but the action begins in the stomach. There, hydrochloric acid denatures (straightens) the protein chain, so that digestive enzymes can more easily access the bonds that hold the amino acids together. An enzyme called pepsin cleaves the protein into smaller chains of amino acids.

These smaller chains (called polypeptides) enter the small intestine, where the real action occurs. Pancreatic and intestinal proteases further digest the polypeptides, clipping the bonds between the amino acids. With the help of other enzymes, they are reduced to the individual amino acids they are composed of.

The amino acids then get absorbed through the intestinal wall and delivered to the liver, and then released into your bloodstream. Cells can then use the amino acids as building blocks. Only a few peptides (chained amino acids) escape digestion and enter the blood intact.

Protein Turnover

Body proteins are constantly being broken down and the amino acids are then recycled to make new proteins. This process is called protein turnover. Each day, more proteins are recycled than are supplied by your diet. For example, of the approximately 300 grams of protein synthesized by your body each day, about 275 grams are made from recycled amino acids. This recycling is the reason we need so little protein in our diet compared to carbohydrate and fat.

Protein Synthesis

A gene is a blueprint that tells your body which amino acids to string together, and in what order, to make a specific protein. The amino acids may come from your digested foods, or from the recycled amino acids that result from the breakdown of body proteins.

When a cell makes a protein, we say that the gene for that protein has been "expressed." Each of us is unique because some of our genes differ, which results in minute differences in the amino acid sequence of our body's proteins. We also differ in the rate at which our genes are expressed or whether an individual gene is expressed at all.

Interestingly, nutrients from our diet can regulate gene expression, and this is one of the large ways in which our dietary habits influence our health. For example, one reason mono-unsaturated fatty acids are beneficial in protecting us against heart disease is because they influence expression of various genes involved in lipid metabolism.

Amino Acid Use

Protein differs from carbohydrate and fat in that we don't maintain stores. All proteins on our body are serving a function. For example, they provide structure to muscle cells and comprise enzymes that allow muscles to contract. Because there is no amino acid storage, we depend on a constant influx of amino acids in our blood, either through dietary consumption or protein turnover.

While amino acids can and do provide us with energy, they serve more important functions in the growth and maintenance of our cells, and your body prefers to shunt amino acids towards their more important roles, as opposed to wasting them as an energy source.

Immediately after a protein-containing meal, the digested and absorbed amino acids in the bloodstream are either shunted towards protein synthesis or can be used as an energy source for the short time that they remain in the bloodstream. Over time, excess amino acids get converted into glucose and stored as glycogen, and if glycogen reserves are filled, the excess get converted to fatty acids and stored in adipose tissue.

At times that we are not digesting protein foods, we still have a constant influx of amino acids into our bloodstream as cells that are comprised of amino acids are constantly being destroyed and re-created. (Some cells only live for a few hours, others as much as a few months.) However, many of these amino acids are quickly recycled for functional purposes, resulting in a fairly constant, though low level, of amino acids in the bloodstream.

How much do you need?

Though protein is critical for our survival, we don't need much, and the average American consumes well in excess of their needs. The idea that we need to get a high level of protein was disproven in the 1970s, although it is a very common belief among the lay public and still promoted by many misinformed professionals.

The World Health Organization, the National Research Council, and the Food and Nutrition Board of the National Academy of Sciences have determined that the very maximum we need is 8 percent of our total daily energy needs [164-166]. Even this 8 percent includes a "safety" factor of an extra 30 percent, and these health agencies have been criticized for pandering to the powerful meat and dairy industries by adding such a large and seemingly unnecessary margin of error [167, 168]. In contrast to the inflated 8 percent recommended by health professionals, the average American gets over 15 percent of their total energy from protein[169].

Since almost all foods get greater than 8 percent of their energy from protein, it is very easy to meet your protein needs and unnecessary to go out of your way to get protein foods in your diet. Even if your diet were comprised of nothing but low-protein sources like bread, pasta, rice and potatoes, you would still get adequate protein to meet your needs (as long as you had sufficient variety to get the full range of essential amino acids - to be discussed shortly - and other nutrients).

The foods that are exceptions to this, meaning they typically get less than 8 percent of their energy from protein, include fruits (which contain about 5 percent of their energy from protein) and many candies and a few "junk" foods. You'd get yourself into nutritional trouble if your diet were limited to these foods.

You practically have to be starving to be protein deficient. It is ironic that we worry about this in our culture of abundance.

Children and pregnant and breast-feeding women need more protein, but that is easily provided by adding green vegetables, lentils, beans, milk or meat to the basic staples.

Getting the right protein

Animal foods and soybeans are called "complete proteins" because they contain ample amounts of all of the essential amino acids. Most plant proteins, on the other hand, are lacking in one or more of the essential amino acids, and there is a persistent myth that vegetarians need to be well educated and choose protein foods that "complement" one another, meaning that the foods make up for the amino acid deficiencies of one another. For example, beans lack methionine and grains lack lysine, but together they contain all of the essential amino acids, and thus rice and beans is a "complete protein."

However, research demonstrates that this is unnecessary, and that both vegetarians and omnivores get sufficient protein, including essential amino acids well in excess of their needs, as long as they are getting sufficient calories [170-172]. Complementary proteins don't need to be consumed at the same meal, and a little dietary variety over the course of a day appears to effortlessly ensure the appropriate mix. Research has clearly discredited the idea that vegetable protein is of lower "quality" and less valuable than animal protein.

Health Effects of Protein Over- and Under-Consumption

Protein Under-Consumption

Because protein plays such an important role in so many body structures and processes, protein deficiency can wreak havoc on effective functioning. Protein deficiency typically goes hand-in-hand with energy deficiency, and the primary malnutrition disease even reflects this in its full name: protein-energy malnutrition. It is a widespread problem in poverty-stricken communities, particularly in developing countries. Protein and energy intakes are often difficult to separate because diets that have sufficient energy typically have sufficient protein.

There are two forms of protein-energy malnutrition: marasmus and kwashiorkor. Marasmus reflects a severe deprivation of food over time and is characterized by a "skin and bones" appearance. Kwashiorkor reflects a more sudden and recent food deprivation, and is more likely to manifest with edema, resulting in a puffy or swollen appearance. There have been no reported cases of marasmus or kwashiorkor in the United States in recent decades.

Protein needs are much lower than most people imagine, and the risk of protein deficiency, in the absence of energy deficiency, is negligible. Even athletes and pregnant or lactating women are at low risk, as ordinary diets supply more than enough to meet the needs of growing bodies.

Protein Over-Consumption

When protein is consumed in excess of the body's needs for growth, it may be used for energy or converted to fat. Protein contains nitrogen atoms, and in either case those nitrogen atoms need to be removed.

The body combines the nitrogen atoms with hydrogen, making ammonia, a compound that many of us know as a household cleaner. Ammonia is extremely toxic, especially to brain cells. To protect itself, the liver converts the ammonia to urea, which is then removed from the bloodstream by the kidneys and excreted in your urine. (When lipid and carbohydrate are broken down for energy, they release only carbon dioxide and water, which are easily tolerated by the body or disposed of, making carbohydrate and lipid "clean-burning" fuels.)

High protein diets therefore require your liver and kidneys to work harder, and it is not surprising to see a well-documented association between protein over-consumption and kidney and liver disease. (However, there is evidence to suggest that the kidney may adapt to higher protein intake, meaning that this association may not be causal[173].) Because increased production of urea triggers dieresis (an increased water loss in your urine), you also lose minerals such as calcium, which explains the well-known association between protein over-consumption and osteoporosis. Given organ exposure to ammonia, a toxic substance, the association to cancer also appears to make sense.

Other diseases that show a well documented association to protein over-consumption include type 2 diabetes and cardiovascular disease. High protein diets may also weaken the immune system.

High protein diets usually entail eating protein from concentrated sources, such as animal products, so they often also contain high levels of saturated fat, cholesterol, oxidants, and low levels of fiber, phytochemicals and antioxidants. This makes it difficult to tease out to what degree these associated factors play the causative role in disease, as opposed to the protein itself. Nonetheless, there is strong evidence to suggest that at least part of the association for all of these diseases is caused by excess protein itself.

Additionally, some amino acids may be disease-promoting while others enhance health, making it necessary to get even more specific about protein when examining the health consequences. A convincing case can be made that animal proteins[174] – independent of other associated nutrients – increase risk for cancer[175-178], atherosclerosis[179, 180], osteoporosis[181, 182], and type 2 diabetes[183]. This was particularly evident in the China Project[103, 179, 180], which is one of the largest and most comprehensive studies ever undertaken to examine the relationship between diet and disease. The data showed huge differences in disease rates based on the amount of plant foods participants ate compared to animal foods.

Vegetarian/ Inadequate protein myths

It's easy to get high quality protein from a vegetarian diet since many plants are by nature rich sources of proteins. Indeed, the world's largest animals are vegetarian: elephants, hippopotamuses, giraffes, and cows.

As discussed earlier, people require very little protein; getting a sufficient amount is hard to avoid if you are getting sufficient calories. As an example, rice alone provides 71 grams of protein and white potatoes 64 grams of protein[184]. Compare this to an average woman who needs approximately 2,000 kilocalories per day. Based on the estimate by the World Health Organizations and others presented previously, she needs 8 percent of it from protein, which translates to 160 kilocalories. Since protein contains 4 kilocalories per gram, her daily protein needs are only 40 grams. (And remember, the 8% estimate contains a margin of error that over-estimates needs!) This calculation shows that even consuming foods considered to be low-protein ensures sufficient protein.

The myths that plant proteins are of lower quality or that vegetarians need to choose complementary proteins, were discussed earlier.

Bottom line? Ignore the warnings. Vegans and vegetarian can easily get their protein needs met. Inadequate protein warnings should go out to those who subsist on candy and junk food regardless of whether they are vegans or omnivores.

The appendix provides more information on vegetarianism or veganism.

The protein/athlete myth

Muscular work builds protein; protein and amino acid supplements do not. Athletes need a diet that provides sufficient energy to protect against muscle wasting, and the typical diet provides more than enough protein to meet the increased needs of athletes. Athletes will be served better by ensuring that they have sufficient clean burning fuel, such as carbohydrate, than focusing on protein. The widely sold protein and amino acid supplements are typically a waste of money, contributing more to diseases associated with over-consumption than to muscular growth or improved performance.

Identifying protein on food labels

The protein section lists the total number of grams.

Action Tips...

Individuals at risk for protein under-consumption are those that don't get enough calories in general, subsist on a "fruitarian" diet, or consume low-protein junk foods that crowd more nutritious foods out of their diet. To ensure that you get enough protein, make sure to eat enough calories in general and to go beyond fruit and candy. Teasing out how much protein may be excessive and disease-promoting is a more thorny issue. But even if the issue of "how much is too much" isn't well-defined, getting the right amount of protein is not difficult.

Eat a varied, nutrient-dense diet, and there is no need to go out of your way to get or avoid protein or specific amino acids or amino acid combinations. It is more important is to pay attention to the other nutrients the protein is packaged with than to concentrate on the protein itself. (For example, is the food high in fiber or low in saturated fat?)

Plant products will typically do a better job of meeting your protein needs than animal products, both because they are often less concentrated sources of protein (making protein over-consumption less likely) and because they are more likely to be bundled with other great nutrients, such as fiber, vitamins, minerals, phytochemicals and healthy fats. However, you do not need to be a vegan to be healthy. If you eat animal products, try using them as an accompaniment to enhance a plant-based meal, rather than building your meal around them.

People would do well to learn more about soy foods and substituting them for some of the animal foods in the standard American diet. This simple change would decrease the saturated fat, and increase the omega-3 fats, fiber and phytochemicals. You would also lower your exposure to environmental toxins. I encourage you to experiment with soy products. There is a wide range on the market, some of which taste terrible and some of which are delicious. But be aware that the more processed the soy food is, the lower the nutritional benefits. For example, "isolated soy protein" may not contain many of the beneficial nutrients found in the soybean.

Get Informed...

The China Study, by T. Colin Campbell, contains a good discussion of protein, with particularly valuable information about the politics behind the misconceptions.

Weight Regulation: An Effortless Process!

Richard Carmona, Surgeon General, the highest government health official, describes obesity as "the terror within, a threat that is every bit as real to America as the weapons of mass destruction"[185]. Six months before he made that grave pronouncement, terrorists had decimated the World Trade Center. The country was on high alert and the fear of continued terrorist action was at the forefront of our minds.

This evening, when your mom ladles that second glop of turkey gravy on your mashed potatoes... when she urges, "Eat, eat! It's good for you!" ... and especially when she puts that second helping of pumpkin pie with whipped cream on your plate, it's time to call 911. Get that woman detained.

Then reflect on the craziness that underlies this "obesity epidemic." Terrorists not only in our cities and our airports, but in our kitchens. Hamburgers and french fries as weapons of mass destruction.

Manufacturing the Obesity Epidemic

At least 400,000 Americans die of overweight and obesity every year, making it soon to surpass smoking as the leading cause of preventable death[186]. At least that's what the Centers for Disease Control (CDC) told us recently.

But an updated federal report acknowledged that the previous analysis suffered from computational errors[187]. In fact, obesity and overweight only result in an excess of 26,000 annual deaths, far fewer than guns, alcohol or car crashes. Furthermore, "overweight" people live longer than "normal" weight people.

What is most striking about this is that the CDC is not publicizing the new results, nor changing their public health message. After all, they used the original study as justification for their war on obesity – why not stop the war now that the evidence has disappeared? The CDC didn't just over-hype a crisis, they helped invent it!

We don't have an epidemic of obesity; our epidemic is one of obesity myths and hyperbole.

- Obesity leads to disease and is life-threatening.
- Weight loss improves health and longevity.
- Anyone can keep lost weight off if she or he tries hard enough.
- Public health recommendations are based on scientific research and in the best interests of consumer health.

For most of us, these statements seem like basic truisms. However, much of what we believe to be true about weight is in fact myth, fueled by the power of money and cultural bias. And public health officials, health care professionals and scientists are complicit (often unintentionally) in supporting and encouraging the lies. The campaign against obesity is not about science or health.

The misconceptions propagated about the most basic research are astounding. Let's take a look at some of them.

Obesity Myths[g]

Myth 1. Obesity Kills.

No obesity myth is more potent than the one that says that obesity kills. It gives us permission to call our fear of fat a health concern, rather than naming it for the cultural oppression it is.

I'm sure every reader has heard the statement obesity kills as it has been a large part of the federal public health campaign. First we were told obesity and overweight killed 300,000 people per

---

[g] This section is drawn in large part from work by Glenn Gaesser, in his book *Big Fat Lies*.

year[188], then it was updated to 400,000 per year[186] and later corrected to 365,000[189]. These statistics, generated by the CDC, have been cited innumerable times in news reports as well as scientific and medical journals[190-193]. As mentioned earlier, the more recent correction to 26,000 received remarkably little federal publicity.

And all along the figures were bogus accounting. It's surprising how weak the verification is for any of these numbers. These numbers rely on a statistical excess of deaths among people who are obese or overweight compared to people who are not, and assumes all excess mortality is due to their fat. Just because someone is portly and dies at a young age, doesn't necessarily mean that their weight was the cause.

While it is well documented that diet and activity patterns can lead to obesity – and to an early demise - there is no evidence that the obesity itself kills. Indeed, there are many factors that are associated with body weight, such as physical activity or eating habits, which could easily be responsible for some or all of the relationship between obesity and mortality. The authors of the initial report later attempted to correct the persistent misrepresentation of their research by stating that "The figure applies broadly to the combined effects of various dietary factors and activity patterns that are too sedentary, not to the narrower effect of obesity alone[194]," but apparently the damage is done, and the statistics now have a life of their own.

Although not well publicized, even government researchers were critical of the earlier reports, stating that the deaths are created by statistics, not science, and urging caution in the use of these statistics[195].

The correction that was published in the Journal of the American Medical Association, reducing the deaths attributable to obesity and overweight fifteen-fold and showing that overweight may actually be protective, is not new news, but is entirely consistent with many other studies showing that a modest amount of "overweight" is good for you, and that obesity itself is relatively benign, except at the extreme.

For example, the largest epidemiological study ever conducted shows that the highest life expectancy is among individuals who are overweight by our current standards, and the lowest life expectancy is among those defined as underweight[196]. What's more, individuals who fit into what is deemed the ideal weight range had a lower life expectancy than those who were obese! Another large-scale study, conducted in Canada, comes to a similar conclusion[197]. Indeed, it is apparent from the research that the health concerns associated with obesity are largely attributable to genetic and lifestyle factors (which at the same time may contribute to the development of obesity).

Epidemiological studies cause statistical deaths

The majority of our knowledge regarding the health impact of obesity is drawn from epidemiological research. Epidemiological obesity research compares groups of overweight and obese individuals with a control group of non-obese individuals who are similar in as many other ways as possible. It is intended to uncover associations which then need further examination. It cannot tell us whether a particular variable causes or even influences another.

For example, epidemiological research indicates a relationship between baldness and heart disease[198]. Because bald men are more likely to get heart disease than men with a full head of hair, does not mean that baldness promotes heart disease or that hair protects against heart disease[h199]. Instead, further research indicates that high levels of testosterone may promote both baldness and heart disease. "Confounding factors" can often serve to further confuse the interpretation of epidemiological research.

---

[h] This example was given by Jon Robison in his article "Risk Factor Frenzy" which describes these ideas at greater length.

Since there are a number of confounding factors that complicate the relationship between weight and mortality (risk for early death), assigning causation is particularly tenuous. For example, it is well documented that heavier people have lower activity levels, and until recently, none of the epidemiological studies on the health impact of obesity controlled for this. More recent studies that control for physical activity levels show that activity – not weight – is much more highly associated with mortality risk[200-205].

For example, research conducted as part of the Aerobics Center Longitudinal Study in Texas found that obese men who are classified as "fit" based on a treadmill test have death rates just as low as "fit" lean men[201]. Furthermore, the fit obese men had death rates one-half those of the lean but unfit men, indicating that fitness is more important than weight in longevity. Similar results were demonstrated for women[202].

That activity and other factors confound the obesity/mortality relationship is well accepted: an editorial that appeared in the New England Journal of Medicine, for example, points out that: "Mortality among obese people may be misleadingly high because overweight people are more likely to be sedentary and of low socio-economic status."[206]

Other research indicates that larger people have a more extensive history of restrictive dieting and weight fluctuation, both of which could also potentially explain the increased mortality risk[87i]. Reduced access to and reluctance to seek health care for fear of discrimination[207, 208] may also confound the picture. The negative effects of weight loss medications, such as amphetamines, could also play a role. (In 1970, 8 percent of all U.S. prescriptions were for amphetamines intended to treat obesity[209]!) And of course, the stress from discrimination may also play a role: larger people are not subject to the same diseases in countries where there is less stigma attached to obesity.

Indeed, the authors of the earlier cited epidemiological study regarding obesity and mortality wrote a disclaimer: "Our estimates may be biased toward higher numbers due to confounding by unknown variables[210]." Of course, many of these variables are not unknown, such as physical activity levels. The authors simply chose to ignore them.

Myth 2. Obesity leads to disease.

Just as the idea that obesity is a large causal factor in mortality (death) risk is a myth, so is the idea that obesity is a large causal factor in excess morbidity (sickness).

Take atherosclerosis, for example. Given that obese people have more fat on their bodies, it has been assumed that they must have more fat in their arteries. Yet the research doesn't substantiate this. Five decades of autopsy studies, for example, consistently show no relationship between body fat and atherosclerosis[211-215]. Ultrasound studies corroborate this [213, 216, 217], and well over half of the angiographic studies conducted between 1976 and 2000 show obesity has no relationship to either the presence of atherosclerosis or its progression over time[213]. The largest, most comprehensive angiographic study examined 4500 angiograms and concluded that every 11 pound *increase* in weight was associated with a 10 to 40 percent *lower* chance of atherosclerosis[218]. In other words, it was the fat men and women that had the cleanest arteries!

Indeed, there is little evidence to support that obesity is the primary cause for any of the diseases for which it is routinely blamed (except osteoarthritis, sleep apnea and uterine cancer). While it is clear that there are several diseases *associated* with obesity, evidence supports several alternative explanations. Similar issues could be raised to those presented in the previous section on obesity's association with longevity.

---

i See Ernsberger's article entitled "Biomedical Rationale..." for a discussion of all of the topics in this paragraph.

For example, some diseases or treatments for diseases may promote obesity. Confounding lifestyle factors may promote obesity at the same time that they also cause certain diseases. Larger people may have higher disease risk because they are more likely to be older, to belong to an ethnic minority, to be of lower socio-economic status, to have less access to quality health care, and to be victims of discrimination. And finally, larger people may be more likely to have tried dangerous weight loss methods and to have gone through damaging cycles of losing and regaining weight. All of these could be major contributors to disease, and any could take center stage.

Myth 3. Weight loss will make you healthier.

The idea that health will necessarily improve with weight loss is dubious at best[213]. No one has ever proved that losing weight prolongs life. In fact, there is an extraordinary amount of controversy regarding whether weight loss is necessary or even desirable for improved health. While it is clear that research indicates a short-term reduction in health risk factors associated with weight loss, there are no randomized clinical studies that have observed the long-term effects of weight loss, and the observational research (epidemiological studies) has typically found weight loss to be associated with dying younger[219, 220].

For example, Gaesser examined the research and found 15 studies published between 1983 and 1993 that show that weight loss actually increases the risk of dying early[221]. This is 13 more than the number of studies published during that same period that showed weight loss reducing the risk of dying early – and one of those two studies in the minority only showed an 11 hour increase in longevity for each pound of weight loss[221]! Even when weight loss intention is considered and subjects with unintentional weight loss (such as might occur with cancer or AIDS) are excluded, the research is ambiguous at best[222-227]. Yet the message that comes through, clearly not supported by the scientific literature, is that we all need to lose weight in order to be healthy.

Note, of course, that just because the research indicates an association between weight loss and decreased longevity, doesn't mean that weight loss *causes* people to die earlier. I suspect the explanation for this lies in the unhealthy methods people use to achieve weight loss, as well as the difficulty in separating weight loss from weight gain[219]. (Many people that do achieve weight loss go through cycles of weight loss and weight gain before finally stabilizing at a lower weight, damaging their body in the process.)

In contrast, there is a great deal of evidence indicating that many of the more prevalent health problems associated with obesity, such as high blood pressure, heart disease, insulin resistance, and type 2 diabetes, can be improved independently of weight loss (through changes in activity or nutritional habits, for example). Health-enhancing changes in activity or nutritional habits may simultaneously result in weight loss, but this is not a given.

Myth 4. Anyone can lose weight if they are disciplined.

Theoretically, all you have to do is eat less than your body needs, and you will lose weight. Associating food with unwanted weight, many people watch their calories closely. When we see heavier people, we assume that they just aren't disciplined enough – or we think that of ourselves if we're holding onto more weight than we want.

Sounds simple, right? Wrong! The ability to lose weight and sustain that weight loss has relatively little to do with willpower or lack of control.

It is well established that diets don't work over the long term. No matter how many times we keep repeating the research, refining our methods, or changing our vocabulary, we get the same results: people who diet eventually regain the weight (and sometimes more). *Not a single study has documented long term weight loss for any but a small minority of participants.*

It's not just that dieting doesn't work. Diet enough, and it actually encourages your body to store extra fat, so that you weigh more than if you didn't try in the first place! Numerous research studies document that people who diet are more likely to gain weight than people who don't[228-234].

Here's a summary of the main points that implicate dieting as a weight *gain* technique. Dieting:

- slows the body's metabolic rate (you use up fewer calories for basic survival needs)
- slows the metabolic rate during activity (when you're active, your body gets stingy with energy use)
- increases food absorption efficiency (you get every little crumb of energy out of your food, digest it faster, and get hungrier quicker)
- causes you to crave fat in your diet
- increases the appetite (like holding your breath, there is only so long you can resist if you are fighting a hunger drive)
- reduces energy levels (you don't have the energy to do as much)
- lowers your body temperature to use up less energy (you feel colder)
- decreases reliability of the feelings of "hungry" and "full" (it becomes easier to confuse hunger with emotional needs)
- decreases the amount of muscle tissue
- increases fat-storage enzymes and decreases fat-release enzymes (all of them ready to go to work storing fat as soon as you eat again)
- decreases the cell's sensitivity to insulin (you need more to do the same job)

So don't blame yourself if you can't stick to your diet. Breaking your diet is not about gluttony or a failure of willpower. Nor is the increase in weight you may have seen as a result of dieting. In fact, most dieters show extraordinary self-restraint, persistence, determination and willpower; just think of all the crazy things that people have done in their efforts to lose weight. They didn't fail; the diet did.

Altering the other side of the energy balance equation, increasing exercise, for example, demonstrates similar results. When formerly sedentary people regularly participate in exercise programs, the research is not showing dramatic weight-lowering benefits. In fact, a meta-analysis of 25 years of exercise programs indicated that training programs only result in loss of 0.2 pounds per week[235]. As an example, 500 men and women participated in a 20 week endurance training program as part of the Heritage Family Study[236]. On average, the men lost less than a pound, and the women lost close to nothing!

In another study, the obese women participating in an intense 6-month resistance training program also did not exhibit any body fat loss or change in body composition[237]. The Midwest Exercise Trial put men and women on a 16-month intensive endurance exercise program[238]. The men were quite successful, losing, on average, about 11 pounds; the women, on the other hand, gained a little over a pound, while losing less than a half pound of body fat!

Many studies have found women actually *gain* weight and body fat with exercise. One study which monitored obese women who did six months of aerobic exercise four to five times a week, found that a third of them gained 15 pounds of body fat, and that the gainers averaged an 8 pound weight gain[145].

Why isn't this information getting out to the general public? Why is this myth of exercise as the ultimate weight control tool perpetuated, in the absence of data to support it? I suppose "Exercise! Lose a pound!" wouldn't make for good headlines.

That most people don't lose weight or sustain weight loss through diet or exercise programs tells us more about physiology and how body weight is regulated, than it does about individual willpower or self-control.

Trust the experts?

Many of our most basic assumptions about dieting and weight are either misleading or blatantly contradicted by what is known by scientists. The conventional wisdom on the danger and cause of obesity and techniques for weight loss have changed little in the past fifty years – despite solid evidence that it is just plain wrong: that the propensity towards weight gain and resistance to weight loss is in large part beyond volitional control, for example, and that the health risks associated with obesity are largely due to other associated factors – such as low fitness level, yo-yo dieting, or perhaps the social stigma – as opposed to fat itself.

In fact, much of the research that supports the view expressed in this book is old news. Fifty years ago, scientists were already aware that body weight was internally regulated in the hypothalamus around a particular setpoint: all that was missing was a detailed explanation of the biochemical supporters and their actions. Since then, particularly in the last decade, scientists have been actively filling in the blanks. The 1994 discovery of leptin was a dramatic advance, giving us a name for the principle biochemical regulator, and allowing us to trace its path. Thousands of studies conducted since have helped in our understanding of the complex biochemistry that drives the mechanism and controls our weight.

The scientific framework expressed in this book is hardly heretical, and is based on compelling research. Why does it differ so much from what is more commonly touted by dietitians and other health care professionals? Why is it that these views have not become commonly accepted by the public, or even by a significant portion of the scientific community? Why are so many intelligent and compassionate people invested in reifying an old paradigm which not only doesn't work, but exacerbates people's difficulty with weight control and wreaks havoc with their self-esteem?

I suspect it is because our views have been shaped by our own personal experiences of managing our weight within a cultural context marked by an obsession with thinness and a belief that success can be achieved through material consumption. No individual can escape the influence of culture. Health care practitioners and obesity researchers are subject to the same bias against fat, and are exposed to the same unrealistic images of bodies and relentless pressure to "purchase beauty" that we all experience in our culture.

From an early age we are taught to despise fat. Our culture tells us – particularly women – that the size of our body defines our merits as a person – and barrages us with images of ideal body shapes that we can never achieve. While this may have begun as a women's issue, it has been increasingly extended to include men. The emotional toll on all of us cannot be calculated. Whether we are fat, believe that we are fat, or fear becoming fat, few people are at peace with their bodies.

The weight loss industry of course has a multibillion dollar interest in promoting the belief that weight can be controlled by dietary manipulation or other consciously applied techniques, and we can't ignore the tremendous power they have had in fueling the cultural hysteria about weight. Body-conscious Americans will spend nearly $40 billion this year to lose weight, and that number is expected to continue to balloon.

We wouldn't be spending that kind of money if we thought we had such limited ability to lose weight. Clearly, it pays for the weight-loss industry to have us believe that losing weight is - with a little help from them - not all that hard. This is obvious in the weight-loss advertisements, where you get the impression that losing flab and keeping it off is easy. The people in these ads are having fun and look happy, especially compared to the way they used to look before they signed up for the program or ordered the "natural" herbal weight-loss pills or bought the diet book.

It pays for the weight loss industry to have us believe that weight has negative health consequences, as is evident in the enormous resources that the pharmaceutical industry has put behind research that exaggerates the health risks associated with weight. Knoll Pharmaceuticals, for example, offers funding to those who "advance the understanding of obesity as a major health problem"[87], as they explicitly state in a call for proposals. After mobilizing concern about obesity, they can profit by selling the cure. The same is happening among physicians, for whom there is a tremendous market in promoting various weight loss methods, particularly surgery.

Obesity researchers are also heavily influenced by cultural assumptions. Though many may be well-intentioned and honest, it is important to recognize that their status, reputation and livelihood are in large part determined by how well they promote the diet and pharmaceutical industries. Career opportunities are limited if they choose not to participate, resulting in little incentive to question the status quo. The result is that cultural bias plays a role in every aspect of research, including our underlying assumptions, what research we choose to undertake and how we interpret scientific data.

The government has played a particularly potent role in propagating the cultural hysteria. Economic interests are favored by government panels when obesity is identified as a major public health threat, when definitions of obesity are set at low standards, when unsuccessful treatments are promoted, and when the dangers of various treatments are minimized. Let's take a look at an example of how this gets played out.

Those who determine public policy and federal grant funding are almost always simultaneously funded by weight loss and/or pharmaceutical companies, thus presenting a conflict of interest. Seven of the nine members on the National Institute of Health's Obesity Task Force, for example, were directors of weight loss clinics[239], and most had multiple financial relationships with private industry[240].

Thanks to this task force, one magical night in June of 1998, 29 million Americans went to bed with average figures and woke up "overweight." Sixty-eight million Americans were overweight or obese on June 16th, but by the next morning America had 97 million fat people. They woke up with a presumed increased risk of type 2 diabetes, hypertension and atherosclerosis and a government prescription for weight loss. And, of course, nobody gained a pound. Instead, the obesity standards were lowered, a change which was obviously favorable for private industry, though not supported by the research.

It is unlikely that many of the people promoting the obesity myths are acting consciously to mislead us, and I am not suggesting a conspiracy. Rather, the myths about obesity are so much a part of our culture, and the penalty for questioning them so high, that assumptions don't even get recognized, let alone challenged. While I am not accusing any individuals of dishonesty, I believe it is important to recognize that public/private conflicts of information combined with the extraordinary financial clout of the weight loss industry may not be conducive to open-mindedness to new ideas or making sure important research gets conducted or reported, nor that the best information gets out to the general public.

Understanding Why You Weigh What You Weigh

Let's get started in our exploration of how body weight is regulated by examining the energy on your body. Suppose you wake up in the morning and weigh yourself (not a recommended practice!). Let's look at what that number on your scale actually measures.

Scales don't measure "substantive" weight

Your body's biggest component is water - about 60% of your weight. You're like a big water balloon: 5 quarts of blood and 40 quarts of other fluids held together by a bag of skin. Your other major components are muscles and bones - what scientists call "lean weight" - and your fat weight.

In a given day, your weight can fluctuate several pounds, primarily due to changes in body water. Considering this, you can see that your scale has limitations; even though it's simple and convenient, the scale is not an effective way to measure *substantive* weight loss. If you doubt this, try eating some salty foods – chips and dip will do – you'll get thirsty, retain water, and "show" more pounds on the scale. Conversely, you can spend a few hours sweating in the hot sun, and manipulate your scale in the other direction.

Water loss won't fool a scientist

Scientists aren't fooled by changes in body water – and neither should you. From the perspective of substantive weight, those day-to-day changes on a scale are meaningless. To study weight regulation with a full deck, scientists use a more precise measure - "energy." Energy skips right past water and refers to fat and lean body tissues exclusively.

Energy weighs you down

Think of your body as a factory that takes in raw materials (food), uses some to produce new products (like hormones) or to fuel operations, routes the rest to storage, and discards the waste. Although you consume fuel only intermittently, the factory never closes; when you run out of food from recent meals, your body zips right over to the storage unit and takes what it needs.

When your combined lean and fat weight is fairly stable, you're in "**energy balance**," despite this dynamic flux. If you're packing on pounds, the amount of food energy you're consuming is exceeding the amount of energy your body is using, which pumps your excess energy into storage; in other words, it ratchets up your fat weight (or, if you are exercising, the energy may get tacked onto your lean weight). Weight loss, on the other hand, means removal of energy from your fat stores (and/or lean energy) to help meet your body's energy needs.

Weight Loss/Weight Gain

Picture this common scenario. New Year's morning arrives, and Maria awakens to a new year filled with hope and promise. She springs out of bed, heads toward the shower, and decides along the way to step on the scale to see whether the holiday parties had taken a toll on her waistline. She looks at the number, and is certain the scale must be broken. She steps off, gives the scale a good shake to get it back in working order, and tries again. As the same number appears, she's stunned by the weight she's put on over the past months, but decides then and there that she will resolve in the New Year's Day spirit to change her ways and lose those extra pounds.

Over the next weeks, she cuts out calories by eating smaller portions and eliminating her early afternoon chocolate fix. She joins a gym and starts to work out regularly. Sure enough, the number on the scale steadily drops. Maria's happy and proud, and feels certain that she's got her weight problem licked.

Sound familiar? Maria's success at losing weight in the short term is not unusual, and perhaps you've even been there. Any weight loss plan that helps you to reduce the amount of energy you eat relative to the amount of energy you spend will result in short-term weight loss.

In the Energy and Metabolism section, we discussed the energy balance equation, which states that body energy is dictated by the amount of energy consumed relative to the amount spent. This equation explains whether you gain, lose, or maintain weight.

The common belief is that all you have to do is eat less food than your body needs and weight loss will naturally follow. Some weight loss programs promote special food combinations, such as high-protein and low-carbohydrate, or low-fat and high-carbohydrate; others advise calorie counting or exercising. But the bottom line is always the same: losing weight and keeping it off is a matter of manipulating the energy balance equation through diet and/or exercise - and *discipline*.

Seems like common sense – and it definitely works on a short-term basis. But it just doesn't pan out in the long run. As much as I hate to burst Maria's bubble, odds are she's going to put the weight back on – through no fault of her own. Though most people believe dieting to be the "right" thing to do, "common wisdom" has sent us down the wrong path.

Instead, an overwhelming body of evidence supports a surprising conclusion: that the contributors to your body weight, such as what, when and how much you eat, as well as how you expend energy (including your inclination to move), are not completely under conscious control.

While the law of thermodynamics is always obeyed, you're not in control. On a short-term basis you can do a pretty good job at manipulating the energy balance equation – and that's why short-term weight loss is relatively easy. On a long-term basis, however, your body can undermine your best efforts, making attempts at weight loss unsuccessful for the vast majority of people.

Within each of our brains lies an incredibly powerful mechanism to control our weight: a body fat control center that works tirelessly to maintain your weight at a level that it (not you!) decides is appropriate: your **setpoint** weight.

Setting the Scene

You are out for an afternoon stroll, enjoying the warmth of the sun on your back. Without any thought or effort, you begin to sweat, which lowers your body temperature and keeps you comfortable. Suddenly, dark clouds sweep over the sun. Again, your body adjusts for you, causing you to shiver, thus raising your temperature. All of this occurs without any conscious effort on your part, right? Now imagine if controlling your weight could be as effortless? Well, guess what? It can be!

Up with biology, down with self-control

Until this recent epidemic of weight gain in the United States, adult weight stability over long periods of time was the norm. One 1970s research study showed that the average weight of a sixty-year-old man was only 4 to 5 pounds more than the average thirty-year-old man[241]. That kind of weight maintenance is no accident.

Your body is strongly invested in helping you maintain a healthy and relatively consistent weight, and it has efficient mechanisms that pull off this amazing feat. Unfortunately, recent lifestyle and environmental changes have resulted in many of us trying to take over the process of weight control. We have undermined our body's ability to take care of us, and the result has been escalating weights, not slimming down. As difficult as it may be to let go of the reins, we would be far better off if we trusted biology to keep off those excess pounds rather than depending on our own ill-fated attempts to control our appetites.

If you "eat normally" and allow your body to regulate around its setpoint, the mechanism will be remarkably efficient. That is why many non-dieters are able to maintain stable weights effortlessly.

Consider, for example, a fifty-year-old man who weighs approximately 5 pounds more than he did when he was twenty. If he eats about 2,000 calories per day, over the course of thirty years, he has taken in about 22 million calories. Five pounds of body fat is the equivalent of about 17,500 calories, which means that his body was only .08 percent off in balancing energy in versus energy out. This amounts to a difference of about 50 calories per month--less than the energy contained in one egg!

Your body is that precise a regulator. So, why not applaud it? Your body can do better than you can at maintaining a healthy weight if you just leave it alone - and quit messing with nature's basic setup-for-success.

Animal research supports this premise[242]. When rats are force-fed, they become obese. However, despite being allowed unlimited access to food after weight gain, they always return to their original weight[243]. Likewise, if their weight is reduced by restricting their food, they lose weight, and then rapidly return to their original weight when food is again made available[244].

Studies with humans show similar results. One of the most famous studies was conducted in Minnesota toward the end of World War II, on a group of 36 conscientious objectors who volunteered for the study as their contribution to our country in lieu of participating in the war[245]. The men were put on a calorie restriction diet until their weight had been reduced 25 percent. When allowed to eat again unrestricted, they quickly returned to their previous weights. (This is a common experience. Even people who are very large react in this same way to a calorie restriction diet, showing initial weight loss, followed by a return to original weight[246].)

Reverse studies have shown surprising results. In one, men were given a very high-calorie diet to *increase* their weight[247], while another study paid men to *gain* weight on their own[248]. In both studies, participants gained weight initially, but when they returned to eating normally, their weight quickly returned to previous levels.

These studies illustrate the important concept of your "setpoint" weight, which is central to your body's weight regulation system. In order to understand this, let's start by examining an underlying physiologic concept: homeostasis.

Homeostasis rules!

Homeostasis refers to your body's innate ability to maintain relatively stable internal conditions, despite constant environmental changes. Without this monitoring system, you would die.

Consider body temperature, for example. Your body must stay within an acceptable temperature range so you can survive; you simply can't tolerate internal extremes of hot or cold. That's why certain physiological mechanisms keep your body temperature hovering in a place that's acceptable.

The hypothalamus is a structure near the base of your brain that monitors the temperature of your blood. When you're exercising vigorously, your body heat increases. The blood courses through the hypothalamus, which senses the increased temperature and triggers the release of hormones and nerve signals that enlarge the diameter of blood vessels in your skin. The volume of blood moving through vessels increases and carries the heat to the surface of your skin, where it dissipates into the environment, resulting in cooling you off.

But what if you go out scantily clad in cold weather and your core temperature drops? Again, the hypothalamus registers this. This time, it sends nerve messengers that trigger shivering, which generates more heat, raising your body temperature.

Many physiological variables (oxygen levels, carbon dioxide levels, blood volume, blood glucose) are tightly regulated. For each, your body will accept a certain range. Redundant physiologic mechanisms keep you humming along and prevent disastrous dips or curves.

Don't underestimate your body's savvy

The concept of homeostasis is especially important when it comes to weight regulation; how much body fat you maintain is also tightly regulated within a certain range by complex physiological mechanisms. Your body truly does "care" what you weigh! (Who would have thought your body was so vain?)

That your body is strongly invested in keeping you at a healthy weight isn't particularly radical or new news from the research laboratories. Over fifty years of research support the homeostatic regulation of body weight, and it's commonly accepted by scientists[249].

Setpoint: your fat thermostat

A section of the hypothalamus (with help from a few other areas) sends out signals that manipulate your eating and activity habits as well as your metabolic efficiency. The range of acceptable weight is called your "setpoint."[j]

Your setpoint is controlled similar to a thermostat. Imagine that you set your home thermostat to 65 degrees. Every thermostat is programmed to maintain a certain acceptable range. Let's suppose that range is four degrees. This means that your temperature control system won't get too aggressive as long as the house stays between 63 and 67 degrees. However, if the temperature drops below 63 degrees, the heat turns on strongly, bringing the house back into the setpoint range. Likewise, if it gets hotter than 67 degrees, the air conditioning comes on.

Your body fat setpoint works much the same way. A certain amount of body fat pleases your brain, and it likes to stay in that ballpark range. Your body fat sends constant signals to the control center that regulates your setpoint, keeping it abreast of the existing state of your fat stores. These signals go out every moment, which means your brain is constantly aware of even tiny fluctuations in fat stores. Your brain pulls together these fat-store messages with other relevant information, and responds by cueing body processes to maintain your setpoint. It's a finely tuned process that really, really works. So why fight it?

Getting a Take on Your Own Setpoint

Want to get acquainted with your setpoint? Here are some of the markers. Your setpoint is:

- the weight that you normally maintain, when you eat naturally
- the weight that results from your body's response to signals of hunger and fullness
- the weight you maintain when you don't fixate on your weight or food habits
- the weight that you keep returning to between diets.

Unfortunately, no physiologic measure can determine your setpoint. Nor can any objective test figure out how tightly yours is regulated. (Scientists estimate that the average person has a setpoint range of about 10-20 pounds[60].) You can zero in on your setpoint only by trying a radical new diet that can be summed up in three words - just eat normally!

When you try to control your weight consciously (by dieting, for example) you disrupt your body's internal regulation signals. If you try to control your weight by watching calories, you're probably above your setpoint, not below. The bottom of your setpoint range is very tightly regulated, and it is very hard to fight your body successfully. On the other hand, although we all have physiologic mechanisms that act at the top of our range, they are not as tightly regulated for most people. Because of this, many people over-ride the signals; they can overeat and gain weight with impunity, rising above their setpoint.

If you're a frequent dieter, the news is worse. You are not only likely to be above your setpoint, but, sadly, you've probably pumped it up a few notches. Repeated dieting not only disrupts the signals, but *increases* your setpoint. Dieting is clearly counter-productive as a weight control technique – analogous to throwing gas on a fire to put it out.

---

[j] Some scientists have suggested using the term "settling point" instead, which more accurately highlights the fluidity that could occur. While this author acknowledges that term as an improvement, this book will continue to use the term "setpoint" as it is more commonly recognized and established.

Your body has super-sized efficiency

Let's examine the conscientious objectors study mentioned on the last page in more depth to get a better sense of how the setpoint works.

Participants were all young adult men of average weight for their height. Because they showed conviction by refusing to serve in a popular war, it's probably safe to assume that they had strong willpower.

During the first twelve weeks of the study, they ate normally, averaging 3,500 calories/day, and participated in daily walks and other forms of physical activity several times per week. Researchers studied their behaviors, personalities, and eating habits. The subsequent six months of the study examined the effects of reduced eating, which meant restricting calories by about 50 percent, with the goal of losing 25 percent of their initial body weight. Researchers chose food and supplements carefully to ensure that the participants got enough vitamins, minerals, and protein.

At first, the men lost weight easily. Then they plateaued, and the same calorie intake no longer produced similar losses. Some stopped dropping pounds altogether, and they had to reduce their calories even more strictly to achieve their weight-loss goals.

Behaviors also began to change in these ways:

- Loss of interest in social interaction and sexual activity
- Difficulty concentrating
- Easily distractible
- Edgy and emotional
- Lethargic and disinterested in activity
- Obsessed with food

Some of the participants fixated on flavor, and many experimented with unorthodox combinations or covered food with spices to intensify flavors. Two men had severe emotional breakdowns and had to drop out of the study. A third chopped off the end of his finger, apparently hoping he would be dismissed from the study.

Eventually, with sufficient calorie reduction, the remaining men managed to lose the weight, and all moved on to the next stage - three months of gradual re-feeding. Surprisingly, when they resumed their normal 3,500 calorie/day diets, they gained weight, even though previously this had been a normal amount for them and hadn't led to weight gain. Also, despite their calorie intake returning to normal, the men's adverse psychological symptoms remained: the men were miserable.

Even after twelve weeks of rehabilitation, when they were presented with unlimited amounts of food, their appetites were out of control. They ate very large meals until they were incapable of ingesting more, and complained that they still felt hungry. Some days their intake was 8,000 to 10,000 kilocalories.

The upshot of this study looks like this:

- When the men plateaued in weight-loss efforts, the same calorie deficit no longer produced the same amount of weight loss. The body has mechanisms that allow it to be more or less efficient with the energy it receives, and weight loss is not simply a matter of reducing the calories consumed. Somehow, your body compensates for taking in fewer calories by reducing the amount of energy expended. This is further supported by the fact that during the re-feeding period, the men gained weight when consuming a calorie count that hadn't caused them to gain weight in the past.
- The men had a minimum setpoint for weight. Though they could temporarily rebel against it and lose weight, the changing efficiency of the body made a large degree of weight loss difficult and facilitated weight regain.

- Some people lost weight more quickly than others. This points to individual variability in response to dietary changes; the same diet will produce different results in different people, depending on a person's innate propensity to gain or lose weight. Some people have strong compensatory reactions to dieting, while others' bodies don't protest as much.
- Individuals responded differently as to when they plateaued and how much they had to decrease calories to continue losing weight after plateauing. This shows variability in terms of how tightly each person's setpoint is regulated.
- Psychological distress wasn't relieved by a return to normal calorie load, but remained until body weight returned to normal. This suggests that the psychological issues weren't just a result of food deprivation, but were instead related to being below their setpoint.

For many dieters, the results of this study are all too familiar: Initial weight loss is followed by a drive to eat that results in weight regain. Many people who have been through this cycle repeatedly also report the disappointing post-dieting weights that are higher than before the weight-loss efforts.

Note, too, that the men in the study weren't binge-eaters or overeaters before the study began, but the diet set those behaviors in motion. In other words, for these men, binge-eating and overeating were not indelible character traits and signs of personal failure; rather, they were results of being below setpoint. This is true for many people. Lack of character and gluttony aren't the cause of bingeing or overeating; those traits are just counter-reactions to attempts to "cheat" biology.

Many people who are heavy believe that they got that way because they overate. If your weight has been fairly stable, however, you're probably not overeating at all, although you may feel like you are. Several studies document that large people eat no more than lean people, despite a popular misconception that large people consistently overeat[250-252]. One review examined thirteen studies, and found the intake of heavier people to be less than or equal to thin people in twelve of them[251]. In one interesting study, investigators unobtrusively observed customers at fast-food restaurants, snack bars, and ice-cream parlors, and found that the overweight customers ate no more than the thin ones. These are only casual observations, of course, but many studies support these results, and few show otherwise[253].

What? You can't gain weight!?!

Results from the reverse experiments are similarly interesting. When four college students were paid to gain as much weight as they could, despite abundant overeating of high-calorie foods, they increased their weight only by 10 percent in three to five months[248]! When the weight-gain attempts ended, they quickly returned to their pre-study weights.

When a group of Vermont prisoners was fed high-calorie, tasty foods for two hundred days, and consumed two to three times what they ordinarily ate, only two gained weight easily[254]. Once they had added 20 percent of their body weight, they could only maintain that weight with continued massive overeating (2,000 calories/day over their previous amount). At their highest weights, the men were lethargic and lacked initiative. After the experiment was over, weight loss was easy for all but the two men who gained weight easily. (Those two were later revealed to have family histories of obesity and/or diabetes.)

Apparently, study participants' metabolism increased to use the extra calories and prevent weight gain. Also, it appears that being above your own setpoint leads to low energy level and mood, similar to being below your setpoint.

Another investigator conducted two studies on British military men, examining how energy gets balanced in non-dieters[255]. Researchers monitored the energy content of everything the subjects ate.

They also kept detailed logs of what the subjects did throughout the day in order to calculate energy expended.

Results demonstrated that the men unconsciously matched the amount of energy they spent with the amount of energy they consumed over the course of the study. In other words, without these people's conscious participation in controlling calories, the body naturally balanced intake and output over time. However, on a day-to-day basis, they seemed to have to work to catch up for the extra energy previously expended. One explanation is that an increased appetite occurs in response to depleted fat stores, as opposed to increased energy usage.

In a study at the University of Pennsylvania, participants drank a liquid diet from a dispenser that tracked the volume consumed[256]. They were instructed to eat normally (meaning to eat whenever they were hungry, and stop when they were full). For the first few days, the participants took too little, but after two to six days, they were able to gauge the amount they needed and drink an appropriate amount to match their energy use.

Without informing the participants, the investigator then manipulated the liquid so that it was half as concentrated but tasted the same. Again, the participants initially drank too little, but after a few days doubled the volume consumed so that they were soon drinking an appropriate amount.

In the last stage of the research, the investigator switched two of the subjects back to the original concentration. As expected, the participants initially took in too much, but after two days each dropped back to the original number of calories. Similar to the previous studies, the participants weren't effective at meeting their caloric needs on a daily basis, but proved to be very effective at matching calorie consumption against energy expenditure on a long-term basis.

Clearly, our bodies do a great job of unconsciously regulating the amount of energy consumed to match the amount of energy expended. Even when the body is over- or under-fed, it tenaciously seeks its setpoint. Eating and energy expenditure are both directed by physiologic mechanisms beyond our conscious control.

Sometimes Your Body Is a Slacker

While all this seems very promising (no more dieting!), the not-so-good news is that your body is very invested in keeping you from losing weight - but not so upset when you gain weight.

The thermostat comparison showed that whenever you lose weight and get to the bottom of your setpoint range, your body has regulatory mechanisms that try to pump up your weight; likewise, when you get to the top of your range, your body's mechanisms press for weight loss. Sadly, for most people, regulation is very tight at the bottom but relatively lax at the top.

From an evolutionary perspective, this makes sense. Not too long ago, at least in terms of evolution, food was hard to find, and people spent much of their day in search of nourishment. Food was a primal drive: they had to eat when they could get their hands on food - or die. It was helpful to have genes that encouraged them to eat and allowed them to conserve energy and store fat, and it makes sense that we developed genes that tell us to eat.

That's why food tastes good. It has to reward us in some way, or we wouldn't keep eating. To better examine this motivation, researchers surgically altered a mouse and completely removed the reward systems in its brain. With no pleasure associated with eating, it lost interest! It had to be fed by tubes in order to survive. So food tastes good. Fat is particularly appealing because it's loaded with calories to sustain us, and sugar is also appealing as it gives us quick energy.

Did you Pump up Your Setpoint?

Other "thrifty genes" have also evolved to help our bodies store fat during time of plenty and conserve energy when food is scarce. When food shortages were common, people at greatest risk were the ones who burned energy quickly and couldn't store fat. So it naturally follows that those who survived to pass on their genes - our ancestors - were the proud possessors of thrifty genes.

Unfortunately, while our genes haven't changed much in the last few centuries, our environment has changed radically. Today, since food is plentiful and more people spend time at a desk rather than gathering food, those fat-storing/saving genes are no longer essential. Those same genes that saved our lives no longer serve us well. The world we have created is very different from the world we were designed for.

Other changes have accompanied increased food availability. In an environment where food is not easily available, hunger drives people to eat. Now that the supply for most Americans is comparatively unlimited, food has taken on different meanings, such as soothing emotional hungers and bonding us socially.

Today, most people eat (or don't eat) based on psychosocial factors, not physiologic ones. Cognitive control of eating behavior is now the norm, whether that means you're consciously trying to control your food intake, and/or eating beyond fullness. Long gone are the days when hunger drove consumption and satiety limited it.

In other words, we now have a genetic propensity to gain weight, though we don't have the food shortages that prevent weight gain. Furthermore, many people no longer physiologically regulate our food intake: we eat in the absence of hunger and physical need, and don't allow feelings of fullness to figure into the equation and push us away from the table.

It gets worse. What we're eating has also changed dramatically over the years. Foods that don't register in our weight regulation system and therefore trigger weight gain – such as those high in saturated fat and certain types of sugar - are now easily accessible and replace foods that are more naturally filling. And to add to our weight-gaining propensity, we're a sedentary society, which makes us less likely to trigger the biochemistry needed to mobilize our fat stores.

Our dieting culture has also spawned an additional weight-gain dilemma. In times of plenty, "thrifty genes" that spur us to store extra fat when food is plentiful, lie dormant. However, your yo-yo-dieting body reacts to dieting like it reacts to starvation. Repeated dieting therefore activates your "thrifty genes," raising your setpoint so that you store extra fat when you go off your diet and there's lots of food around. Dieting is one of the quickest routes to long-term weight gain.

With all of the evidence stacked against us, it's easy to see why so many of us are above our setpoints, or raising these setpoints - leading to our bulging waistlines. These environmental and lifestyle changes have resulted in the fattening of America, and the increasing prevalence of diseases related to diet and activity habits. It is currently estimated that 70 percent of Americans die of nutrition- and activity-related illnesses.

It will take thousands of years before our genes catch up with these environmental changes. Until that happens, many individuals will face illness and early deaths due to the interaction of their eating and activity habits with their genes.

But don't worry...

A bulging waistline doesn't mean that you have failed. On the contrary, it simply shows that your body is very good at protecting your fat stores and has a finely calibrated system for weight regulation. You can harness this power to your advantage.

Clearly, we don't want to give up good-tasting food - and there's no reason we need to. Beneath the excess weight spawned by these cultural changes, our bodies still have internal mechanisms for regulating a healthy setpoint weight. The answer lies in ceasing our habit of overriding these failsafes - and getting back to the basics of letting our body do the job of regulating intake.

The key is in switching goals: instead of continuing the deprivation-waging, frustration-inducing uphill battle called dieting, make it your new intention to support your body in healthy weight regulation.

Checking out Your Setpoint

Why do we all have different setpoints? There are two components to your setpoint, genes and lifestyle. While you can't exactly change your genes (it's too late to choose your parents!), you can tweak your lifestyle and have an influence on how your genes act.

Blame it on your parents?

Researchers separate the effects of genes from lifestyle habits by studying families. How the study was conducted and the kinds of relatives that are studied vary between studies, resulting in wildly different estimates. For example, the two most comprehensive studies, using twins, adoptees, and nuclear family data, suggest that genetics alone accounts for 25 to 40 percent of the weight variance between individuals[257-259]. (This means that of factors that influence our weight, genetics alone represents a third of the total influence.) Many studies attribute an even larger role to genetics, suggesting that it accounts for 50 to 90 percent of the variance[260]. Not only is how much fat your body maintains inherited, but where and how you carry your fat is also inherited[261].

Some studies try to tease out the effects of genetics versus environment on weight. Adopted children have weights very similar to their biological parents, but there's little or no correlation between the weight of the adoptees and their adoptive parents, showing biology as a bigger player than upbringing[262].

Indeed, the commonly held belief that anyone can lose weight if they eat less and exercise more is at odds with compelling scientific evidence that weight is to a significant extent genetically determined. In fact, the heritability of obesity is considered to be greater than that of almost any other condition [263-265] – greater than breast cancer, schizophrenia, heart disease, etc.[60]

Check out this study as an example that supports this idea: researchers put 28 pairs of identical twins on a 6-week high-fat/low-carbohydrate diet, followed by a 6-week low-fat/high-carbohydrate diet. In each pair, one twin ran an average of 30 miles per week more than the other[266]. Despite the extreme difference in physical activity, each twin had very similar changes in weight and blood cholesterol. Getting more exercise didn't result in a weight difference – the body has a genetic setpoint which it maintains. Consistent with other studies, there was a lot of variability when the men were compared to men who weren't their twins, again demonstrating the power of genetics.

Although genes have a large influence on your weight, they of course don't present the entire picture, however. For example, one study compared twins separated at infancy and raised in different homes. The identical twins had similar, but not identical, body sizes and shapes[264]. Even with identical genes, weight can vary, sometimes dramatically.

It is estimated that lifestyle factors can explain an average weight gain of 7-10 pounds over the past decade in the United States[60]. However, it is genetics, not lifestyle, which accounts for the large proportion of why we all differ so much in weight and body type.

Increasing Your Gene-Sense

One of the most common misconceptions about genetics is that there are genes for certain things, for example breast cancer, shyness, or obesity. But it's not as clear-cut as that. Yes, we all have genes that regulate a tendency to get cancer, or to be shy or to get fat. But just having a gene doesn't mean it's active. For example, suppose two siblings have a gene that predisposes them to melanoma (skin cancer). One spends extensive time in the sun, which triggers expression of that particular gene, and increases the likelihood that she will get skin cancer. However, her brother limits his sun exposure, and though he has the gene, it remains dormant. As a result, he never gets skin cancer.

Another misconception is that traits arise from single genes. In fact, most traits are the result of multiple genes. Many genes play a role in obesity, and your specific combination, as opposed to any individual gene, determines your proclivity for weight gain. Except in rare cases, no single "obesity gene" is a precursor of getting fat.

The genetic heritage you receive from your parents sets the stage. However, the activity of those genes is malleable. What affects gene activity most is your lifestyle – and the two most influential aspects are your eating and activity habits. Nutrients from the foods you eat can turn on and off genes, and change the speed at which they work. Activity, stress, and other lifestyle factors can also stimulate the production of hormones and neurotransmitters that regulate how your genes are expressed.

The message is this: You have some degree of power to regulate your genes, though not as much as most people believe. Both nature and nurture play a role in how you look.

How can you alter gene expression?

Resetting your Setpoint: Living Well is the Best Revenge!

First, face the simple fact that not everyone on the planet can be thin. You may be genetically hard-wired to be fat, with genes so powerful that they resist lifestyle changes.

Or you may be soft-wired for obesity in that your genes aren't stubborn - they respond well to lifestyle changes. For most of us, the truth lies somewhere in between: our genes permit a limited range of body size, and our lifestyle habits let us choose where we will be within that range.

The best evidence that our way of living definitely counts is the recent epidemic of weight gain in the United States. The number of overweight and obese people has skyrocketed in the last few decades. Genes certainly don't evolve that quickly. Something has clearly changed in the American lifestyle.

The Pima Indians provide good evidence to substantiate this. The Pimas originated in Mexico, and about 1,000 years ago, some moved to Arizona, establishing a community there. The Mexican Pimas are of average weight, while the Arizona Pimas have the world's highest reported prevalence of obesity[267]. Clearly, genes alone aren't enough to tip the scales. If they were, both sets of Pimas would be of similar sizes.

Nor is environment the single answer because if that were true, everyone in Arizona would be obese and everyone in Mexico, average. It is the combination that counts. Apparently, the "fat genes" carried by the Pimas are "set off" when these people live in Arizona. In other words, a person genetically wired to get fat may actually defy fate if she eats a certain diet or has certain activity habits; on the other hand, this same individual will be very likely to live up to her "fat gene" destiny if she is sedentary and relies on fast food as a dietary mainstay (like the Arizona Pimas).

Synching up Genes and Lifestyle

Instead of asking whether nature or nurture determine obesity, it's more accurate to look at obesity, like other complex traits, as inheritable *susceptibility*, which only manifests itself under certain conditions.

Even if you do try to go against nature's plan for your body, your degree of effectiveness at making lifestyle changes is affected by your genetics. Watch two people on a weight-loss program, eating the exact same diet and exercising the same amount; one of them may lose weight while the other stays the same. In the past, experts believed that differing degrees of compliance were behind these mixed results. No matter what the non-loser reported, others speculated that the one who failed to shed pounds just didn't follow the program. But today, that blame-laying is on shaky ground. Now experts recognize that the way in which people respond to weight-loss regimens is also genetically determined. Given the same weight loss program and full compliance, people will show substantial variation in results.

Consider, for example, a study in which scientists overfed a group of twelve pairs of identical male twins, adding an extra thousand calories to their daily diet six days a week for one hundred days[268]. Since each man was overeating the same amount and they weren't consciously changing other factors that affect weight, one would expect to see each man store the same amount of energy on his body, resulting in identical weight gain. It is true that each man's weight gain was similar to that of his twin, thus showing the importance of genes in weight gain/loss and response to changed eating habits. Each pair of twins was also consistent in the way the distribution of their body fat changed. However, when comparing the men who were unrelated to one another, there was tremendous variability. In one set of twins, each man gained only nine pounds, while in another, each gained approximately 29 pounds!

(Incidentally, they re-measured these same men four months later and then again five years later. The men had all gone back to their weight before the overfeeding; in other words, when they returned to their normal diets and lifestyles, they returned to their setpoints.)

In other experiments, identical male twins exercised on stationary bicycles twice a day, nine of ten days, over twenty-two days[269] or one hundred days[270]. Diets were consistent, and the exercise caused them to spend an extra 1,000 calories. Just as the above-mentioned study revealed, these experiments showed that each man's weight loss and change in bodyfat distribution was similar to those of his twin, although there was large variability when the sets of twins were compared.

Listen to your genes, not the fashion designers!

In other words, even if you follow all the guidelines, you don't get a guarantee that you'll get the weight outcome you want nor an outcome similar to your friends'. But the good news is that even if you don't lose the weight you want to, lifestyle changes like those advocated for in this book will have a very positive effect on your overall health and well-being. This translates to a win-win; make changes and your body will stabilize at its natural weight – regardless of whether you shed pounds, you have the benefit of improved health.

Reclaiming Language

Throughout this section, I've used the terms "overweight" and "obese," because they are common medical terms. To determine whether someone fits into these categories, a formula is used, called the Body Mass Index (BMI), which is defined as weight (in kilograms) divided by height (in meters) squared. A BMI less than 25 is considered "normal," between 25 and 30 is considered "overweight," and 30 and above is classified as "obese."

However, these categories are meaningless in determining someone's health status, and the terms "overweight" and "obese" miss the mark. Over what weight? There is no precise weight beyond which you will be unhealthy! And the etymology of the word "obesity" mistakenly implies that a large appetite is the cause.

Using these terms medicalizes and pathologizes weighing over a certain amount, and now that we're better educated, I'd like to leave those terms behind and use a more appropriate term: fat. There is a growing movement that seeks to reclaim the term "fat" as a descriptive term, stripped of all its pejorative implications. This change is supported by many fat acceptance activists and the National Association for the Advancement of Fat Acceptance, a "human rights organization dedicated to improving the quality of life for fat people." NAAFA argues, rightfully so, that fatness is a form of body diversity that should be respected, much like diversity based on skin color or sexual preference.

If you find the word "fat" upsetting, that's your cultural bias talking. Would you similarly flinch when someone calls you blonde or brunette, or names your ethnic group? It's not surprising if you are uncomfortable with using the term "fat," as our culture associates it with "bad." It may not be easy to retrain yourself to just see it as a simple descriptor, but I encourage you to consider it as an important step in making peace with fat, a fact of life.

The New Peace Movement: Health at Every Size

What is now known should be sufficient to end our war against fat – which is simultaneously a war against fat people and against anyone who wishes to be at peace with their bodies[60]. It's time for a new peace movement: one which supports people in making healthy lifestyle choices, regardless of their size.

Join the new peace movement: it's called "Health at Every Size."

Health At Every Size (HAES) Basic Guiding Principles*:

- Acceptance of and respect for the diversity of body shapes and sizes.
- Eating in a manner that is attuned to individual cues including appetite, pleasure, hunger and satiety.
- Enjoyment of individually appropriate physical movement.
- Maximizing physical, social, spiritual and emotional health and well-being for both individuals and communities, despite experiences of illness, disability or trauma.

*As drafted by members of the San Francisco Bay Area HAES Think Tank and Show Me the Data international listserv.

Trusting your body to guide your eating

What would it be like to not have to think about weight control or what you eat? Young children are great examples of this principle: they eat when they're hungry – only what they want – and stop when they're satisfied. Research shows that when young children are given a wide variety of foods and free reign to choose what they want, they instinctively choose a balanced diet containing appropriate energy. This skill is innate and within all of us.

Our ideas about what we're supposed to eat, and how much, result in our disconnection from our bodies and our distrust of our body's needs around food. Many of us come to believe that our body signals need to be ignored and our desires controlled.

Giving yourself permission to eat whatever you want – attentively and without judgment – is an important aspect of eating "normally" and healthfully.

It takes time and patience to reestablish this trust, and courage to face our fears around letting go of control. But it can be done. And the rewards are immense. Food can become effortless and pleasurable.

HAES works: the evidence

My own research demonstrates that people can make significant health improvements when they stop dieting and learn to trust their bodies, and that it is more effective than dieting[271-273]. My colleagues and I compared obese women on a typical diet with others on a HAES program. The HAES program supported the women in accepting their bodies and listening to internal cues of hunger and fullness. After two years, the HAES group sustained improvements in blood pressure, total cholesterol, LDL, and depression, among many other health parameters. The diet group, on the other hand, showed initial improvements in all of those parameters (and weight loss), but returned to starting point at study end[273]. The HAES group improved their self-esteem and reported feeling much better about themselves at program end, while the dieters' self-esteem worsened. Also noteworthy, 41 percent of the diet group dropped out of the program (typical of diet programs), while almost all (92 percent) of the HAES group stayed with the program.

Eat what you want and get healthier?

The idea that you can stop watching your calories and eat what you want when you want is so contrary to current ideas that it evokes tremendous fear. Some health care practitioners and researchers express concern that these aspects will result in indiscriminate eating and increased obesity. One of my colleagues was so doubtful that she insisted we test the participants' blood lipids and blood pressure three months into the study, and be prepared to stop the research if we noticed worsening in these measures. As I expected, the research shows this concern to be unfounded.

I believe this is true because once participants realized they could eat whatever they wanted and were supported in choosing foods that were truly delicious, food stopped holding as much power over them. For example, they didn't have to binge on the ice cream because they knew that it would be available to them whenever they desired it. They could put it away when their taste buds toned down and it stopped tasting as good, which resulted in eating smaller quantities (which is more consistent with stable blood sugar regulation).

They also were choosing foods that helped them to feel better. For example, most started out with typical fast food habits, and like many Americans, were frequently constipated from the lack of fiber and felt the bloat and tiredness commonly experienced from energy-dense meals. After experimenting with a higher fiber diet, they realized that it made them feel better – bowel movements were more comfortable, and they felt more energized and mood-stable throughout the day. This motivated them to make better choices.

Also, participants got more creative while shopping, in the kitchen, and in restaurants, experimenting with different foods and food preparations, finding wholesome foods they loved. It's easier to make changes when you are choosing foods you desire as opposed to avoiding foods you consider off-limits.

The research clearly shows that it is possible to dump the obsession with food and weight, and the self-hatred and shame about your body. You can reclaim the joy in eating - and it can markedly improve your health and how you feel!

Action Tips...

Putting it all together: weight change

Step one: Don't try! Accept your body as it is. This is not about giving up; it's about moving on. Shift your emphasis to happiness and healthy living, things that *are* achievable. If weight change is possible for you, it will be a side effect since the techniques for healthy living are identical to those that are optimal for weight control.

Improving body image:
- Throw away your scale.
- Think about how you treat your body. Then compare this to how you would treat a friend. Be kinder to yourself! Pamper yourself: hot baths, massages...

- Talk to your friends about your feelings. You'll find that you're not alone.
- Enjoy your body. Use it. Find activities that are fun for you.
- Take the time and money you would have spent on dieting and spend it on positive, supportive activities instead.
- Identify what you've been putting off until you're thin. Start doing them now!
- Go to an art gallery and look at all the beautiful images of larger people. Surround yourself with images that reflect your body size. You don't have to buy into a culture that tells you that there is something wrong with you!

Step two: Eat intuitively

Shift control to your body
- Dump the diet mentality and all notions that some outside expert can tell you what to eat.
- Eat when you are hungry.
- Take care to get the food you want and enjoy.
- Stop when you are full or the food stops tasting as good.
- Be flexible.

This is a slow learning process. Focus on:
- How you feel
- Your satisfaction level
- Choosing appropriate foods to hold you over until your next meal or snack

Address Emotional Eating
- Ask yourself, am I physically hungry? If the answer is no:
  - What am I feeling?
  - What do I need?
  - Do it! (Take special care of yourself. This is a time to be kind to yourself, not come down on yourself.)

Step three: Get moving!
- Old model: *work* out for weight control.
- New model: move for the fun of it!
- Find the joy in play and activity.

To gain health benefits, activity:
- doesn't have to be vigorous
- doesn't have to be continuous

Suggestions to be more generally vital:
- Walk more
- Make up contests for suburban walks: find the cleanest windows, tackiest paint job
- Take the stairs instead of the elevator
- Have walking meetings
- Socialize with activities (hiking, tennis) rather than over coffee or food
- Dance with your vacuum cleaner
- Race your child from the car to the house
- Make a family walk and talk a nightly ritual

- Chase your dog when playing fetch
- Garden

Step four: Nutrition

All of the changes suggested for optimal health are identical as those for weight control. So review the previous sections!

- Eat more whole (unprocessed) plant foods
- Choose foods that are high in nutrient density
- Choose foods that are high in fiber
- Choose foods that enter the bloodstream slowly
- Minimize added sugars, particularly high fructose corn syrup, and refined grains (replace with less processed sugars and starches)
- Minimize saturated and trans fats (replace with mono-unsaturated fats)
- And remember to mediate quantity with internal cues

Other advice: Food should be fun and nurturing. Don't allow your knowledge about a food's impact on weight or health over-ride enjoyment. Happy people make healthier choices!

Step five: Stress

Calm down, relax! (Stress hormones send input to your weight regulation system.) And be sure to get sufficient sleep. (Several research studies show a relationship between sleep deprivation and decreased release of hormones that help regulate your weight.)

Get Informed...

This section was excerpted from Bacon, Linda, *Health at Every Size: The Surprising Truth About Your Weight,* Benbella Books, 2008.

For more information debunking the obesity myths, check out:
- *Big Fat Lies*, by Glenn Gaesser
- *The Obesity Myth,* by Paul Campos
- *Fat Politics,* by J. Eric Oliver

For help with eating intuitively, check out:
- *Intuitive Eating,* by Evelyn Tribole and Elyse Resch
- The Hugs Program also provides good support, both on-line and through books: www.hugs.com

For help with body image: check out www.bodypositive.com

For developing "fat pride" and an otherwise fun read, check out *Fat!So?* by Marilyn Wann and the website www.fatso.com.

The National Association for the Advancement of Fat Acceptance (NAAFA) provides support and information about the fat acceptance movement (www.naafa.org).

Eating Disorders

Given that eating disorders often begin with a desire to change one's weight, it seems appropriate to tackle the subject of eating disorders next.

The current "anti-obesity frenzy" distracts attention from the seriousness of eating disorders – and is in fact fueling their prevalence. For example, if you compare the childhood eating disorders data from the National Institute of Mental Health versus data from the Center for Disease Control on children who have type 2 diabetes (the most common illness associated with childhood obesity), you find that the average child today is several hundred times more likely to have an eating disorder. Yet which hits the news more?

And what are we doing in our anti-obesity crusade? Well, in Arkansas, they're forcing public school students to stand on a scale, and then sending a note home to parents about the child's Body Mass Index with instructions on managing calories for weight control. Texas is attempting to ban elementary school students from bringing cupcakes to celebrate a birthday. And there are current laws being debated in Congress to allow teachers to rifle through lunchboxes and seize contraband such as potato chips and candy bars. These policies make us more obsessed about what we shouldn't eat rather than supporting us in enjoying a healthy relationship with food and our bodies, doing more to promote disordered eating than combat obesity.

Eating disorders just don't seem to elicit the cultural concern that is warranted. A recent conversation that I overheard illustrates this point: Several women were sitting in a campus dining room talking about eating disorders. One woman casually commented: "Oh, I wouldn't mind getting anorexia. I could be happy getting rid of these saddlebags!" The other women giggled in agreement.

In fact, eating disorders compromise the quality of life for many people, and are sometimes even life-threatening. We need to be talking more seriously about them, and we need to be concerned about the cultural attitudes and public "health" policies that encourage them.

I'm going to use the term eating disorder more loosely than its clinical definition, to include everyone whose eating habits or attitude toward their body interferes with their enjoyment of life. You don't need a medical diagnosis to feel the distress associated with an eating disorder. If you are excessively concerned about your body size, the impact of the food you eat on your weight, if you feel guilty or ashamed of your eating habits, if you strictly avoid certain foods because you believe they are fattening, use laxatives, diuretics, make yourself vomit, or excessively exercise, these are all clues that you need some help.

Don't come down on yourself if the above describes you; within our cultural context it's hard not to develop an eating disorder! We all get enormous pressure to conform to unrealistic cultural standards of beauty. Advertising of many commercial goods functions by cultivating our body insecurity or hatred in order to sell products. If we all believed we were attractive as we are, we would have little need for most commercial beauty products. Other industries are equally insidious: cars, for example, aren't sold on their own merits, but on their ability to make the owner seem sexy.

Women in particular are taught that their self-identities are hinged on how closely they resemble the cultural ideal. Most of us feel inadequate and that we can never measure up. And it seems as if advertisers have recently realized that they were so busy exploiting women's insecurities, that they'd forgotten half the population. So now they're doing their best to make men feel equally horrible about themselves. Buying into these images doesn't benefit anyone but the advertisers.

While this context is tough, not everyone develops an eating disorder. The key issue that distinguishes those that do from those that don't - or where you are on the continuum - is your degree of self-esteem. Self-esteem refers to how you feel about yourself. If you have high self-esteem, you value who you are – as you are. The lower your self-esteem, the more you measure yourself up against an outside standard – a standard you can never meet – with painful ramifications.

I'm hesitant to give precise definitions of the specific eating disorders, because labeling yourself won't tell you too much. The issues may resonate with you regardless of whether you have a clinical diagnosis. Wherever you fit on the spectrum, if you feel uncomfortable - label or not - start talking about it and reaching out for help.

It's easy to get caught in a destructive cycle and the sooner you catch yourself, the easier it is to break the cycle. You start dieting, which can lead to feeling out of control around food and to binge-eating, which makes you feel worse about yourself and wreaks havoc on your self-esteem, which leads to more dieting, binge-eating and a greater sense of losing control. A full-blown eating disorder can result.

Here's some info about the most common eating disorders:

Anorexia Nervosa

Anorexia nervosa is identified by extreme thinness from food restriction. Most anorexics don't recognize how underweight they are, and still feel fat though they may look emaciated to others. Or, they may know they are emaciated, but still be intensely fearful of food and weight gain.

Bulimia Nervosa

People with bulimia experience periods of uncontrollable binge eating (past the point of physical discomfort) followed by some form of purging to get rid of the unwanted calories. Purging can take the form of vomiting, laxative abuse, excessive exercising, or fasting. (Yes, exercising is included on this list. Exercise abuse is particularly insidious because of the social affirmation given to those whose eating disorders are hidden in their exercise routines.)

Binge-eating disorder

Also known as compulsive eating, binge-eating disorder includes uncontrollable binge-eating. It differs from bulimia in that it is not followed by purging.

Orthorexia Nervosa

Orthorexia refers to an obsessive concern about the health content of food. It is particularly insidious because its victims, affectionately called "health food junkies," may receive social support for their obsession, and its dangers are not as apparent.

Orthorexia is not a currently recognized clinical diagnosis, and its place as a bona fide eating disorder is being debated among health care professionals. Regardless of whether it meets the classic criteria for an eating disorder, orthorexia is helpful to consider in this section, as a rigid fixation on "eating right" can be just as painful as the other eating disorders.

Do you wish that you could just enjoy eating and not worry about its health implications? While many people experience this discomfort to some degree, it turns into orthorexia when it limits your ability to develop relationships and other interests.

How to save yourself

There is no magic formula that will help everyone to heal from an eating disorder – it is a very personal path.

The first step is to shore up your self-esteem. Recognize your value and respect your uniqueness. Be proud of who you are. The more you cultivate your internal resources and recognize your value, the less others can infiltrate your world.

Your primary source of power lies in changing your relationship to the images that get presented. The less you measure yourself against the images, the less they can serve to trigger your insecurity and your drive for a different body. The marketplace would be powerless at promoting self-hatred if we didn't buy into it – and enforce it against one another.

Note that I am not saying that it is wrong to care about your appearance. Your appearance is another aspect of who you are – but your appearance is just one of many traits, and a relatively unimportant one. What you do to improve your appearance – whether you dress up or dress down, wear make-up or shave – is less important than the intent behind it. If you perform your beauty rituals out of a belief that there is something wrong with you, it is a problem. If you can't go out in the morning without putting your face on, you have absorbed the beauty standards and they are harming you. When you dress in vertical stripes to hide your curves, those beauty myths are taking their toll. But when you dress to celebrate your individuality and other characteristics, the same act can be seen as positive.

Define your own beauty standards – and make sure they include you! Beauty is about uniqueness. Your special combination of attributes makes you gorgeous. (Repeat after me: "I am beautiful just the way I am.")

And show some compassion towards yourself. It is hard to accept your body when you are constantly bombarded with messages that you need to change – and this is particularly difficult the more you deviate from the social ideal. It's not easy going against the grain, and there is remarkably little social support for individuals to develop a healthy self-esteem and challenge the beauty standards. But you'll need that social support – and a place to talk about your feelings – in order to heal. Supportive friends and a good psychotherapist or psychologist can do wonders.

Emotional Eating

Do you find yourself attacking the ice cream when you're lonely, depressed or merely bored? Can ice cream really cure that broken heart?

Food allows us to cope with our emotions, whether those emotions are positive or negative, extreme or neutral. Eating temporarily soothes us. Whether the emotion we are experiencing is happiness or anger, boredom or excitement, eating tempers the emotion and temporarily gets us back on an even keel, bringing us to a more familiar and comfortable state.

The drive to eat when you are not physically hungry means that you want something, though it isn't food. This is not a time to come down on yourself! You reach for food as a way to take care of yourself, not to hurt yourself.

Acknowledge that if you are an "emotional eater," to some extent, eating has been good to you. For example, when I was younger and feeling lonely, I didn't have the emotional skills to take care of myself. Eating was very effective at diverting me from the loneliness. It helped me get through tough times, and was generally pretty dependable.

But then my obsession with weight surfaced. And suddenly food wasn't as effective in helping me. Sure, it tempered the feelings in the moment. But this was only a quick and short-lived comfort, followed by a more intense and longer lasting guilt. The weight I gained served as evidence of my failure and another reason to come down on myself.

This is where most of us get stuck. We recognize the short-term comfort or pleasure we get from food, and without other skills to take care of ourselves in the moment, we depend on it for an instant feel-better fix. But doing so does not mitigate our feelings in the long run, and gives us the added burden of guilt and anger about our eating habits and their ramifications on our weight. Studies show that although you might receive immediate emotional comfort from eating, the associated guilt overpowers any emotional support you receive.

What can you do when you feel the drive to eat and you know that you are not physically hungry? Start by showing appreciation for the help you have gotten from food. Acknowledge how important it is to take care of yourself. Without food or another technique, life could have been pretty difficult and overwhelming.

Explore your emotions more thoroughly and try to identify what you are really looking for and what it would take to satisfy your need. Address those feelings more directly. If you tell your mother you are angry at her, does that change your drive to eat? If you write a letter to her, even if you never intend to give it to her, does it change the drive to eat? If you sound off to a friend, does that help? If you take a furious walk down the hall, will that be more effective for you than eating? If you bring a book to read while waiting for your appointment, does that seem more fulfilling than the candy bar?

Learn other skills to take care of yourself so that food is only one of the many tools in your arsenal for handling your emotions. This allows you to move on. Your emotional eating can decrease – not because of your self-control, but because you don't have use for it anymore.

Sometimes you may also choose to eat. You are not a bad person if you do this; you are deciding in the moment that it is the best way you know to take care of yourself. This is another wonderful learning opportunity. Take advantage of it! Pay attention to whether or not it is effective, and if it is effective, how long that lasts. Try to lay off the judgment. Instead, keep your focus on whether the food is accomplishing what you want it to accomplish.

If you learn that food is not relieving your pain – and in fact, that it causes more pain – you may choose a different option next time. The drive to eat becomes irrelevant because you recognize what you need and that food is not going to help you get it. Of course, it may take many times of noticing this before your behavior changes, so be patient.

I cannot emphasize enough how important it is to lighten up around the despair you may feel about your body and your weight. The despair evokes the concern that there is something wrong with you: you are not entitled to the food that you want, and you need to deprive yourself as punishment for your "overweight." It can cause a powerful retaliatory appetite! Being judgmental about your weight can be quite distracting from becoming an intuitive eater. However, it is important to acknowledge that this is the body you currently have, and move on. The more comfortable you feel in your body as you are, the less you will be driven to overeat.

Your appetite can be a wonderful gift: it lets you know that you are experiencing feelings you don't know how to handle, and gives you an opportunity to react differently and grow emotionally (rather than physically). Labeling our behavior as self-destructive won't help us to understand or change it. Instead, this judgment gives us another reason to engage in the behavior. So be kind to yourself.

Chances are you will continue to eat for emotional reasons. Everyone does sometimes. If you put less of an emphasis on judging or changing the behavior, and more of an emphasis on understanding what you need, taking care of it, and feeling compassion for yourself, you will find that your behavior can shift naturally. So try to be patient, and enjoy the journey to knowing yourself better and learning how to be more kind to yourself.

If we can learn to be kinder to ourselves, our drive to eat for emotional reasons will decrease. You were looking for comfort when you felt compelled to eat. Give it to yourself!

Change the Culture

Repeat after me: "My weight is not a problem. Society's problem about weight is the problem." The true heroes among us are not those that have lost weight. They are the people who move on with their lives, who live proud despite and regardless of their weight.

The single most powerful act available to you is to own your body - to walk proud and let others see you enjoying your body. Self-love is a revolutionary act! A person who is content in their body –

fat or thin – disempowers the industries that prey on us, telling us we are unacceptable and need their products to gain acceptance.

We don't have enough visible heroes in large bodies. One of the myths related to weight is that larger bodies are a sign of personal failing, and many fat people tend to deal with their struggles silently and independently. Having learned about these issues and fortified your defenses, people of all sizes can take another step which will both help you to solidify your new identity and make the path easier for others: walk proudly and tell your story so that others can benefit. Challenge the myths about weight whenever you hear them. Write letters, make phone calls, SPEAK UP.

It is possible to make peace with ourselves and transform the culture. Indeed, personal transformation is exactly what is necessary to inspire cultural change.

Get informed…

Check out the National Eating Disorder Information Centre at www.nedic.ca and Something Fishy at www.somethingfishy.org.

For a personal touch, visit http://www.andreasvoice.org/index.htm, a wonderful resource created by Doris and Tom Smeltzer in honor of their daughter, Andrea, who died of an eating disorder. Check out a book entitled *Andrea's Voice … Silenced by Bulimia: Her Story and Her Mother's Journey Through Grief Toward Understanding*, by Doris Smeltzer with Andrea Lynn Smeltzer.

Action Tips…

Take the Pledge … today and every day. Photocopy it and keep it handy.

<u>Live Well Pledge</u>

Today, I will try to feed myself when I am hungry.
Today, I will try to be attentive to how foods taste and make me feel.
Today, I will try to choose foods that I like and that make me feel good.
Today, I will try to honor my body's signals of fullness.
Today, I will try to find an enjoyable way to move my body.
Today, I will try to look kindly at my body, and to treat it with love and respect.

Signed: _____

Micronutrients: Vitamins, Minerals, Phytochemicals and Supplements

We increasingly rely on processed convenience foods that have been stripped of many beneficial nutrients, while other nutrients and compounds – some beneficial and some not – have been added. When compared to their whole counterparts, processed foods are typically much lower in nutritive value. One of the ironies of modern life is that as the technology of food production and transport has "improved," the nutritional value of food is often diminished.

Substances in food exist in an astonishingly complex balance. Many foods contain dozens of different compounds that work together to provide a health-enhancing benefit, making the whole package much greater than the sum of its parts. The array of compounds in food, and their interaction with one another, cannot be reproduced in a pill or dietary supplement, and is typically absent in a heavily processed food.

Eating a wide variety of fresh, whole foods – particularly plant products which are rich in phytochemicals – is the best way to obtain all the benefits that food offers. No special diet that emphasizes a limited number of foods can do this. Sure, broccoli and carrots are nutritious, but if all you ate were broccoli and carrots, you would be deficient in several nutrients.

Note that some people speak about the "wisdom of the body" and suggest that your body will cause you to crave certain foods to ensure nutritional adequacy. As comforting as the theory may be, there just isn't scientific evidence to link most cravings to nutrient requirements, though theories abound. There's actually a documented desire to consume laundry detergent and cigarette butts, which have been associated with iron deficiency! On the other hand, there is no scientific support for the common belief that a desire for meat accompanies iron (or protein) deficiency. While it is true that the body regulates your *energy* - and sugar craving could be the result of low blood sugar, for example - your cravings may not lead you to obtain all of the micronutrients you need. When you're low on zinc, it's unlikely that you'll crave zinc-rich foods.

Micronutrients

The term "micronutrient" refers to nutrients that we only need or use in small (micro) amounts. In contrast to the macronutrients, the body uses them without breaking them down.

Vitamins

A vitamin is an organic compound that your body requires to help regulate functions within cells. Organic, in this usage, refers to substances that contain carbon and come from materials that are living, such as plants and animals, or that were once living, such as petroleum or coal.

Most vitamins are essential (translation: you have to get them from food), although a few can be synthesized by your body. Each of the 13 different vitamins has a special role to play. They affect a wide variety of functions in your body, such as promoting good vision, forming healthy blood cells, creating strong bones and teeth, and ensuring healthy functioning of your heart and nervous system.

Some vitamins are water-soluble (Vitamin C and the B vitamins – Thiamin, Riboflavin, Niacin, Folate, Vitamin B12, Vitamin B6, Biotin, and Panthothenic Acid). Water-soluble vitamins are absorbed into the bloodstream and travel freely in your blood. If not used, they get filtered into your urine and excreted. (Ever notice that your urine is yellow after taking a vitamin supplement? This is the result of excreting unused vitamins. Americans sure have expensive urine!) Because water-soluble vitamins aren't stored on your body, you need to be sure to get them regularly.

Other vitamins are fat-soluble (Vitamins A, D, E and K) and are found in the fats and oils of foods. Once absorbed into our bodies, fat-soluble vitamins get stored in the liver or other fatty tissue.

As a result, you don't need to take them as regularly. The downside, however, is they can more readily build up in excess amounts and become toxic, when consumed in excess.

Freshly picked raw foods usually have the highest nutritive value, although in some rare cases cooking allows you to absorb more nutrients. Most vitamins are sensitive to varying degrees of heat and light, and there is always some loss of vitamins when food is stored, handled and cooked. Cooking at moderate (rather than high) temperatures, using small amounts of cooking liquids, and for short times, all help to preserve the vitamin content of cooked foods.

The Vitamin/Energy Myth

The body does not break down vitamins and release their energy, so it's a myth that popping vitamins will give you an energy boost. While vitamins don't directly supply energy, however, some of them help facilitate the chemical reactions that extract energy from the macronutrients. Nonetheless, if you are low on energy, it is likely that you need calories, not vitamins. You'll get that from the sugar in your smoothie, not the "B vitamin boost."

Minerals

Minerals come from the earth, and in contrast to vitamins, they are inorganic (don't contain carbon). Each mineral is a chemical element. They are absorbed into water and taken up by plants through the water or soil, and transfer to animals that consume the mineral-laden plants and water. Humans get minerals through drinking water or eating plants or animals that contain them.

Minerals help with many vital body functions, such as bone formation or effective functioning of the heart, nervous and digestive systems. Because minerals are inorganic, they are indestructible and don't have to be handled with as much care as vitamins. For example, heating foods doesn't destroy minerals, and minerals don't break down after a plant is harvested. However, minerals can be processed out of foods or lost during cooking when they dissolve in water that is discarded.

The terms "hard water" and "soft water" describe a water's mineral content. Hard water rises to the earth's surface from underground springs. It contains many minerals (particularly calcium and magnesium) that it picks up as it moves through the ground. Soft water is "surface water," the run off from rain-swollen streams or rainwater that falls directly into reservoirs, and has fewer minerals.

The mineral content of water has relatively little impact on your health, although soft water can more easily dissolve harmful metals from pipes, such as cadmium and lead. Many consumers dislike the residue that forms around faucets from hard water, and install water softeners.

The one mineral that receives the most attention is sodium, so here are a few words on the sodium controversy. Salt contains two essential nutrients: sodium (40 percent) and chloride (60 percent). Its essential for us – and its even more essential for the food manufacturing industry. Salt enhances other flavors and reduces bitterness – in other words, it just helps foods taste good. It also extends shelf life, binds water, and minimizes discoloration. And its cheap.

So salt is a major ingredient in all processed food. And our tastes buds adapt to it. Without salt, many people find food bland.

Despite the vast amount of scientific research on the topic, there is still little agreement as to the value of reducing salt in one's diet[274]. The largest study of U.S. adults , which included nearly 100 million people, reported "a robust, significant, and consistent significant inverse association between dietary sodium and cardiovascular mortality." Translation: the more people consumed, the *less* likely they were to die from cardiovascular disease.

In some people excess sodium increases blood pressure, raising the risk for cardiovascular disease and stroke. How many people are affected in this way? It's not apparent. Some scientists estimate about 30 percent of the population. How do you know if you're one of them? You don't, although your family history can give you some indication.

Given that few people know whether they're among the unlucky for whom salt is problematic,the government has established salt recommendations for all: less than 2,300 mgs per day. This is no problem if you do your own cooking and don't add much salt. But if you eat processed foods, it's hard to comply. Labels are required to list sodium content, so at least you're informed.

The good news is that your taste buds adjust to a lower salt diet in just a few weeks. (But its much easier to get used to increasingly saltier foods than less salty foods.) So if you want to kick the processed foods habit, you will start to enjoy a wider range of foods, if you can just be patient through the transition.

Phytochemicals

Phytochemicals are found in plants. They have health-protective benefits, but unlike vitamins and minerals, are not essential for life. There are thousands of different phytochemicals. You might be familiar with some of their names, such as lycopene (found in tomatoes and other red fruits), anthocyanin (which gives blueberries their color), or allium (which accounts for the strong smell of garlic).

Plants contain phytochemicals because they protect the plant in some way. For example, an orange has a few hundred phytochemicals - some help resist bacteria and fungi and others prevent damage from the sun, among many other protective functions. When we eat the plants, the phytochemicals bestow on us many similar benefits, reducing our risk for heart disease, cancer, diabetes, and hundreds of other diseases.

Micronutrients Naturally Occurring in Foods

The micronutrient content of foods varies tremendously, with leafy green vegetables topping the list and processed sugars and fats at the bottom. The Appendix contains a handy nutrient-density list so that you can get a better sense of which foods are rich sources of micronutrients. An easy rule of thumb for plant foods is that rich colors and strong smells are often indicative of high nutrient density.

Micronutrients Added to Foods

Refining grains typically removes many nutrients. For example, wheat flour has about 55 percent of the folic acid, 43 percent of the calcium, 25 percent of the iron, 17 percent of the niacin, and 13 percent of the Vitamin B6 found in the original whole wheat it was made from. It is also stripped of fiber and many other micronutrients.

The term "**enriched**" describes the process of adding some nutrients back, and U.S. law requires refined grains to be enriched with these five nutrients. When a product is enriched, the nutrients aren't added back in the same quantity or quality and are sometimes less easily absorbed.

The term "**fortified**" is used when nutrients are added that might not have originally appeared.

How much do you need?

It is important to get the right amount of vitamins and minerals; too much or too little can be problematic. The recommended dietary allowances (RDAs) established by government are based on prevention of deficiency diseases, not on promoting optimal health or treating specific medical concerns, so merely using the guidelines may not be optimal. Intake of several vitamins in quantities above the RDA may prevent heart disease, cancer and numerous other chronic diseases.

And of course, obtaining phytochemicals is not a standard recommendation; they are helpful, but not necessary. We are a long way from knowing how much of each is beneficial, and how all the nutrients interact.

Furthermore, politics play a role in influencing the RDA. The RDA for calcium, for example, appears to be excessively high due to strong lobbying from the dairy industry.

Women's needs for certain nutrients are different than men's, and everyone's needs change throughout the life cycle. Additionally, you may have different needs based on your lifestyle habits: smokers, for example, require more Vitamin C to fight the oxidation caused by the smoking. Medications may also affect your need for specific nutrients.

Supplementation: Dietary insurance?

Believing that there are shortcuts to good nutrition or that foods may be deficient in meeting their micronutrient needs, many people are taking vitamin/mineral pills or other supplements.

Advice from the government is that supplements are unnecessary for healthy adults who eat a wide variety of fresh, whole foods. When USDA researchers analyzed the estimated intake of a person who ate a diet based on the recommended Dietary Guidelines for Americans (2005), they determined that Vitamin E is the only nutrient that may be a challenge to get in sufficient amount[275]. (Of course, not many of us have diets that conform to the Dietary Guidelines.)

While it is clear that most Americans consume diets that contain enough vitamins and minerals to prevent the classic signs of deficiency, some scientists argue that many Americans exhibit subclinical levels of deficiency, meaning that although they don't have classic deficiency symptoms, they do have metabolic abnormalities (some of which can be identified through laboratory tests). Furthermore, research has clearly demonstrated the additional benefits of consuming nutrient-rich foods beyond prevention of deficiencies, although the recommended dietary allowances are calculated only to prevent deficiency.

I believe that the government recommendation that supplementation is unwarranted fails to account for the research which shows that the vast majority of us are deficient in some nutrients. For example, USDA records indicate that the average meat-eater is deficient in 7 different nutrients (calcium, iodine, vitamin C, vitamin E, fiber, folate, and magnesium)[276]. And when similar standards were used to analyze the average vegan diet, they were determined to be deficient in 3 nutrients (calcium, iodine, and vitamin B12)[277].

It also contradicts my own experience of analyzing my own diet as well as thousands of diet records from students and participants in my research studies, all of which demonstrate that almost all of us have at least minor deficiencies when our diets are compared to the RDAs. It also doesn't address the issue that the RDAs don't identify amounts that promote optimal health.

Furthermore, it's interesting to note that vitamins, minerals and phytochemicals can't be patented, which I expect plays a role in why encouraging a nutrient-dense diet seems to play second fiddle to prescribing drugs and surgery.

In light of this, I do advise that people take a daily vitamin/mineral supplement. But don't fool yourself into thinking that this will save you from an unhealthy diet. When it comes to obtaining all the nutrients your body needs, there is no substitute for good food. Scientists are increasingly recognizing that there are a lot of compounds in food that serve as powerful disease-fighting or disease-preventive agents, beyond the stuff that gets into supplements.

Also, you usually can't beat nature's packaging. Nutrients are typically absorbed best from foods as they are dispersed among other ingredients to help their absorption. In contrast, when nutrients are taken in pure, concentrated form, they are likely to interfere with the absorption of other nutrients.

We are a long way from being able to replicate (or even identify) the exact substances and combinations that are most effective.

And while we know some benefits of many individual nutrients, many research studies have failed to document that taking those nutrients in the form of supplements yields the advantages of getting the nutrient from food. For example, while it is clear that antioxidants play a large role in preventing or reversing heart disease or cancer, two major reviews of trials of taking antioxidant supplements indicate little or no benefit for these diseases[278, 279]. And a third comprehensive review found no evidence that antioxidant or B-vitamin supplements influence the progression of atherosclerosis[280].

Fortunately, eating a richly varied diet which includes vegetables, fruits, whole grains, and beans is a tasty prescription to receive! The easiest way to ensure a nutrient-dense diet is to consume fiber-rich foods as the fiber, great stuff on its own, also tends to get packaged with lots of other beneficial nutrients.

I'm not a big fan of taking pills. And there isn't sufficient scientific evidence to convince me that taking a multi-vitamin/mineral supplement is beneficial. Nonetheless, I do take a daily multi-vitamin/mineral supplement. I consider it a possible extra insurance policy – and a cheap one at that. (A standard vitamin/mineral supplement costs will put you back about $40 a year.) As long as I don't get nutrients in excessive quantities, I figure it can't hurt - unless you let it fool you into thinking you can get away with a low-nutrient diet.

How to choose a vitamin/mineral supplement

First, always remember: supplements will never save you from the dangers of an inadequate diet. Use them to supplement good eating – not as a substitute. Used wisely, they may (or may not) be part of an overall health strategy to optimize your body's potential, along with more important stuff, such as consuming nutritious food, being regularly active, enjoying supportive friendships, managing your stress…

Research shows that cheap versions of supplements are fine: price isn't a good indication of quality. Be sure that your vitamin/mineral supplement is made specific for someone of your sex as men and women have different nutrient needs. (For instance, women lose iron during menstruation and require more; men lose zinc during ejaculation and require more.)

And don't fall into the over-consumption trap: just because a little is good, doesn't mean a lot is better. Don't take anything in excessively high quantities as some vitamins and minerals can reach toxic levels. You are unlikely to get more than you need from eating real food, but you may be getting too much of certain nutrients if you take mega-doses, unbalanced amounts, or eat a lot of fortified food. For the most part, a multi-vitamin/mineral supplement which meets 100-150 percent of the RDA for most nutrients is a safe bet. Vegans should also make sure to supplement additional Vitamin B_{12}. (These days our plant foods are too clean to contain the Vitamin B_{12} made by bacteria, that was previously found on many plant foods!)

Make sure to buy your vitamins in an opaque container, as they are subject to oxidation. And be sure there is an expiration date and that you are getting them fresh: vitamins lose their potency over time. Lastly, make sure the label states that it meets USP (United States Pharmacopeia) standards; these standards aren't much, but do indicate that the product is represented as complying fully with all the requirements (purity, potency, content uniformity, dissolution etc.).

And I need to re-emphasize this point: While supplements may provide you with extra insurance, this isn't well established, and they will certainly never make up for an unhealthy diet. From a nutritional perspective, your best bet for a long, healthy life is to eat a wide variety of nutrient-dense foods.

Other supplements

Numerous dietary supplements are available, beyond just vitamins and minerals. These include other less familiar substances, such as herbals, botanicals, amino acids, and enzymes. They may be purchased in a variety of forms, such as tablets, capsules, powders, energy bars, or drinks. Most of them provide more hype than help, and you are well advised to educate yourself before spending your money. You'll find that competent research rarely indicates that supplements meet their claims. Although certain products may be helpful to some people, there are also circumstances when these products can pose unexpected risks and dangers. Many supplements contain active ingredients that can have strong effects in the body. Think twice about chasing the latest headline; sound advice is usually based on research reproduced over time, not the latest sexy study touted in the popular media.

Supplement Regulation and Safety

Unfortunately, supplements are very loosely regulated, making it hard to judge their safety or efficacy. There are no requirements that a manufacturer has to prove safety or effectiveness. Congress codified that when it passed the Dietary Supplement Health and Education Act (DSHEA) in 1994. Before DSHEA, if the Food and Drug Administration (FDA) questioned a supplement's safety, the manufacturer had to prove it. But now manufacturers are in the driver's seat and it's up to the FDA to prove if they believe a supplement is dangerous. And even when the FDA considers something unsafe, it typically issues a consumer advisory – but doesn't prohibit the company from selling the product. In other words, the FDA can bark, but it can't bite! Whether consumers ever hear the advisories is unclear as the FDA doesn't monitor that.

There is of course no incentive for companies to study the safety of their products. That information could cause them to not be able to market their products, but would never support them in being able to bring them to market. And there are no warnings required when potential side effects or dangers are known. For example, beta-carotene supplements are unlikely to warn smokers that high doses (at least 25 mg or 42,000 IU) may increase risk for lung cancer.

Supplement and food manufacturers regularly mislead us. Numerous labels make statements like V8 does on their Strawberry Kiwi Splash: "Vitamin A is essential for vision and healthy skin." True, if you have severe Vitamin A deficiency you are likely to get skin lesions and go blind. But extra Vitamin A won't do a thing for the average American's skin or sight. And sure, "Vitamin C is needed for healthy bones, gums and teeth." If you get scurvy - unheard of in recent decades in the U.S. - it can help your bleeding gums and weak bones. But it won't help the average American's gums or bones. And when Tropicana claims that Twister Mango Tangerine Mambo has "FruitForce energy releasing B vitamins," look hard to find the small amount of fruit. The B vitamins they add do indeed help cells convert food to energy, but don't be deceived into thinking that they'll make you feel more energetic.

When purchasing supplements, caveat emptor (buyer beware).

Action Tips

To best ensure that you obtain all of the micronutrients to optimize your health, eat a wide variety of fresh or minimally processed nutrient-dense foods.

Water

Why is water important?

Water is the lifeblood of our planet, and our existence is intimately connected with the amount and quality of water available to us. Your body is predominantly composed of water, about 60-75 percent of your total body weight. Your brain is about 85 percent water, your blood about 90 percent water, your muscles about 75 percent water, your liver about 82 percent water; even your bones are about 22 percent water. Every part of the human body is dependent on water. Without water, you would die in a few days.

Water is a solvent, meaning that many compounds inside your body dissolve in it. Not only is it essential to body functioning, but even getting rid of it is good for you, flushing out contaminants and preventing mineral deposits. Among its many functions, water:

- Acts as a medium for chemical reactions to occur.
- Helps regulate body temperature.
- Fills cells, the space between them, and acts as a lubricant.
- As a major portion of blood and urine, helps to carry nutrients to cells and remove waste.
- Aids digestion and the movement of nutrients through your gastrointestinal tract.

Water intake

When we think about water intake, the first aspect that comes to mind is drinking liquids. Of course, this is a large component, but surprisingly, it amounts to only about 55 percent of the total water an average person consumes in a day. Another 30 percent comes from eating. (There is a lot of water in food: lettuce, for example, is 90 percent water; hamburger is 50 percent water; and cheeses range from 30-75 percent water). An additional 15 percent is created by your body as a by-product of chemical reactions involved in digesting and metabolizing your food.

Water Output

You lose water constantly. The gases you breathe are humidified by water as they pass through your respiratory tract, resulting in water loss through your **breath**. The water loss through your **skin** occurs after water diffuses to the skin surface and then evaporates into the environment. Together these two are called "insensible water loss," and typically amount to about 28-40 ounces per day, which is about 30 percent of your total water loss. More water is excreted as part of your **feces** (about 2-7 ounces per day), and the largest portion is excreted in your **urine** (generally about 20-53 ounces per day).

Because water leaves your body constantly, you have to replenish your body water frequently.

How much water is enough?

There are many complicated factors that play a role in how well you absorb and retain water (including the climate, the amount of exercise you get, the types of food you eat, the speed at which you drink, etc.), so there is no accurate method to calculate how much water you need to drink.

Under normal conditions, thirst is a fairly accurate indicator of when it's time to drink. You can confirm by paying attention to the color of your urine. It should be clear or pale yellow. (Sometimes substances in foods can confuse you, however. High quantities of Vitamin C, for example, will make your urine yellow even if you are well hydrated.)

The thirst mechanism can be compromised when you sweat during sports as you sweat out proportionately more water than minerals compared to their ratio in our body. The concentration of sodium in sweat is about one-third that of blood plasma. So as you sweat, the concentration of minerals in blood plasma may actually increase, which triggers the body's thirst mechanism as it tries to maintain mineral balance. This mechanism is too slow and inefficient to help you stay properly hydrated while you are exercising and can hamper your performance.

What's the best way to stay hydrated?

Drink water! Most beverages will also help with hydration, and the fewer calories they have relative to their liquid content, the more effective they are.

Note that caffeine is a diuretic, which means that it triggers the release of hormones that make you urinate more. Caffeine-containing drinks may still help to meet your hydration needs, but not much.

Alcohol is a diuretic as well, and since it additionally requires about 8 ounces of water to metabolize every ounce, it can really serve to dehydrate you. In fact, dehydration is a partial cause of hangovers.

Can you drink too much water?

Unlikely, but not impossible. Drink too much too quickly and you could end up with "water intoxication," where the water dilutes the sodium level in your bloodstream, resulting in an imbalance of water in your brain. (The scientific name for this is hyponatremia.) In one well-publicized fraternity hazing, a young pledge was forced to drink massive quantities in a short period of time and eventually died.

Hyponatremia has also occasionally occurred in athletes competing under very hot and humid conditions. While exercising, they lose a lot of water and salt in their sweat, but only replenish the water, resulting in a similar imbalance. Hyponatremia is unlikely to occur under most exercise conditions, but those competing in long events, such as marathons, and under hot conditions, should be careful to replace electrolytes along with water. A little salt is enough to do the trick – or you could go for the pricy sports drinks.

What's in your drinking water?

Of course, the water you drink contains more than just hydrogen and oxygen. A lot happens to the water on its way to the tap or a bottle.

For example, it can pick up minerals from rocks and soil. The principle mineral contained in water is sodium. "Hard water" and "soft water" are terms that describe water's mineral content. **Hard water** rises to the earth's surface from underground springs and contains a lot of minerals (particularly calcium and magnesium) that it picks up as it moves through the ground. **Soft water**, on the other hand, is "surface water," the run off from rain-swollen streams or rainwater that falls directly into reservoirs, and contains fewer minerals. The chief mineral in soft water is sodium.

Whether you have hard water or soft water won't have much of a health impact, although the reduced sodium content in hard water provides a small advantage. Soft water makes more soap bubbles with less soap, and tends to do a better job cleaning clothes. Hard water, on the other hand, leaves residue around faucets and tubs. Soft water tends to be preferred by consumers and some people install water softeners.

One disadvantage to soft water is that it can also more easily dissolve certain harmful metals, such as cadmium and lead, from pipes. People who install water softeners in their homes may be better off connecting them to their hot water lines for washing and bathing, and use cold, hard water for cooking and drinking.

Fluoride is a mineral routinely added to public water supplies, and more than half of the United States regularly drink fluoridated water. Fluoride combines with other minerals in your teeth and makes the minerals less soluble (harder to dissolve). This reduces your susceptibility to cavities. Overall, drinking fluoridated water cuts the rate of tooth decay 18 percent to 40 percent, according to a 2001 analysis by the Centers for Disease Control and Prevention. Some people describe fluoride as the "real tooth fairy."

Because fluoride concentrates in bones, there is question as to whether fluoridated water increases the risk of bone cancer. The National Academy of Sciences (NAS) reviewed the evidence and concluded that it is plausible but that there is insufficient evidence to make a determination. In addition to bone cancer, elevated levels of fluoride are also associated with bone fractures, IQ deficits, thyroid function losses, and Alzheimer's disease, and NAS recommends that additional research is warranted.

Another concern that is expressed about fluoride is that over-exposure during tooth-forming years can result in dental fluorosis, which damages tooth enamel, making teeth look mottled. Fluorosis is predominantly a cosmetic concern. Fluorosis has increased over the past 30 years, and research supports that some children who drink fluoridated water are at risk for fluorosis[281].

A March 2006 NAS report indicates that the current legal levels of fluoride in drinking water are dangerous and should be lowered. However, it is likely to take years before that might happen. Though they express concerns that the legal limits don't adequately protect us, the NAS report does indicate that the vast majority of Americans - including those whose water supply has fluoride added - drink water that is within safe limits.

Consumers can learn how much fluoride is in their tap water by asking their local utility. Those with high fluoride levels can reduce their exposure by using a home filtration system. Since filtration systems vary in their ability to remove fluoride, be sure to do your research.

Bottled waters can have fluoride too. If the fluoride in bottled water is naturally occurring, it is likely to be in safe limits, and won't be listed on the label. Some bottlers add fluoride, but even so, the amount added is still likely to keep the level within safe limits.

Contaminants

Hundreds of contaminants have been detected in public water, including disease-causing bacteria; viruses from human wastes; toxic pollutants from highway fuel runoff; spills and heavy metals from industry; and pesticides from agriculture.

All public water must be tested regularly for contamination, and home-owners receive an annual "right to know" statement that names chemicals and bacteria in their water. This list is also available upon request from your local water utility.

Water Treatment

Before the water gets to us, it undergoes treatment, which typically involves both filtration and disinfection. Treatment can remove or detoxify some contaminants. (Private well water is usually not treated.)

Chlorine and chloramine (a combination of chlorine and ammonia) are common disinfectants added to water; chloramine is currently used in San Francisco and in many counties in the Bay Area. Both chlorine and chloramine react with other compounds in water to form "disinfection by-products," some of which are known carcinogens, or can increase risk for miscarriages, birth defects, and liver disease. Chloramine is considerably less toxic of the two.

Several studies show an association between drinking water with chlorine by-products and increased cancer risk[282, 283]; one study by the Environmental Protection Agency suggests that chlorinating water may account for up to 700 cancer deaths annually.

Although the dangers are acknowledged, government officials suggest the benefits of chlorination outweigh the risks. Others suggest that we should be using alternative methods of disinfection that don't introduce the risks, though these may be more costly. The National Resources Defense Council, for example, recommends that different treatment be used, such as ozone or UV light, which have the advantages of eliminating some pathogens unharmed by chlorine and also don't yield the chlorination by-products. They also recommend using activated carbon, which can further reduce contamination.

The taste of chlorine can also be detected in drinking water, which is another reason that some people dislike its use.

How safe is our water?

Tap Water

The National Resources Defense Council (NRDC) evaluated the quality of drinking water in 19 cities and found that although water purity has improved slightly during the past 15 years in most cities, overall tap water quality varies widely from city to city and many cities are not adequately ensuring the safety of their water supplies[284].

San Francisco was one of five cities (also Albuquerque, Boston, Fresno, Phoenix) that was rated "poor," meaning that the drinking water was sufficiently contaminated so as to pose potential health risks, particularly to vulnerable populations (such as the elderly, children, pregnant women, and those that are immune-compromised). Since that report was issued, San Francisco has switched from using chlorine to chloramines, but this change is unlikely to have an impact on the concerns raised. The report also indicated that "in many cases, right-to-know reports have become propaganda for water suppliers."

Bottled Water

Americans spend massive amounts of money for something that is readily available for free: water. Why do we shell out the money for bottled water rather than drinking our less expensive tap water? Perhaps because we believe the marketing and advertising hype that bottled water comes from pristine springs and lakes. Or maybe because we prefer its taste or we have the perception that bottled water is better regulated, safer or purer than tap water.

The bottled water companies have worked hard to undermine public confidence in public water utilities through their marketing, even though their water may come from municipal sources (that they then mark up hundreds of times the original cost). According to government and industry estimates, about one fourth of bottled water is bottled tap water (sometimes, but not always, with additional treatment). Dasani, for example, made by Coca Cola, is bottled tap water, as is Aquafina, made by PepsiCo. Both companies clean the water a bit and add some minerals.

Labels are not required to name the source, but often do clue you in. For example, the label may tell you that it's spring water or that it's bottled from municipal sources (like tap water). But don't fall for the pretty pictures or wholesome names. Glacier Clear Water, for example, does not come from a glacial source, but from municipal sources – in other words, tap water. And while Everest Water features a pretty picture of Mount Everest, inside the bottle you will find treated municipal tap water from Texas.

Furthermore, don't assume that spring water is any more pure than tap water: there's no telling if that spring is near an agricultural area with a lot of pesticide run-off, for instance. Additionally, while most cities regularly disinfect their water and test for parasites, bottled-water manufacturers are not required to.

NRDC conducted 1,000 separate tests of more than 100 brands of bottled water, and concluded that bottled water is not necessarily any purer or any safer than city tap water[285]. Some bottled water is of very high quality and very pure; other brands of bottled water contain elevated levels of arsenic, bacteria, or other contaminants. Two-thirds of the bottles tested were found to be "good quality," while the other third were considered contaminated - including many bottles from popular brands, some of which contained "bacterial overgrowth." Another study, reported in the Archives of Family Medicine, compared 57 samples of bottled water to the tap water in Cleveland and found that while 39 samples of the bottled water were cleaner than tap, more than a dozen had at least 10 times the bacterial levels found in the city's water[286].

One advantage to bottled water is that most are chlorine-free. Most water bottling plants disinfect their water with ozone, which leaves no taste and doesn't yield the toxic by-products that chlorine does. (Even if tap water is used, the chlorine is often removed before sale, though the more dangerous by-products may remain.)

Sparkling water contains carbon dioxide (sometimes naturally occurring, sometimes added) to make it bubbly. Seltzer is carbonated tap water that is filtered. And club soda is seltzer with minerals added.

The bottles, usually made of polyethylene, are designed for one-time use, as the polyethylene can be damaged over time. The plasticizers used to make the bottles soft are "endocrine disrupters," meaning that they interfere with hormones. Over time, they leach into the water and could be responsible for fertility problems and several types of cancer. However, it is unclear how significant a risk they pose. The chemicals diffuse out more easily when the plastic is heated, so best to keep your bottles out of the sun and the microwave.

I wouldn't suggest that you re-use the disposable water bottles as they can become contaminated with bacteria from your hands and mouth. One advantage to tap water is that you can leave tap water out and bacteria won't grow due to the chlorine. On the other hand, if you leave bottled water uncapped and out for a day in the sun, bacteria may thrive.

Also of concern, the bottles pose dramatic environmental consequences. Our landfills continue to grow at enormous rates and a plastic bottle will take hundreds of years to break down. Recycling is dismally under-used and even if the recycling rate increased, it's not an ideal solution. The plastic we recycle doesn't turn into more of the same plastic dropped in the recycling bin, but has to become lower-quality plastic that has limited applications. And of course the energy required to manufacture and transport the bottles takes its toll on our limited fossil fuel supplies and exacerbates global warming. Is it really necessary to ship water from Fiji when rain delivers it direct to your neighborhood?

Thinking outside the bottle

Reconsider tap water. It's often as pure as bottled water, it produces much less waste and its free. Also, its simple enough to filter your water and take it to another level of purity.

Blind taste tests have found that most people can't distinguish tap water from bottled anyway[287]. If taste is your primary criterion, I encourage you to set up a tasting with friends before jumping to the assumption that bottled is better. You may be surprised by the results. You'll probably have a good time - and fortunately, there's no danger of a hangover (unless of course you use wine to clean your palate between sips).

Choosing a water treatment system

The list of contaminants in public water is concerning, and you may want to use a home water treatment system. (Don't trust me on this; get the list from your public water utility.)

There are four basic models. Carbon-filter models use carbon to adsorb impurities as they pass through the system and are effective at removing chlorine by-products and some impurities. These are the cheapest and are generally pretty effective. Reverse osmosis systems push water through a semi-permeable membrane, which acts like a filter. Some systems combine carbon filters with reverse osmosis. Another model uses UV light in combination with carbon filters and very effectively removes contaminants; however, home units may cost around $700. Distillers are the least practical, and they rely on boiling and condensing water.

If you are thinking about getting a filter for your home, there are several things to consider.

First, home purifiers vary a lot in the contaminants they remove. Make sure you get a filter that removes the contaminants of concern in your tap water. There is no one good home purifying system as the type of contaminants vary widely from place to place. (See your city's annual water quality report for information.) And note that some only improve the taste, but do not remove contaminants. Be sure to do your research!

Second, be sure the filter is independently certified by NSF (or a similar independent organization). They verify that the manufacturer's claims about reducing specific contaminants are true, that it doesn't add harmful substances, that it is structurally sound, and that the advertising and information provided do not mislead.

Third, maintain the equipment and change the filter as often as the manufacturer recommends.

Action Tips

- Of course, the best way to protect our water supply is to minimize pollution in the first place. Be sure to read the Ecology section for more information on water pollution (and water scarcity).
- Find out what's in your local water supply by contacting your local water utility and asking for their annual consumer confidence report (drinking water quality report). Or, you could access your local municipality's report here: www.epa.gov/safewater/dwinfo.
- Find out what's in your home's water. Lead, for example, may be leaching from your pipes. Lead is a neurotoxin and pregnant women and children are particularly susceptible to its health dangers. For a list of lead-testing labs, see www.epa.gov/safewater/faq/sco.html, or contact your local health department.
- If you have a private well, make sure you have tested for contaminants. For more information, check out the Water Systems Council at www.wellcarehotline.org.
- Home water filtration is probably a good idea. If you do filter your water, maintain your equipment and make sure to change filters regularly.
- Bottled water may not be any better for you than tap water and poses environmental concerns. However, if you do choose to purchase it, consider these tips:
    - Steer clear of plastic water bottles that release chemicals along with their water.
    - If there's a hint of a plastic smell, don't drink it.
    - Keep water bottles away from heat and out of microwaves.
    - Don't store bottled water for too long.
    - Don't re-use water bottles intended for single use.
    - Choose rigid reusable containers.

Get Informed...

NRDC reported on the results of testing 103 brands of bottled water. Check out their results at www.nrdc.org.

NSF International tests and certifies home water treatment systems. Verify that your system is NSF certified. Find their info at http://www.nsf.org.

Maternal, Infant and Child Nutrition

(with minor notes for Paternal Nutrition too!)

Getting off to a healthy start

Who has a better chance of giving birth to a live child: a pregnant woman in Singapore or the United States? You may be surprised to learn that the U.S. infant mortality rate is substantially higher, despite our great wealth and purportedly more advanced health care[288]. The U.S. infant mortality rate was 7 deaths per 1,000 live births, which is well above that of other "developed" countries, such as France (4), Germany (4), Singapore (4) and Japan (3)[288].

Why is our infant mortality rate so much higher than that of other developed countries (almost double!)? No one has a clear answer to this. While it may have something to do with more precise measurement, something else is going on as well.

What we do know is that there are huge gaps in infant mortality rates within the country between different racial and ethnic groups. Black infant mortality rates, in particular, are exceptionally high, and the relative gap between black and white infant mortality rates has been increasing over time.

The higher rates in minority communities likely represent economic inequities and differences in access to health care. Universal access to quality health care would undoubtably improve our infant mortality rate – not to mention our health status throughout our lives.

Do take special care of yourself. See a health care provider before considering pregnancy, and stay in close contact throughout the pregnancy. Competent medical care throughout pregnancy can save lives – and help the baby off to a healthy start.

Pre-conception

It's important to start out right. A growing fetus gets its nutrients from the mother's diet as well as her bones and tissues – which is one reason why a mom-to-be should be eating well long before conception.

At no stage in life is good nutrition more critical than during fetal development and infancy. Our bodies are developing at a phenomenal rate during that time, and our ability to reach our physical and intellectual potential as adults is in part determined by the nutrition we receive during this time.

To give an example of the gravity of a nutritional deficiency, consider folate. Folate is a B vitamin found in some foods and added to many vitamin and mineral supplements in the form of folic acid. Folate is needed both before and in the first weeks of pregnancy and can help reduce the risk of certain serious and common birth defects called neural tube defects, which affect the brain and spinal cord.

The tricky part is that neural tube defects can occur in an embryo before a woman realizes she's pregnant. And most American diets are deficient in folate. That's why the government strategy is preventative: encouraging all women of childbearing age to include folate in their diets. Fruits, dark-green leafy vegetables, dried beans and peas, among other foods, are good sources of naturally-occurring folate, and many cereals and grains are fortified as well.

Fortunately, there has been a decrease in the incidence of folate-related birth defects over the past few years. This is probably due to government regulations, enacted in 1998, requiring that U.S. grain products be fortified with folic acid.

If you are trying to get pregnant, be safe: make sure to get plenty of folate (>400 mcgs) in your diet. Any vitamin that claims it contains a "women's formula" will have the necessary amount of folic acid. Even if you aren't trying to conceive, if you are capable of becoming pregnant, it may be advisable to take a vitamin for extra insurance.

Pre-conception Concerns for Men

The man's nutrition prior to pregnancy is important as well; malnutrition could lead to abnormalities in sperm. And guys, if you're trying to help conceive, you may want to stay away from hot tubs and saunas, which can overheat your testes and cause damage. Running a fever could have the same result. Hard bicycle seats are not recommended, as they may cause circulatory and neurologic difficulties that can affect functioning[289]. And while some experts report that tight shorts and pants may reduce blood flow in the groin and adversely affect sperm production, I couldn't find research to support this.

Nutritional Considerations when Pregnant or Lactating

Healthy eating during pregnancy and lactation is not all that different than at other times – its just that the quantity you need increases and the implications of the quality of your diet get intensified. Here are some basic tips:

- Hunger and fullness should still serve as an effective guide to the amount to eat.
- Smaller meals spread more frequently throughout the day will help smooth digestive concerns, nausea, and energy levels.
- While your need for protein increases (to an RDA of 60 grams), if you eat a well-balanced diet you should still get more than enough. That amount is easily supplied in typical American diets consumed by non-pregnant women.
- Getting sufficient essential fatty acids, and in a good ratio, is particularly important to nourish the baby's growing brain.
- Because the body's ability to handle toxic substances is not well developed until later in life, it is particularly important to minimize the fetus's exposure. So cut down on foods laden with pesticides, mercury and other contaminants.
- The need for many miconutrients increases during pregnancy. For extra insurance, take a pre-natal vitamin/mineral supplement. Be sure to avoid high-dose supplements.

Alcohol and pregnancy just don't mix.

No one knows exactly what harmful effects even the smallest amount of alcohol has on a developing baby. While a minority of experts says moderate drinking during pregnancy is okay, it is much more commonly accepted to believe that taking even one drink is like playing Russian Roulette with the baby's health. Public health officials in the United States recommend that mothers-to-be play it safe by steering clear of alcohol entirely, and they're joined by experts at the American College of Obstetricians and Gynecologists and the American Academy of Pediatrics.

Drinking endangers the growing fetus in a number of ways. First, it increases the risk of miscarriage and stillbirth. Even as little as one drink a day is associated with increased odds for low birth weight and increased risk that the child will develop problems with learning, attention span, and hyperactivity. And some research has shown that expectant moms who have as little as one drink per week are more likely than nondrinkers to have children who later exhibit aggressive behavior.

The most severe result of alcohol use is fetal alcohol syndrome (FAS), a permanent condition characterized by poor growth, abnormal facial features, and damage to the central nervous system. Babies with FAS may also have abnormally small heads and brains, and heart, spine, and other anatomical defects. The central nervous system damage may include mental retardation, delays in physical development, vision and hearing problems, and a variety of behavioral problems.

Whether caffeine is safe during pregnancy is controversial.

Some studies suggest that caffeine intake of less than two average cups of coffee per day presents a slight risk to the embryo or fetus, but others do not. There is stronger evidence that larger daily amounts of caffeine during pregnancy may increase the risks of miscarriage, preterm delivery and low birth weight, but no solid proof. Though the research isn't conclusive, it makes sense to cut back.

Some studies have found that pregnant women who consumed large quantities of caffeine (five or more cups of coffee a day) were twice as likely to miscarry as those who consumed less, while fewer or no effects were seen at lower levels of caffeine consumption[290, 291].

Food Cravings

Many pregnant women experience intense food cravings or aversions. No one is sure whether they are motivated by nutritional deficiencies; there just isn't scientific data on the subject. It is clear that hormonal shifts during pregnancy intensify sense of smell (which heavily influences taste) and are powerful enough to affect food choices. That pregnancy causes shifts in metabolism and need for particular nutrients is also a driving force.

Your cravings aren't necessarily a problem if they don't cause imbalances in your diet or prevent you from eating other important foods, so my suggestion is to enjoy the motivation to explore new foods and combinations.

A more serious type of craving, called pica, in which women crave nonfood items, like dirt or laundry starch, can be dangerous and even fatal. Several theories have been proposed as to what causes pica, from a deficiency of calcium or iron, to the ability of certain nonfood items to quell nausea and vomiting. However, there has never been any medical reason determined. Needless to say, cravings of this nature are best not indulged; check in with a physician if they come up.

What to feed an infant?

You can't beat breast milk as the perfect food for a newborn, although certain diseases, maternal drug use, or other concerns may make it inappropriate for some. Don't buy the "technology improves on nature" argument for infant formula – scientists are a long way from figuring out how to recreate the wonderful benefits of breast milk. It's interesting that the composition of breast milk is sensitive to the baby's needs, even changing the relative percentages of fat and protein while a baby nurses.

For the first six months or so, it's best to limit your baby to breastmilk (preferably) and/or baby formula. While cow's milk is the perfect food for baby calves, don't be tempted to feed it to your baby: its nutritional composition just isn't well-suited to human growth needs.

How to feed and infant?

Fortunately, babies are born with an innate drive to get their nutrient needs met. So you don't have to work too hard at figuring out amounts – you just need to be attentive to their desires. Let your child call the shots: he or she will tell you when it's time to eat and how much is an appropriate amount. Feeding and nurturing infants are one and the same.

How long to breastfeed? There's no clear-cut answer here, so best to go with the mother's and child's preferences and comfort. Considering that you can't match the nutritional benefits of breast milk, carry on as long as is comfortable.

The transition to solid foods should be based on what your baby can do, not on how old she or he is. A baby is ready for solid foods when they can sit up, open their mouth for the spoon, close their lips over the spoon, keep most of the food in their mouth, and swallow – and of course shows interest. If any of these are missing, hold off!

Helping Kids Establish Nourishing Eating Habits

Although kids have different nutrient needs than adults, I don't have different general suggestions for what to eat. The same general recommendations that work for adults will also support kids in getting their nutrient needs met.

Kids, particularly when young, do need to eat more frequently than adults, however. Their energy needs are high and their digestive tracts less developed, and frequent eating is the best way to keep their bodies with a steady energy supply. Three meals a day just isn't enough for them – at least not without a couple snack times in between.

The key rule of thumb, from infancy on through adolescence, is the following: the adult's responsibility is to provide food, your child's is to decide whether he or she wants it and how much. Always provide them with a variety of options to choose from, so they have the opportunity to choose foods they like and develop their own tastes. You will experience less and less control over your child's exposure to foods over time, and your best bet is to support them in learning how to make good choices and take care of themselves. Always hard for a parent to let go of controlling their kids, but it is in the child's best interest in the long run. Only they know best when they are hungry and how much they need to eat.

Know that little kids mimic what they see around them. What you eat sets the stage for your kids' taste preferences. If you like and regularly eat vegetables, odds are they will too. So the best advice to instill good habits in your kids is to cultivate good habits for yourself.

Children - often even more so than adults - are easily seduced by intense flavorings and mouth-feel, like the sugar, salt, and fat often found in processed foods. When their diets are centered on processed foods, it dulls their ability to sense and appreciate more subtle and wider-ranging flavors, a trait they will carry on into adulthood.

Exposing them to a wide variety of whole foods when they are young will make them less interested in fast foods and processed foods. This isn't to say that they will lack interest in processed foods, but they are more likely to achieve a healthier balance.

There's no need to be rigid around less nutrient-dense options. Moderation is a lesson they'll need to learn and depriving them of foods they like won't allow this growth opportunity. Setting limits – supporting them in enjoying moderate amounts of sweets - is likely to be much more successful than deprivation. Be sure to set those limits so that the less nutritious options are viewed in a positive light. In other words, convey the idea that desserts can be fun and tasty and are meant to be enjoyed, but moderation is helpful so that they don't crowd out more nutrient-dense choices.

Know that children, particularly when they are young, may hesitate to try new things. This is normal. In fact, there's even a scientific name for this phenomenon: neophobia, or fear of new things. Don't expect your child to accept foods right away, but do make sure to offer a wide range of foods to help expand their range of tastes. Present foods positively and don't pressure your child to eat. And continue to offer previously refused food as repeated exposure often helps kids open up.

Given our cultural fear of fat, you may be tempted to limit or withhold food if you have a pudgy kid. Don't. Kids of all sizes need to learn how to regulate their food intake – you won't always be around to control them. And besides, withholding food just doesn't prove helpful in controlling weight anyway.

Pudgy kids will be feeling plenty of cultural prejudice. They don't need more hassling from you – they need your support. Better to shore up their self-esteem: reinforce the idea that kids come in a wide range of sizes and that every body is a good body. Similar to the earlier advice given for adults, it will be a lot easier for them to develop healthy eating and activity habits with a more positive attitude towards themselves.

Food Safety

Public concern about food safety is increasing. Stories about Bird Flu and outbreaks of E. coli and Salmonella routinely grab headlines. We now have the added concern of terrorists poisoning our food and water. Clearly, we no longer trust our food supply.

Of course, food safety has dramatically improved over the years. For example, in the decades before the Civil War, milk was delivered unrefrigerated in the same wagons that carried out cow manure; the milk was so contaminated that newspapers accused the dairies of murder[292]. Poor food preservation techniques, poor sanitation, and various contaminants in the food supply caused serious illnesses like typhoid and cholera, which fortunately have essentially been wiped out – or at least greatly minimized - through government intervention and food safety regulations.

Despite these dramatic advances, however, our current concern about food safety is not unwarranted. Changes in how we produce, process, and distribute food have made food a vector for pathogens. The Centers for Disease Control (CDC) reported in 1999 that food-borne diseases cause approximately 76 million illnesses, 325,000 hospitalizations, and 5,000 deaths in the United States each year[293]. This is over twice as many illnesses as were estimated by a task force convened by the Council for Agricultural Science and Technology (CAST) five years earlier, and cited by the CDC for comparison[294], so the situation may be worsening.

Seventy-six million of us get food poisoning every year! That's about one in every four Americans. Frightening as this figure may be, it becomes particularly concerning when you consider that it was derived from government data – and the government is known for its conservative estimates. (To be fair, estimating this stuff is tough. Do you visit the doctor every time you get stomach upset? Even if you do visit a physician, testing for food-borne disease is rarely conducted as the testing is expensive and patients will typically recover before the results are determined. And when a diagnosis of food-borne disease is given, doctors are not required to report it to the CDC and frequently don't. As a result, the statisticians don't have detailed information to work with, as the CDC acknowledges as a limitation of their analysis.)

I believe that the government has been largely ineffective in adequately protecting us from dangers in our food supply. As Dr. Michael Greger comments, if 19,000,000 pounds of ground beef contaminated with E. coli bacteria were distributed to half the population by terrorists, we'd be going berserk[295]. But when it is distributed by a major corporation (ConAgra, in July 2002)[296], it's just business as usual. We have come to expect it.

The government even heard about the tainted meat well in advance of the aforementioned crisis, and refused to investigate[297]. Not that the government could do much about it anyway: the regulatory agencies responsible for inspecting and regulating food safety don't even have the power to order recalls of contaminated food, but must ask food companies to *voluntarily* remove food[296]. (Can you believe this? The government can recall a teddy bear with a plastic eye that may possibly become a choking hazard, but can't recall tainted meat that could be lethal?) In addition, recent lawsuits brought by the meat industry have limited the government's ability to close plants producing contaminated meat[296].

Microbial Contamination

How often have you had the stomach flu? Okay, that was a trick question. The stomach flu doesn't actually exist[298]. Influenza is a respiratory disease, caused by a virus, which primarily affects your lungs - not your digestive tract. Most likely, if you had diarrhea, stomach cramping and/or vomiting, you contracted a disease caused by a bacteria, virus or parasite found in your food or water. Food poisoning is extremely common. Odds are you've experienced it – numerous times.

The common manifestations of food-borne disease have changed over time. Symptoms of cramps, vomiting and diarrhea usually appeared shortly after eating contaminated food (typical signs of "staph" poisoning). But pathogens common now – such as E. coli – may not result in symptoms until two to seven days after exposure, making it difficult to connect the illness with the food. Most diners blame the last place they ate, but tracing the source of contagion is rarely that simple.

Let's go back to those conservative figures presented by the CDC and put them in perspective. The U.S. population is about 290 million[299]. That means that every year there is a 1 out of 900 chance that you will be hospitalized for a food-borne illness. And in that year, 1 out of 59,000 people will die from a food-borne illness. These are not good odds!

Contracting food-borne illness can happen anywhere. It is common in restaurants, for example. In fact, government data show that consumers are twice as likely to report food poisoning caused by restaurant food than from food prepared at home[300]. When a home cook fails to observe safe food handling techniques, it may affect their household, but when an individual in a restaurant does the same thing, hundreds of people can suffer. In 1993, four children died and more than 700 people became sick in a food-borne illness outbreak linked to E. coli O157:H7 bacteria which contaminated Jack-in-the-Box hamburgers. The outbreak was a wake up call to consumers and government officials, and in 1995 new standards were implemented to improve inspection and testing[301].

However, consumer advocates express concern that the new standards are grossly inadequate and food safety regulations and enforcement have actually become more lax since that outbreak[302, 303]. Government assessment on this topic is particularly frightening. For example, a detailed study of fast food restaurants by the Food and Drug Administration on compliance with food safety regulations showed that in 42 percent of incidents observed, restaurants failed to properly control temperatures to minimize bacterial risk[304]. Poor personal hygiene (31 percent), chemical contamination (28 percent), and contaminated equipment/protection from contamination (22 percent) also had notable out of compliance percentages.

Schools are also vulnerable. In fact, the Center for Science in the Public Interest (CSPI) has identified at least 67 documented outbreaks since 1990, with more than 4,000 illnesses, in schools[296]. And a Congressional study indicated that the number of school-related outbreaks reported to the Centers for Disease Control and Prevention doubled over the last decade and generally increased by about 10 percent per year[305].

Food-borne illness is also entering our home kitchens. For example, USDA inspections show that more than 97 percent of turkey carcasses are contaminated with pathogens capable of causing disease in the humans that eat them[306]. Ninety-seven percent! Frightening, isn't it?

That high level of contamination isn't an anomaly, but shows up consistently in the research. Take a look at some of the more common bacterial contaminants. Campylobacter bacteria, for example: one government study showed contamination in more than 80 percent of the carcasses of broiler chickens[307], while a random sampling of turkeys on supermarket shelves by CSPI found that 90 percent were sufficiently contaminated to cause illness[308].

Many animal products are contaminated with Salmonella bacteria as well[309]. Every year, approximately 40,000 cases of salmonellosis are reported in the United States[310]. Because many milder cases are not diagnosed or reported, the CDC estimates that the actual number of infections may be thirty or more times greater: 1,200,000[310]. That's over a million cases, and – as mentioned earlier - the government is known for its conservative estimates!

Another government study showed that greater than 99 percent of broiler chickens carcasses had detectable E. coli[311]. Since the CDC estimates 250-500 deaths from E. coli O157 every year (and ground beef is the primary vehicle), that amounts to a daily death due to eating a hamburger.

The frequency of food poisoning in the U.S. today makes it evident that our current food safety system needs improvement. In March 2003, Ann Veneman, who at the time was the USDA Secretary of Agriculture, described the USDA as "working under a Meat Inspection Act that pre-dates the Model T."[312]

Time Magazine quotes a former USDA microbiologist, Dr. Gerald Kuester, on chicken: "The final product is no different than if you stuck it in the toilet and ate it."[313] The situation is so bad that research shows higher levels of coliform bacteria (from feces) in American kitchens than on the rim of their toilets[314]! This didn't surprise food-borne disease expert Dr. Nicols Fox, who comments, "The bathroom is cleaner because people are not washing their chickens in the toilet[302]."

Factory Farmed Disease

Conditions on factory farms and in slaughterhouses are responsible for a large proportion of food-borne disease.

Crowding large numbers of animals in small spaces forces them to wallow in manure and contributes to quick and easy spread of bacteria. It also means the animals share common sources of food and water, which again means that large numbers of animals can quickly be exposed to a food or water-borne pathogen.

Additionally, large populations of animals create more manure than can be converted to fertilizer. With lesser numbers of animals, on the other hand, the wastes can be composted and returned to nurture the soil, a process that also generates heat which helps to kill bacteria.

At the slaughterhouse, even greater numbers of animals are commingled, also allowing easy spread of pathogens. A little contamination can go a long way. Health officials estimate that just one infected cow can contaminate eight tons of ground beef! In fact, investigators once traced the origin of a single lot of hamburger meat to slaughterhouses in six states and 443 individual animals[315].

Research clearly indicates that current legislation is inadequate to protect the environment from E. coli contamination from untreated wastes spread to land[316]. As Dr. Marion Nestle comments, "it is difficult to imagine a system better equipped to promote the spread of disease – and to obscure the source of illnesses or outbreaks."[3] Nestle alerts us to a dramatic example: a 1994 Salmonella outbreak that sickened more than 220,000 people in 41 states[317]. (The origin was ice cream that was contaminated in a truck that had previously carried liquid eggs.)

No one disputes that factory farming conditions play a large role in the extensive food contamination. Yet amazingly, there is no current requirement that farms be tested for pathogens! The U.S. meat industry has aggressively fought any legislation that would require testing.

E. coli O157-H7 (the more virulent strain) provides an example of the worst of factory farming. It is a by-product of grain-based feeding to dairy and beef cattle in an attempt to fatten them up quicker and at a lower cost. The cow's digestive system (and acid balance) evolved to break down grass, not grain. A grain-based diet creates a highly acid environment in the cow's stomachs, allowing the deadly bacterium to thrive. Research documents that almost half of U.S. cattle host the deadly E. coli bacterium[318].

There is no reason for anyone to get E. coli poisoning. It's a direct by-product of producing cheap, unhealthy cattle. It is a totally avoidable problem. Yet we've come to accept it. And we blame ourselves. We didn't cook the shit out of our food! (Actually, that's not literally true – you are still eating feces; it's just that when cooked it's less likely to harm you.)

Many Americans are well-schooled in the fact that raw animal foods pose dangers – we've heard the warnings to avoid eating raw cookie dough or Caesar's dressing, to pass on the rare burgers, to sanitize our cutting boards. But until recently, we didn't worry about our salads. Lately, however, there have been a number of outbreaks from fruits and vegetables – and many of them from my home state of California, not the imports.

In fall of 2006, more than 200 people in 26 states were sickened and three people killed by spinach contaminated with E. coli O157:H7. Soon after, at least 183 people in 21 states got salmonella from tainted tomatoes, followed by more than 160 people in New York, New Jersey and other nearby states getting sickened with E. coli after eating at Taco Bell restaurants.

The contamination problems with plant foods can often be traced back to fecal contamination originating in animal agriculture. The raw waste brings pathogenic bacteria into contact with plant products that aren't usually contaminated with those organisms, making them susceptible to causing outbreaks of food poisoning. For example, in the recent outbreak of contaminated spinach, which sickened at least 200 and killed three, federal investigators traced the source to a local animal farm.

Because E. coli infections originate with farm animals, and because the vast majority of E. coli poisoning can be pinned on the feeding practices, gross over-crowding and disease conditions found in factory farming and slaughterhouses, cleaning up our farms and food processing plants will go a long way toward cleaning up the problem.

So far, private industry has done little to take responsibility – and the government has done little to encourage them. Government prevention campaigns have focused on educating consumers to cook and handle foods carefully, shifting responsibility from food producers to consumers. While it is certainly valuable for consumers to practice food safety in their homes (for example, washing their hands, chilling leftovers promptly, cooking animal products thoroughly, avoiding cross-contamination), this is not enough to solve the problem. Sunny-side up eggs shouldn't be a biohazard. In countries where animals are more humanely treated and raised in cleaner conditions with more space, food-borne disease is significantly less than the United States. The contamination incidents described above are fully preventable (as discussed in detail by Nestle)[3].

Fortunately, we can be less concerned about organic agriculture. (Minutes after the FDA's 2006 spinach warning, proponents of industrial agriculture were blaming the outbreak on manure-based fertilizers used in organic production. Yes, the contaminated spinach was packed at a plant that also bags organic produce, but the infected product was not organically grown.) Organic growers are required to follow strict rules for heating manure to kill any harmful bacteria and for storing treated manure until it is safe to use. They are also inspected to ensure they follow those rules. Conventional crops, on the other hand, are not subject to any regulations on the use of manure.

Antibiotic Use

Antibiotics are medications used to kill bacteria. When farmers started using them on animals, it was for good intentions. Just as with humans, when antibiotics are given to animals sick with bacterial infections, they are very effective at killing certain (not all) bacteria and curing disease. However, farmers noticed that the antibiotics were useful in other ways as well, including helping the animals to grow more quickly and need less food (for reasons not well understood). Given the disease-promoting conditions on factory farms, and the added advantage of growth stimulation, many factory farms started to routinely administer antibiotics to their animals, regardless of whether they were sick.

Antibiotics are helpful medicine, but the more they get used, the more the bacteria build resistance to them. Now, not only do we need to be concerned about bacterial infection, but we also need to be concerned that food-borne bacteria are becoming dangerously resistant to antibiotics. Research reported in the New England Journal of Medicine indicates that 84 percent of supermarket meat packages (pork, beef, and chicken) contained antibiotic-resistant bacteria, which can then get transferred to a person eating them[319]. If that person gets sick, the antibiotics would be useless. Food poisoning is not our only problem. Now we have to worry that we are losing our tools to fight the food poisoning[320].

Many antibiotics - like penicillin - are now helpless against the infections they used to cure. For this reason, antibiotics have been banned for routine livestock use in most countries (but not the U.S.), a practice strongly advocated by the World Health Organization. Both the American Medical Association and the American Public Health Association also oppose their routine use in healthy farm animals. Interestingly, routine antibiotic usage is supported by the American Veterinary Medicine Association. It has been suggested that AVMA holds this position because of the extensive financial support they receive from Bayer Pharmaceuticals, a maker of antibiotics who stands to lose a great deal if they are banned[8].

Indeed, the increasing emergence of antibiotic resistant bacteria is a large global health threat. Infections resistant to antibiotics are now the eleventh leading cause of death among Americans. About 70 percent of bacteria that cause infections in hospitals are resistant to at least one of the common drugs used to treat infections – and some organisms are resistant to all approved antibiotics[321].

Given that 70 percent of the total U.S antibiotic production is put in animal feed[322], banning their routine use could make a very strong dent in solving our antibiotic crisis. Instead, the government has put their energy into a campaign to encourage physicians to be more circumspect in prescribing. Although valuable, this tactic is clearly much less helpful than going after the meat industry, where antibiotic abuse is much more prominent and has a larger impact.

Industry claims that antibiotics are necessary to keep the costs of food production down. However, the National Academy of Sciences estimates that a total ban on the routine use of antibiotics to farmed animals would raise the price of poultry anywhere from 1 to 2 cents per pound and the price of pork or beef 3 to 6 cents a pound, costing the average meat-eating American consumer up to $9.72 a year[323]. Is this going to break your budget?

Consumer advocates are now actively putting pressure on industry. Tyson Foods, the nation's largest chicken producer, responded to this pressure: since June 2007, it has been producing all of its fresh grocery chicken without antibiotics and will market these products with a label saying "Raised Without Antibiotics."

But don't get fooled by manufacturer claims such as "antibiotic-free," "no antibiotic residues," "without added antibiotics," and "no subtherapeutic antibiotics." In fact, no meat sold in the U.S. is allowed to have antibiotic residues, so therefore it is all "antibiotic-free." The problem is not antibiotic residues in the meat. It's in the resistant bacteria that contaminate the meat.

Perchlorate Contamination

Perchlorate the explosive chemical in rocket fuel, has severely contaminated the nation's food and water supply, according to an analysis of Centers for Disease Control data conducted by the Environmental Working Group. It has leaked from military bases and defense and aerospace contractors' plants in at least 22 states, and has been widely detected in milk, lettuce, produce and other foods. In an alarming study, the CDC found perchlorate in the urine of every person tested. Perchlorate interferes with thyroid function. Since small changes in thyroid hormone levels during pregnancy are associated with decreased intellectual and learning capacity in childhood, perchlorate contamination has huge implications for public health. There is a large consumer campaign pressuring for clean-up, but so far little or nothing has been done.

Growth Hormones

Another health concern relates to the hormone implants that are given to more than 90 percent of all U.S. beef cattle[324]. Hormone implants have been banned in Europe since 1995 because of concerns that they may cause cancer and reproductive disturbances in humans who eat the cattle[325]. There have been no long-term studies of the human health effects, and many international organizations disagree with the European Union's assessment. However, others contend that in the face of uncertainty, precaution should rule.

A disturbing political dilemma has resulted from the European ban on hormone implants, as it means that they can no longer accept imports of hormone-tainted beef from the U.S. The loss of income that this entailed for the U.S. beef industry prompted the U.S. to bring a case to the World Trade Organization (WTO), claiming that the European ban posed an unfair limit on free trade. The WTO ruled in the U.S.'s favor, declaring that Europe's ban on hormone-tainted beef was illegal. Europe has since elected to pay regular fines to the U.S. rather than lift the ban.

New fears...

Anyway, cook your food at high temperatures, and you can eliminate bacteria such as Campylobacter, Salmonella – even Listeria and E. Coli – or you can combat them with pharmaceuticals (though this won't be true for long, given increasing antibiotic resistance).

But what if there were a pathogen that defied all attempts at destruction? Something that could invade the immune system, riddle your brain with holes, and cause a cruel and painful death? And what if modern food processing resulted in exposing much of our population to this lethal pathogen? If it caused disease so slowly that many of us could be exposed to it before there was much awareness of its presence?

No, this isn't the plot to a bad science fiction movie. It's a potential reality – and its called Mad Cow Disease.

Mad Cow Disease

Mad Cow Disease has previously been called the biggest food scare in history (although it has lately been dwarfed by fears of an avian flu epidemic). Known to scientists as bovine spongiform encephalopathy, or BSE, it's an infectious disease that derives its name because it riddles the cow's brain with holes, making it look like a sponge.

Mad Cow disease is caused by prions, which are infectious proteins. Researchers have traced the outbreak of Mad Cow Disease to factory farming's cost-cutting practice of mixing bits of sheep's neural tissue into the feed of cows[326]. It is believed that the sheep were infected with scrapie, the sheep form of spongiform encephalopathy, and the prions were able to cross the species barrier. The practice of feeding (infected) cow parts to cows furthers the spread.

The first known infections of BSE were in the United Kingdom. The epidemic peaked there in January of 1993, with almost 1,000 new cases per week. By the end of 2005, more than 180,000 cases of BSE had been confirmed[327].

A series of steps were undertaken to eradicate BSE. Most notably, in 1988, England banned the feeding of cow parts to other cows, and in 1996, preemptively slaughtered nearly four and a half million asymptomatic cattle[327]. Eventually, the epidemic receded.

Prions are virtually indestructible: cooking, digestive enzymes, irradiation – anything you can think of - are all ineffective. If you eat a food that contains prions, they can be transferred to your body, causing new variant Creutzfeldt-Jakob disease (nvCJD), a human spongiform encephalopathy whose symptoms typically involve a painful deterioration as brain tissue gets destroyed. nvCJD is always fatal. So far, over 120 people have died of nvCJD in Europe.

Only three cows with Mad Cow Disease have been reported in the United States. However, it is possible that others exist, and that we just don't know the extent of the problem[328, 329]. Mad Cow Disease has a long incubation period[330], and most cows are slaughtered before it would even show up on the type of test we use in the United States[331, 332].

Given current factory farming methods, we are at risk for epidemic exposure. A quick lesson in conventional agriculture will help you understand this. Cows are ordinarily herbivores. Their digestive tracts weren't designed with effective mechanisms to digest animals. However, we've turned cattle into carnivores. Until very recently, we fed them "protein concentrates," a euphemism for the stuff left at the slaughterhouses that couldn't be sold: primarily ground up meat, bone, blood and other by-products of the slaughtered animals. Supplementing their diets with protein concentrates results in much more meat on cattle, and increased milk production in dairy cows. (The same result could come from plant products such as soy or corn, but those are more expensive.) So we not only turned cows into carnivores, but we made them cannibals as well.

So let's imagine there are cows with Mad Cow Disease, even if they are relatively few. Toss their remains into the rendering pot to make the protein concentrates, and now those prions get spread to all the cows that eat those concentrates. It's like unsafe sex and the spread of AIDS. You're not just having sex with one person, but it's as if you're having sex with every partner they've had, and every partner of those individuals. It spreads exponentially. Every quarter pound burger you eat could actually be made from the meat of hundreds or thousands of different cows! It is this recycling of rendered cattle pieces that scientists believe is responsible for the epidemic in England[333].

It took a while, but in 1997, the U.S. government implemented some safeguards – like a ban on feeding most cattle parts to other cattle – but many express concern that there are too many loopholes in the law and problems with enforcement, and we still haven't gone far enough[334-336]. For example, blood, a known infectious agent[337], is not excluded, yet it is routinely fed to calves as part of their "milk replacer."[336, 338] (That prions are transmissible through blood is well-accepted; the Red Cross, for example, will not accept donations from individuals who have lived in most parts of Europe, precisely because of their concerns of nvCJD infectivity[339].) Also, it is still legal to feed sheep and cows to pigs and to feed chickens and pigs to cows[334, 336], despite research documenting that encephalopathies can cross species barriers. And chicken litter, which contains chicken feces and uneaten feed containing cow parts, is exempt from the ban and routinely fed to cows[334, 340].

In other words, there is a fairly easy route for infected cows to cycle through other animals and into the human food supply. In fact, the United States is violating all four concrete recommendations laid down by the World Health Organization to prevent the spread of BSE into the human population[335]. The Food and Drug Administration is currently considering closing some of these loopholes, but whether it will be accomplished remains to be seen.

Even when standards are in place, they are not always followed and rarely enforced[336]. For example, according to a 1997 ban, cattle feed is not supposed to contain the nervous tissue of other ruminant animals. Yet a review by the Government Accountability Office in 2001 found that 20 percent of American feed companies had no systems in place to prevent the contamination of cattle feed[341]. According to the report, more than 25 percent of feed manufacturers in Colorado weren't even aware of the Food and Drug Administration rules to prevent mad cow disease, three years after their introduction. A follow-up study the next year showed that the FDA's "inspection database is so severely flawed" that "it should not be used to assess compliance" with the feed ban[342].

And our inadequate testing of U.S. cattle may be missing cases of BSE. The European Union, for example, for a long time assured their citizenry that BSE had not been detected in their cattle, which was true because relatively few cattle had been tested. Once they began widespread testing, its existence was clear. The U.S. is presently testing only a tiny fraction of our cows; Dr. Stanley Pruisner, winner of the Nobel Prize in Medicine for his discovery of prions and considered to be the world's expert on prion diseases, describes the number of tests done by USDA as "appalling."[343] Dr. Pruisner estimates that the cost for testing all cattle slaughtered for human consumption is just a few extra cents per pound of meat[344].

In other words, there is some question that the reason the United States doesn't have more confirmed cases could be due to our inadequate detection system[345] – and perhaps we're eating the evidence. As others have said, our Mad Cow strategy appears to be "Don't look, don't find." Thirty-six countries have expressed their concern by banning the import of beef from the United States.

Given the long incubation period in cows, some experts are concerned that we wouldn't even know if we were in the midst of an epidemic here in the United States. The incubation period in humans was previously believed to be up to 30 years[346], and people may be unknowingly incubating prions[336]. A more recent investigation suggests an even longer estimate for the incubation period: 50 years[347].

Also, we may be seeing CJD already and not know it[348]. Inadequate testing of the brains of people dying with dementia may be missing hundreds of cases of CJD. Since symptoms are very similar to Alzheimer's there is no telling if many of the people diagnosed as suffering from Alzheimer's actually had CJD. We just don't know the extent of the problem.

Nonetheless, though some trumpet these fears, that we're not clearly seeing an epidemic right now may be telling. Perhaps we are doing a good job of keeping it out of our population.

The meat industry and some governmental bodies feel confident that we are well protected. For example, the Harvard Center for Risk Analysis, a group sponsored in part by the meat industry, conducted a study commissioned by the United States Department of Agriculture[349]. Their conclusion? "Our analysis finds that the U.S. is highly resistant of any introduction of BSE or a similar disease." These investigators believe that U.S. policies are effective, and that "The new cases of BSE would come primarily from lack of compliance with the regulations... Even if they existed, these hypothetical sources of BSE could give rise to only one or two cases per year." They conclude that "the disease is virtually certain to be eliminated from the country within 20 years after its introduction."

I hope they're right.

Other government investigators are not so optimistic. For example, the Government Accountability Office has been sharply critical of U.S. policies on inspection, testing and enforcement: "While BSE has not been found in the United States (this was written in 2002, shortly before the first case was detected), federal actions do not sufficiently ensure that all BSE-infected animals or products are kept out or that if BSE were found, it would be detected promptly and not spread to other animals... or enter the human food supply."[342]

The bottom line? No one has the answers as to the level of risk of contracting CJD, but it is clear that some level of risk exists. We don't treat our animals well or adequately protect them from contracting Mad Cow Disease. And there are just too many loopholes in the laws and problems with compliance. That said, I do, however, expect that the risk is quite low.

If you are concerned, know that you have options. Of course, you can choose to pass on that hamburger. If you want to eat beef, you can limit your risk by avoiding the foods more likely to carry mad-cow disease: brains and processed beef products that may contain nervous-system tissue, such as hamburger, hot dogs, and sausage. Organic or 100 percent grass-fed beef carries the least risk, as these cattle are not fed any animal remains. Steak and hamburger that's ground while you watch are also lower risk, as they don't contain meat from multiple animals. Be wary of anything that contains broth made from meat, such as gelatin.

Avian Flu

It seems you can't read a paper, or turn on television, radio or computer right now without hearing about the "Bird Flu." The highly pathogenic H5N1 strain of avian influenza has grabbed headlines because of its ability to infect humans who have come in close contact. Among those who have been hospitalized with the disease, about half have died. What has public health professionals most worried is the potential of the virus to mutate into a form that can be passed from person to person.

To understand the threat, let's discuss the birds first. Wild birds can carry the avian flu virus, although they usually don't get sick. Infected birds shed the flu virus in their saliva, nasal secretions, and feces, and, unfortunately, it is very highly contagious. This means that wild birds can easily infect domesticated birds (including chickens, ducks, and turkeys). The domesticated birds that contract the virus do get very sick – and die. Factory farm conditions are also a vector for quick spread of the disease: if one bird is infected, it could shortly spread to millions.

It is unclear why domesticated birds exhibit symptoms while wild birds don't, but a possible explanation is the decreased immunity that results from confinement and factory farm conditions. There are no currently documented cases of avian flu in domestic birds raised in organic, pastured, free-range conditions.

Outbreaks of avian influenza H5N1 occurred throughout Asia (Cambodia, China, Indonesia, Japan, Laos, South Korea, Thailand, and Vietnam) during late 2003 and early 2004. At that time, more than 100 million birds either died or were killed in order to try to control the outbreak, and by March 2004, the outbreak was reported to be under control. Since late June 2004, however, new outbreaks were reported by several countries in Asia (Cambodia, China [Tibet], Indonesia, Kazakhstan, Malaysia, Mongolia, Russia [Siberia], Thailand, and Vietnam). Infection has also has been reported in Turkey, Romania, and Ukraine, and among wild migratory birds in China, Croatia, Mongolia, and Romania, indicating that we're not doing a very good job at controlling its spread.

So what does this mean for humans? As of November 29, 2006, 258 cases have been reported in people, 154 of them fatal. Most cases of avian flu infection in humans have resulted from contact with infected poultry or surfaces contaminated with secretion/excretions from infected birds. So far, the spread of H5N1 virus from person-to-person has been rare and has not been confirmed to continue beyond one person. Seven confirmed cases of H5N1 avian influenza in a family in Indonesia involved "close and prolonged exposure" to another infected person, prompting the World Health Organization (WHO) to suggest (but not make a definitive conclusion) the possibility of person-to-person transmission.

Nonetheless, because all flu viruses have the ability to change, scientists are concerned that H5N1 virus one day could be able to infect humans and spread easily from one person to another. Since viruses like H5N1 do not commonly infect humans, there is little or no immune protection against them in the human population. If H5N1 virus were to gain the capacity to spread easily from person to person, an influenza pandemic (worldwide outbreak of disease) could begin. So scientists are on alert.

Can I get infected from eating poultry or eggs?

Currently, avian flu has not been detected in U.S. birds or the U.S. food supply. If and when it does enter the U.S., know that the vast majority of human cases of avian flu have arisen from direct contact with infected birds, making those involved in the slaughtering or manufacturing process at higher risk than consumers. The virus is sensitive to heat, and is destroyed through adequate cooking. Even if it does enter our food supply, there is no evidence that you can get infected from eating properly cooked poultry or eggs. So protect yourself: make sure that you fully cook all parts of poultry (no "pink") and eggs (no "runny" yolks).

How best to protect myself?

Consumers' best protection is not difficult, given that many of us are disconnected from the source of our food: stay away from potentially infected birds. Next, be sure to cook your poultry and eggs well. And lastly, maintain a healthy immune system: eat well, be active, sleep well, develop caring relationships, enjoy life...

Industrial Contamination

Other food safety concerns relate to industrial waste chemicals, such as heavy metals, mercury, dioxins and polychlorinated biphenyls (PCBs), which contaminate the air, water and land, and enter our food and drinking water.

Mercury, predominantly the result of air pollution that comes from coal burned in power plants, seeps into the ocean, contaminating fish and shellfish. It is considered the most dangerous environmental poison of all the toxic heavy metals (see below)[350]. Dioxins, which are spewed out of municipal incinerators burning PVC plastics, are said to be even worse: "the most dangerous substance ever produced." And PCBs, previously made for use in electric equipment, are also extremely damaging[351].

Industrial contaminants are known to concentrate in animal fats, particularly fish, meat, milk, and milk products.

Fish from Troubled Waters

Seafood tends to be particularly high in toxins, and many experts recommend that certain fish be excluded from our diets altogether, while others only be consumed in limited quantities. Big predatory fish typically have higher pollutant levels since toxins get concentrated as you go up the food chain. (Animal products have higher toxin content than plant products for this same reason.) Fatty species of fish are particularly contaminated. Also, farmed fish tend to have higher levels of contamination than wild[352]. (The Appendix provides details on toxin levels in specific species.)

Mercury Contamination

Mercury is probably the biggest concern for fish eaters. Surprisingly, mercury by itself is not very toxic. If you eat it straight, you probably wouldn't absorb very much through your digestive tract. However, when it gets into the water, microorganisms "methylate" it, turning it into methylmercury. Plankton absorb the methylmercury, get eaten by small fish that also absorb some of the methylmercury, and it continues up the food chain until it gets to humans. And in that form, it's easily absorbable.

Symptoms of methylmercury poisoning are vague and hard to pin down, including muscle weakness, fatigue, headaches, irritability, difficulty concentrating, perhaps numbness and tingling. Many of these symptoms could be caused by other disturbances, making diagnosis difficult. There is certainly question that many of the kids diagnosed with Attention Deficit Hyperactivity Disorder (ADHD) could actually be suffering methylmercury poisoning, perhaps as a result of high consumption of canned tuna.

The Institute of Medicine encourages everyone to minimize consumption of the fish that are highest in methylmercury, especially tilefish, shark, tuna, and swordfish – and suggests that pregnant or lactating women and children avoid them entirely.

Canned tuna is particularly popular in many American households. According to FDA tests, albacore tuna is particularly high in mercury. Most canned "light" tuna has only 1/3 as much mercury as albacore, making it a generally better choice. However, some (6 percent) "light" tuna contained at least as much mercury - in some cases more than twice as much - as the average in albacore, a level that the FDA judges unsafe for pregnant women. The FDA has not warned consumers about those occasionally higher mercury levels. According to a Chicago Tribune investigative report[353], a top FDA official admitted they wished to 'keep the market share at a reasonable level." That's comforting, isn't it?

All seafood is contaminated with methylmercury, although amounts vary widely. The appendix will help you sort out the ones with higher amounts.

Pesticides

Insects have been around much longer than humans: probably about 350 million years compared to our meager 2 million years. During this time they have developed an amazing ability to adapt to their environment. Like us, they need to eat. And they often share our favorite foods.

Pesticides are poisons, used against the insects and other animals that eat our crops. Agriculture is the heaviest user of pesticides[354]. The human body isn't immune to their effects: most of them are poisonous for us as well as the pests[355].

While pesticides are certainly effective at killing insects, mass killing does not seem to be a very effective long-range plan, given our dependency on insects. Wiping out insects entirely means the destruction of our species as well. We need insects for many reasons, probably the largest being that they help pollinate our plants. Pollinator loss is a costly side effect of pesticide use, and now growers often must resort to artificial means of pollinating their crops[356].

The insects are also too smart: they simply build resistance and come back. Genetic adaptation happens quickly when an animal has such a short life span! In areas where pesticides have been used longest and heaviest, insect damage to crops is now worse than before farmers started using them[356]. Even though the use of insecticides increased 10-fold from 1945 to 1989 in the U.S., crop losses from insects nearly doubled in the same time period, from 7 percent to 13 percent[356]. So pesticide usage also doesn't seem to address the problem of pests.

In addition, the number of insects resistant to pesticides increased dramatically over the same time period[356]. As pesticides become less effective, many growers are increasing the quantities of chemicals they use[356].

The damage pesticides pose to wildlife is well-documented. As an example, an estimated 672 million birds are exposed to pesticides every year in the United States from agricultural pesticide use alone. An estimated 10 percent, or 67 million of these birds, die from this exposure[356].

"Body burden" data (tests that evaluate pesticide loads in humans) gathered by the Centers for Disease Control[357] show there are many pesticides in our bodies that are well above officially permitted thresholds established by health and regulatory agencies[355]. One pesticide was so far above permitted levels, that vulnerable populations (which includes women, children and the elderly) exceed the officially established "acceptable" dose for chronic exposure[355].

Clearly, ingesting pesticides isn't good for humans, but how damaging are they? No one really knows the answer to this question, but many suspect the answer is "pretty bad!" One reason we don't know the answer is because it's hard to clearly document cause and effect in the etiology of many of the disease processes that may be related to pesticides. To what extent we can attribute pesticide usage to cancer, for example, is unclear, as there are many other contributors to cancer which can't be adequately separated out in the research.

Along with their cancer risk, pesticides can cause a myriad of other health problems, including reproductive concerns, such as disruption of our hormonal systems, decreased fertility, low infant birth weight, and birth defects[358, 359]. As an example, research documents a 40 percent decline in sperm count over the last half of the century[355], and while there is no widely agreed explanation, some studies have linked this to pesticide exposure[360, 361].

Currently, at least 5,000 agricultural workers from Nicaragua, Costa Rica, Guatemala, Honduras and Panama have filed five lawsuits in this country claiming they were left sterile after being exposed to the pesticide known as DBCP[362].

Research also suggests that a number of degenerative diseases which are on the rise, such as Parkinson's Disease and Amyotrophic Lateral Sclerosis (otherwise known as Lou Gehrig's Disease), may be due to toxic injury to parts of the brain from increasing pesticide usage[363].

Another complication in cataloguing the effects of pesticides is that it is difficult to understand the impact of dosage. It is clear, for example, that pesticides are to blame for the extremely high rates of cancer and birth defects among farm workers[364]. One study compared Hispanic California farm workers with the general Hispanic population, and showed that the farm workers were more likely to develop certain types of leukemia by 59 percent, stomach cancer by 70 percent, cervical cancer by 63 percent, and uterine cancer by 68 percent[364]. However, we don't know if that means that they are dangerous in the low doses many of us are exposed to through eating. (That they are damaging to workers should be reason alone to reconsider their use, of course. Unfortunately, we tend to view agricultural workers as disposable, rarely considering protections for their health or human rights.)

Government standards on "acceptable" levels of pesticides in food aren't reassuring. Most standards are based on acute toxicity (that is, immediate harm, not chronic exposure) of single compounds. It seems logical that chronic exposure affects us differently[365], but this is not considered. And farmers typically use numerous pesticides, each up to their legal limit. The combined toxic load caused by consuming legal amounts of multiple toxic residues simultaneously could easily be more than our body defenses can handle[366], although again, this is not considered. Longer term tests for carcinogens are conducted on rats and mice; there are obvious difficulties in extrapolating these results to humans.

Even more alarming is that most of the toxicity testing is conducted by the manufacturers. To get an idea of what's behind the curtain, a professor of developmental endocrinology at the University of California-Berkeley, compared several previous experiments performed by others on the effect of atrazine, a popular corn pesticide, on frogs' sexual differentiation[367]. Seven of the studies were paid for by Syngenta, the manufacturer; nine others were funded by independent sources. Every one of the Syngenta-funded studies concluded that atrazine did not affect amphibian gonads, while all but one of the independent studies found that the chemical did have an effect. His conclusion: the Syngenta studies didn't falsify data; they were simply designed to find "no effect" by exposing both the control and experimental groups to insufficient atrazine. This hardly makes me feel secure!

Also, government regulation doesn't protect us against many known carcinogens. For example, several pesticides that are banned for use in the United States are commonly used in other countries which then export the pesticide-laden produce to us. There have been multiple instances where U.S. manufacturers were producing pesticides that were later banned; they continued to sell these pesticides to other countries after the ban[368]. This contributes to what is known as a circle of poison: we recognize a pesticide as carcinogenic, ban it, import food grown with it, and consume it on our food.

Not that the United States is overly tough when compared to other countries in regulating pesticides. In fact, several of U.S. agriculture's most popular herbicides and pesticides, including atrazine, endosulfan and aldicarb, are illegal or restricted to emergency uses in other countries. Industry groups say their products have undergone rigorous reviews in the United States and are not only legal here but safe. They say some governments, particularly the European Union, have overreacted and banned chemicals with little or no evidence of a human health threat.

Herein lies the difference: The European Union has banned many substances, in response to consumer concerns, by invoking the precautionary principle, which is codified into law. Precaution prescribes that protective steps be taken when there is scientific evidence of risks to public health or the environment. Unlike EU policies, U.S. law requires the EPA to prove a toxic substance "presents an unreasonable risk of injury to health or the environment," consider the costs of restricting its use and choose "the least burdensome" approach to regulate industry" [quotation from the Toxic Control Substances Act][369].

Pesticides are particularly concerning when it comes to the health of children[355]. When the EPA sets a pesticide tolerance for the pesticides found on foods, it is based on their estimate of what an adult male can tolerate, which they then reduce by a factor of ten to accommodate the greater sensitivity of women and children[355]. The factor of ten is clearly not enough to protect infants and children. They are particularly vulnerable as they don't have as well developed body defenses to fight off toxins, and also because they take in a lot more food relative to their body weight than adults do[355]. (At ages one through five, kids eat three to four times more food per pound of body weight than adults!) Centers for Disease Control data shows that young children carry particularly high body burdens, with some pesticides registering at nearly twice that of adults[355].

The National Research Council of the National Academy of Sciences (NAS) issued a report in 1993 which stated that pesticide residues set for adults could cause permanent loss of brain function for fetuses and children[370]. NAS warns that children may be ingesting dangerous levels of carcinogens, even under current EPA "allowable limits."

The question of how bad pesticides are when considering the health of the environment is clear: they are devastating. Pesticides persist in the environment – in water, for example – with disastrous effects on other animals, such as frogs, fish and birds.

Given how threatening the increasing interest in organics is to conventional agriculture, it is not surprising that there is an active dis-information campaign. The Hudson Institute, for example, funded by large agribusiness corporations such as Archer Daniels Midland, Cargill, ConAgra, and Monsanto, denies that they are an environmental disaster, a danger to wildlife, and a hazard to human health. Oh, please! While research can't quantify the dangers posed by pesticides, that they're harmful is certainly not up for debate, regardless of whether you are a scientist or just use your common sense.

Don't worry: the government is protecting us?

Even the staff of the Environmental Protection Agency finds our poor pesticide regulation appalling and dangerous. The union representing the views of nine thousand EPA scientists wrote a strongly worded letter to the head administrator of the EPA, protesting that "industry pressure" is compromising the "integrity of the science upon which agency decisions are based."[371, 372] The letter objected to the imminent approval of dangerous pesticides without completing adequate hazard evaluations and called for a ban on pesticides known to be highly toxic. The letter stated that they believed that under priorities of EPA management, "the concerns of agriculture and the pesticide industry come before our responsibility to protect the health of our nation's citizens."

Political influence at the Food & Drug Administration (FDA) is also deeply concerning. Nearly one-fifth (18.4 percent) of the FDA scientists who responded to a survey conducted by the Union of Concerned Scientists said that they "have been asked, for non-scientific reasons, to inappropriately exclude or alter technical information or their conclusions in a FDA scientific document."[373] Forty percent fear retaliation for voicing safety concerns in public. More than a third of the respondents did not feel they could express safety concerns even inside the agency. This fear, scientists say, combines with other pressures to compromise the agency's ability to protect public health and safety.

Avoiding/Minimizing Pesticide Consumption

Our best goal is to peacefully coexist with insects, which is what organic farmers strive for. Organic crops are grown without synthetic pesticides. Organic farmers use methods such as crop rotation, and planting nonfood crops nearby that lure pests away from food crops. Releasing sterile fruit flies into orchards is another helpful method: because fruit flies don't produce offspring when they mate with sterile partners, the overall fruit fly population drops. Buying organic foods is your protection against pesticides.

When purchasing conventional foods (meaning non-organic foods), understand the principle of bio-magnification: pesticides (and other toxins) get concentrated as you go up the food chain.

Consider what occurred with DDT, a pesticide that was originally considered to be safe and was used for over 25 years before it was finally banned. When it was sprayed on farm crops, some of it ended up in rivers, lakes and oceans. Plankton absorbed it, and then when shellfish ate the plankton, they became contaminated too. Bigger fish ate the shellfish, seals ate those bigger fish, and killer whales ate the seals. And of course when animals eat smaller animals or plants, they don't just eat one or two, they may eat thousands or millions throughout their lifetime.

By the time the DDT gets into the killer whale, it is millions of times stronger than when it first contaminated the plankton. This is because toxins can get stored and accumulate in fatty tissue of animals. When animals eat other animals, they're also ingesting the toxins stored in their prey's fat. Due to biological magnification and being at the top of the food chain, it's the whale that suffered the most from DDT poisoning – and whale pups in particular. Young animals (including humans) typically take in more food relative to their body weight than adults, and additionally don't have as well developed defenses.

And who else is at the top of the food chain? Humans, of course. And the most vulnerable humans are kids. Also vulnerable is anyone with a compromised immune system. So if you want to protect yourself, when you do consume conventionally produced foods, eat lower on the food chain.

When considering plants, it helps to recognize that pesticides are differentially applied to different crops. The appendix provides a list of the more contaminated crops; you may want to compromise and go organic for these. Also, be aware that domestic pesticide restrictions are often tighter than those found in many other countries, making crops grown in the U.S. typically a little safer.

Washing and rinsing produce will help reduce pesticide residues, but it does not eliminate them entirely. Peeling will eliminate some of the residue, but valuable nutrients will go down the drain with the peel. Also, many fruits and vegetables contain wax on the peel, which helps to seal in some of the pesticides. The best option is to choose organic when possible, wash all produce, and avoid waxed products or peel them.

And don't let pesticides scare you away from fruits and vegetables. Ultimately, you're better off eating produce with pesticide contamination than not eating produce.

The "USDA Organic" label holds foods to a rigorous standard and independent certification. Trust it! (While it may not guarantee that a product was grown sustainably, a topic to be discussed in the next chapter, it does provide assurance that the product was grown without synthetic pesticides.) Other trustworthy labels include TransFair USA's "Fair Trade Certified, and Northeast Organic Farming Association's "Certified Organic." Do not trust the "Earth Friendly, Farm Friendly" seal. This was created by the Center for Global Food Issues, which is an offshoot of the Hudson Institute, a group funded by agribusiness, chemical and pesticide manufacturers, the biotechnology industry and others. They oppose organic farming.

Food Additives

Would you like some butylated hydroxyanisole (BHA) with that? Given this option in a restaurant, you'd probably flinch. Yet BHA is a common preservative and odds are you're consuming it regularly if you eat cereals and potato chips or chew gum.

Food additives have become increasingly more commonplace in our foods. The good news is that the vast majority are benign. Additives like sugar, salt, and baking powder, for example, have been used for years and appear to have no deleterious effects when used in moderation.

However, there are clearly some additives for which caution is recommended, BHA among them. The Center for Science in the Public Interest includes the following on a list of compounds that are unsafe or are poorly tested: acesulfame potassium, artificial colorings: blue 1, blue 2, green 3, red 3, yellow 6, butylated hydroxyanisole (BHA), potassium bromate, sodium nitrate, and sodium nitrite. Please see their report for more details on these and a more comprehensive listing: http://www.cspinet.org/reports/chemcuisine.htm.

The safety of each of the additives is probably less important to consider than the question of why an additive is being used. Additives are typically markers for low-nutrient processed foods.

Afterward

Food safety is clearly much more than practicing good hygiene and cooking foods well – some issues are beyond our control. This section highlights inadequacies in protecting our food supply – and makes the point that we can't trust that our food supply is safe and that our government is sufficiently protecting us. Economic interests play a large role in determining what gets to our plate – with consumers' best interests often trailing dismally behind. The greatest tragedy of food-borne illness is that it is largely preventable.

Writing this section proved particularly difficult. As I was examining government documents and scientific research, my concern about food safety mounted and I found myself increasingly paranoid about everything I ate; I was viewing food as a biohazard as opposed to a vehicle for nurturing myself.

What can you do to facilitate viewing your hamburger as food and not a biohazard? First, recognize that food safety is often a relative term – and only you can determine if a food seems safe enough for your standards. You can't live life risk-free. Every time you cross the street you do so with the belief that any dangers associated with the risk of getting hit by a car are far outweighed by the advantages of getting where you want to go. Hopefully, you do what you can to minimize the risk, looking in both directions before you step out.

I want to encourage you to learn more about the issues – and decide for yourself the benefits and risks that are involved in eating different foods. You may find that you believe my interpretation of some of the risks to be exaggerated, for example, and that I err too much on the side of caution (and outrage). A lot of my concerns are about the unknown: for example, how prevalent is Mad Cow Disease in our cattle?

Next, I want to encourage activism. There are plenty of ways to make yourself heard by government and industry – and the more they know we care, the more it becomes in their best interests to prioritize our health and safety. And don't underestimate the power behind your purchases. Buying organic food, for example, will not only get you healthier food and a host of other benefits, but it supports the organic movement (which will eventually make organic foods cheaper), and takes money out of the pocket of the pesticide industry.

There are plenty of wonderful consumer groups that can support you in making change. You *can* make a difference.

Action Tips...

Bacterial Contamination (Note: Looking at, smelling, and even tasting our food, rarely tells us if it is tainted. Protect yourself!)

- Wash hands/foods/cutting surfaces well.
- Practice safe handling techniques and avoid cross-contamination.
- Cook foods (meats/poultry/eggs/fish) adequately.
- Keep hot foods hot, and cold foods cold.
- Refrigerate leftovers.
- Eat lower on the food chain.

Industrial Contamination

- See the appendix to learn about the contamination of specific fish species.
- Choose foods lower in fat.
- Don't microwave most plastics or plastic cling wraps as this can induce the plastics to leach chemicals into the foods.

Pesticides

- Go organic!
- Compromise: If you don't want to choose completely organic products, choose organic for products that are more contaminated. (See the appendix for a guide to contamination levels in produce.)
- Wash produce well (although this won't eliminate most pesticide residue).
- Buy unwaxed products or peel waxed products.
- Reduce your consumption of animal products.

Antibiotic-Resistance

- Choose products produced without antibiotics. Many producers that do not use antibiotics have been certified organic. Others raise livestock according to animal welfare standards set by private organizations, and approved by the USDA. On meat and poultry, labels that say "raised without the use of antibiotics" or "no antibiotics administered" assure buyers that the animals didn't consume any antibiotics. More common are labels that indicate the producer has limited how antibiotics were used. For example, products labeled as "Certified Humane" indicate that animals weren't given antibiotics subtherapeutically; they may, however, have been treated therapeutically.
- Choose GMO-free products as antibiotic resistance markers are inserted when genetically modifying foods.

Mad Cow Disease

- For the best possible protection, stop eating meat and meat by-products.
- If you want to eat beef, here are some strategies to limit your risk:
  - Choose organic or 100 percent grass-fed beef.
  - Avoid cow brains and processed beef products that may contain nervous-system tissue, such as hamburger, hot dogs, and sausage.
  - Have your steak and hamburger ground while you watch.
  - Avoid foods that contain broth made from meat, such as gelatin.

Bird Flu

- Cook chicken and eggs well to prevent contracting it from food, in the event that it gets into our food supply.
- The larger concern down the line is contracting it from an infected person. In this case, flu protection techniques are valuable, such as washing your hands well.

The Global Picture

Most suggestions above are individual solutions. However, we also need to fix, in the words of Marion Nestle, "our highly dysfunctional food safety system."[374] Prevention has to be part of our game plan. The current system produces large quantities of food at low cost, but it does so at steep price, one not included at the checkout stand. The lack of regulation and regulatory power of government agencies is appalling; industry is essentially left to voluntarily regulate itself – and they are clearly not doing an effective job.

Educate yourself on the issues. Have an opinion? Talk to your friends and get the word out! There are also plenty of ways to support efforts to influence lawmakers. The Get Informed section will give you some leads to get connected with others concerned about these issues.

Get informed...

The best general book on food safety issues is Marion Nestle's *Safe Food, Bacteria, Biotechnology and Bioterrorism*. Eric Schlosser's *Fast Food Nation* also has some relevant chapters.

The industry perspective is easily accessible in traditional textbooks. You can also check out the largest meat and poultry trade association, the American Meat Institute, at www.meatami.org, or another trade organization for the meat industry, the National Cattlemen's Beef Association (http://www.beef.org/) for their perspectives on issues such as Animal Cruelty, Mad Cow Disease, Food Safety, and Antibiotic Use. Enjoy the pictures of happy cows and wide open grazing meadows.

The Center for Disease Control gives you the government's perspective on food safety issues: http://www.cdc.gov/ncidod/diseases/food/safety.htm.

Here are some sample websites for more alternative views, most of which provide you with additional links:

The organization, Safe Tables our Priority, wrote a good report on **food safety** issues, which can be accessed at: http://www.safetables.org/pdf/STOP_Report.pdf.

Check out Center for Science in the Public Interest's Guide to **Food Additives**, http://www.cspinet.org/reports/chemcuisine.htm) which provides an easy to use database of additives and their safety. Their "Chemical Cuisine" database provides a convenient summary of the research on many food additives.

The Institute for Agriculture and Trade Policy (www.iatp.org) has a Smart Fish Calculator to help you learn levels of **toxins** in different species of fish. They also provide great information on **antibiotic resistance** through their Antibiotic Resistance Project: http://www.iatp.org/foodandhealth/issues_antibioticsanimals.cfm. Their Eat Well guide can help you find foods produced without antibiotics: http://www.eatwellguide.org/.

For more information about **pesticides**, check out the Pesticide Action Network North America at http://www.panna.org.

The best resource on **Mad Cow Disease** can be found at the Organic Consumers Association, http://www.organicconsumers.org/, which is moderated by Michael Greger, M.D.

Dr. Greger also wrote a book called *Bird Flu: A Virus of Our Own Making*, available for free download at: www.birdflubook.com.

Mad Cow USA, by Rampton and Stauber, is a great book you can download for free at http://www.prwatch.org/books/madcow.html.

John Robbins' book, *The Food Revolution*, covers most of the topics in this section.

Biotechnology

Biotechnology refers to using living things to make or modify new products.

Let me acknowledge my bias up front. I'm a big fan of biotech. Some of the stuff biotech has allowed us to do is amazing. Think of the simple act of using yeast to make bread. Yeast is alive. Put some of these living organisms into a mix of flour and water, feed them a bit of sugar, and they're happy. As they exhale carbon dioxide, the dough rises. Biotech in action. This is good stuff. And how many of us really want to forgo beer, which depends on fermenting bacteria? Or deny safe insulin - which is produced in genetically engineered bacteria - to people with diabetes?

Of course, sometimes biotech gets a bit more ethically complex than rising bread or fermenting beer. Consider genetic modification. Is it okay to genetically modify chickens so that they become pharmaceutical factories for human medicines? To implant human genes into plants (which we then eat)? What about giving animals growth hormones – with the result that their "meat" grows larger in proportion to the organs that support them?

So far, the biotech industry has given us three major tools to "improve" our food supply: pesticides, food irradiation and genetic modification. We've already discussed pesticides, and in this chapter we'll address the controversial topics of food irradiation and genetic modification. You'll see that as much as I'm a devotee of biotechnology in general, I don't believe that it has served us well in nutrition.

Food Irradiation

For lunch today someone bit into a hamburger that had been exposed to a very high dose of radiation: the equivalent of 150 million chest x-rays - and sprinkled with spices treated with the equivalent of 1 billion chest x-rays[375]. Sounds serious, doesn't it? Wonder what happens to the food?

Well, first, to dispel a common myth, you can rest assured that the food – and the packaging - is not radioactive[376]. The gamma radiation that is utilized doesn't elicit neutrons, which are the subatomic particles that make substances radioactive. Simple tests conducted with a Geiger counter verify that irradiated food is not radioactive. So no need to don your lead apron next time you chomp down on that irradiated burger.

When food is irradiated, it is subject to a blast of ionizing radiation which disrupts the DNA of bacteria, parasites, mold and fungus; this kills them or renders them incapable of proliferating. After reading the food safety section, I'm sure you've got a heightened awareness of how badly contaminated our food is and how beneficial that could be.

In the process, the food's shelf life also increases. Irradiating strawberries, for example, can extend their shelf life from the usual 3 to 5 days to approximately 22 days[377]. Again, I'm sure you can imagine how beneficial that can be: it certainly makes it much easier to get those strawberries to market before spoilage.

While irradiating foods poses some advantages, it also has some limitations and drawbacks. One limitation is that irradiating food doesn't wipe out the problem of pests entirely. At the level it is conducted on food, for example, it can't kill the bacteria responsible for botulism (clostridium botulinum)[378]. Because it doesn't kill all bacteria, the hardier bacteria can breed, which may eventually result in the increasing prevalence of radiation-resistant bacteria.

Nor does it inactivate dangerous toxins which have already been produced by bacteria prior to irradiation. In the case of C. botulinum, it is the toxin produced by the bacteria, rather than the bacteria itself, which poses the health hazard.

Another disadvantage is that helpful bacteria that aid digestion and may alter the nutritional value of a food are also killed in the process[378].

Food irradiation also damages nutritional content[378]. For example, vitamin B complex is particularly vulnerable and can be up to 96 percent lower than is commonly found in the same non-irradiated foods. (Most vitamins are much less vulnerable and show minimal decrement.) As shelf life increases, more nutrients are lost.

It is also evident that irradiation creates known carcinogens like benzene[379, 380] and formaldehyde, other toxic chemicals[381], as well as new and unidentified chemicals that have not been tested for safety[382, 383]. While the long-term health consequences are unknown, many speculate that these carcinogens are created in such small quantity as to be irrelevant.

Irradiation also changes the taste of some (not all) foods. In August 2003, Consumer Reports described that professional taste tests found irradiated meat to have a "scorched "taste and a smell reminiscent of singed hair[384]." Numerous studies corroborate that it can result in an off-odor, taste or texture[385-389].

Irradiation is also expensive. The USDA estimated that it may add between 13 and 20 cents per pound to the cost of ground beef[390]. When they actually obtained bids for the National School Lunch Program they found that this estimate had vastly underestimated the cost[391]. The cost differential in the retail marketplace is even higher[392].

And of course, the food can be re-infected between the time it is irradiated, shipped, sold and prepared by the consumer. For example, irradiation is unlikely to eliminate E. coli, since E. coli is often re-introduced after irradiation.

Nor does it address the range of food safety concerns: for example, it does not kill viruses (like hepatitis) or prions (that cause Mad Cow Disease).

But the largest complaint posed against irradiating foods is that it does nothing to change the conditions that cause the rampant contamination in the first place, or to prevent the contamination. "After all," writes food safety advocate Carol Tucker Foreman, "sterilized poop is still poop."[393]

In other words, food irradiation is a Band-aid for a much larger problem of food sanitation – and not a very effective one. Cleaning up factory farms will go a long way toward minimizing the bacterial contamination. And adequate attention to food safety can keep you protected after the fact. (Cooking meat sufficiently is more effective at killing harmful bacteria than irradiation.)

The agricultural industry strongly supports food irradiation. Because irradiation extends the shelf life of food, food lasts longer and can be shipped longer distances. Food can be grown in other countries, where labor is cheap and environmental and regulatory laws are not as strict. It also shields industry from addressing the issue of why contamination is so widespread in the first place, and the need to clean up factory farms.

The meat industry is actively engaged in trying to increase public acceptance of irradiation and is pushing for a new term to be used, "cold pasteurization," as they are concerned that "irradiation" has negative associations within the general public and that calling it what it is will limit its acceptability.

Many foods are already government-approved for irradiation, and it is increasingly more commonly conducted. You have already eaten irradiated food, although it is unlikely that you have been informed. Though labeling laws require irradiated foods to be labeled, there are many instances in which you won't be informed.

For example, labeling laws apply only to irradiated *whole* foods. This means that if you eat it in restaurants, schools, or in processed foods that contain irradiated ingredients but aren't irradiated themselves, you may never know. (Most irradiated hamburger and chicken is going directly to restaurants, not consumers – and many processed foods contain irradiated ingredients. Canned soups, for example, may contain irradiated potatoes, onions or spices – and won't be labeled.)

When it is noted on a food label, it will be accompanied by the radura symbol (which to me resembles a stylized flower, hardly the image that irradiation conjures up for me). Apparently, the petals are intended to represent the food, the central circle the radiation source, and the broken circle the rays from the energy source.

Bottom line? I'm not too concerned about the dangers of irradiated foods. But I am concerned that it distracts us from more appropriately addressing contamination problems earlier. Irradiation is a cheap attempt by industry to avoid taking responsibility for cleaner practices. And while I understand that extended shelf-life may benefit large scale producers, I'd much prefer to buy fresher, tastier, more nutritious food from a small local farmer. All told, what it really comes down to is this: I'd rather eat clean food than sterilized feces.

Genetically Modified Organisms (GMO)

Genetic modification of food is also quite controversial. While industry promotes it as the ultimate tool to fight anything that ails consumers, farmers or the environment, many consumer advocates and environmentalists challenge their contentions.

What is genetic engineering?

Genetic engineering is not a new concept. We have altered the genes of almost every food we eat, over almost 10,000 years of selective breeding. For example, farmers have re-planted seeds from their best crops, or cross-pollinated (mixed the seeds) the seeds from different plants which had desirable traits. When we mix all of a plant's tens of thousands of genes, getting a desired trait is akin to winning a lottery – making this type of engineering a long, slow process.

Today, we can produce changes by selecting a gene that may result in a desired trait and inserting it directly into the plant. (However, it should be acknowledged that we don't have as much control as that sounds and a lot of trial and error – and luck - is still required.)

Genetically modified organisms (GMOs) contain a gene that has been artificially inserted instead of the plant (or animal) acquiring it through pollination or breeding. The term "transgenic" is used interchangeably (or GMO foods are more derogatively referred to as "Frankenfoods").

One way this differs from traditional breeding is that in traditional breeding, genes of only closely related organisms (such as a wheat plant and its wild relatives) can be exchanged. Through artificial insertion, on the other hand, the gene can come from an unrelated plant (e.g., a disease resistance gene can be transferred from rice to wheat) or a different species (e.g., a cold tolerance gene can be transferred from a fish to a strawberry). Nature may not have allowed a fish to mate with a tomato, but laboratory techniques allow us to break this barrier.

That means that genetically engineered foods can carry traits that were never previously in our foods. There is even some current research being conducted on transferring human genes into plants. Japanese researchers, for example, have recently inserted a gene from the human liver into rice to enable it to digest pesticides and industrial chemicals. The gene makes an enzyme which is particularly good at breaking down harmful chemicals in the body. Critics complain that the partially human-derived food is a move towards cannibalism.

A U.S. firm also recently reported successfully implanting human genes into chickens so that they lay eggs carrying vast numbers of antibodies that fight cancer[394]. If this research further develops, chickens could essentially become pharmaceutical factories with wings.

The biotechnology industry makes grandiose claims regarding nutritional advantages provided by GMOs. For example, much media attention has been given to "golden rice," a variety of rice that has been engineered to contain higher levels of beta-carotene, a substance which the body can convert to Vitamin A. The new rice was heralded as a miracle cure for vitamin A deficiency, a condition which afflicts millions of people in developing countries.

Vitamin A deficiency can cause partial or total blindness, and less severe deficiencies weaken the immune system. Each year, it is estimated that deficiency causes blindness in 350,000 pre-school age children, and it is implicated in over one million deaths.

At first glance, then, golden rice would seem to be magic. But more scrutiny reveals that the magic has been limited to public relations for the biotech industry. Most of the media neglected to inform us that a child would have to eat at least 12 pounds of the stuff a day to get a day's minimum dietary requirement of vitamin A[3]. Even then, they may not be able to absorb the nutrient, because in order to convert the beta-carotene to vitamin A, the body needs sufficient dietary fat and protein, which is not something malnourished children who eat only rice are likely to have.

There is tremendous potential for GMOs to have nutritional advantages, and research has been conducted on engineering potatoes to absorb less oil when fried, higher fiber corn, oils with less saturated fat, and added vitamins and minerals in several foods. Unfortunately, none of these have hit the market yet. In other words, the promise of GMOs is more about potential than reality.

Private industry claims that growing GMOs will conquer world hunger. The reality is that we already produce much more food than is necessary to feed the entire world population: the problem is one of distribution rather than insufficiency[395]. (See the World Hunger and Food Insecurity chapter for more details.) Furthermore, genetically engineered crops have not been found to increase crop yields[396-399]. These and many other issues combine to make it much more likely that GMO crops will continue to increase starvation rather than solve the problem.

What's really going on is that despite the lip service being given to improving the food supply, agricultural biotechnology has been profit-driven rather than need-driven[400]. In fact, the majority of GMOs grown today have been engineered to be herbicide-tolerant (nearly 80 percent!) or pesticide-resistant[401].

An herbicide is a poison that can kill plants. It is frequently sprayed on weeds to prohibit them from taking important water or nutrients from the soil, thus supporting the growth of the crops that the farmer intends to grow. Ordinarily, herbicides also kill the intended crops, so they need to be used judiciously in order to kill the weed, but not the crops that you are intending to grow.

When a plant is genetically modified to become herbicide-tolerant, the plant is engineered to resist an herbicide. This means that farmers can spray massive amounts of herbicide to kill the weeds, without concern that they will also kill their intended crops. While private industry told us this would reduce herbicide and pesticide usage, the opposite has occurred: since farmers know that they can't damage their crops by spraying herbicides and pesticides, they use them in even greater quantity[402]. And of course, there is a huge side benefit to industry: the companies making the GMOs also make the herbicides, and selling the GMO seeds increases herbicide sales.

Indeed, many crops have been genetically engineered to be resistant to Roundup (an herbicide), and Roundup is now the third most commonly reported cause of illness among California farm workers and the top cause among landscape workers. It has also been documented to cause many environmental problems, including damage to plants and wildlife. As an example, the U.S. Fish and Wildlife Service found 74 plant species that are potentially endangered by glyphosphate[403], the active ingredient in Roundup.

And of course, when herbicide is applied, a few hardy weeds survive; they multiply while the others die. Soon the hardy weeds dominate - and farmers find themselves without an easy way to manage the new weed problem. It is only a matter of time before Roundup-resistant weeds develop in our food crops. This has already occurred with Monsanto's genetically-engineered cotton, and farmers are hurting.

Also concerning is that some genetically engineered foods, such as potatoes and corn, are engineered to produce pesticides in every cell so that the pesticide will kill the pest that indulges[401]. Because the pesticide is not a food, it is exempt from regulation by the Food and Drug Administration. For example, the New Leaf potato was deemed a pesticide and mandated to be regulated by the Environmental Protection Agency (EPA)[404, 405], not the Food & Drug Administration (FDA) which regulates food, even though it was produced for human consumption. Given that safety testing in the EPA is not as strict as the FDA, this is clearly problematic. (The New Leaf potato is no longer on the market.)

How necessary is it to breed plants that tolerate chemical herbicides or produce their own pesticides? Do they really deliver genuine benefits to consumers? Or is it another cheap shot to bolster large agribusiness – at a cost to consumer/environmental safety?

Not that much scrutiny is given to safety testing in the FDA anyway. In fact, the FDA does not require safety tests on genetically modified foods. They justify their position by stating that "The agency is not aware of any information showing that foods derived by these new methods differ from other foods in any meaningful or uniform way"[406] How they came to this position is entirely unclear as documents made public from a lawsuit revealed that FDA experts had actually previously agreed that genetically modified foods are different and might lead to allergens, toxins, new diseases or nutritional problems[407]. These FDA experts testified that they had urged their superiors to require long-term safety studies, but were ignored.

A peer-reviewed article in *Biotechnology and Genetic Engineering Reviews* identified numerous health risks of GM foods that are not being tested for, and cited "serious deficiencies in both regulatory oversight and corporate testing procedures."[408] While there are many opinions about the safety of GM foods, there is little data[409].

And here's some wonderful irony that I have to share with you. Staff at the British headquarters of Monsanto, the largest producer of GM seeds, eat only non-genetically modified products on their lunch breaks[410, 411]. Apparently the contractor that maintains the canteen is said to be concerned about health risks.

On another note, imagine having a kid who is allergic to Brazil nuts. You scan food labels carefully to ensure that there are no Brazil nuts in her foods. Well, GMOs could bring new allergens into foods that you would not know to avoid. This isn't just theory. A study by scientists at the University of Nebraska shows that soybeans genetically engineered to contain Brazil-nut proteins cause reactions in individuals allergic to Brazil nuts. Since no labeling is required, a parent would never know.

Scientists have limited ability to predict whether a particular protein will be a food allergen if consumed by humans. The only sure way to determine whether a protein will be an allergen is through experience. So we're gambling, and when people die, then we'll know to take it off the market. This hardly seems like sound science!

There are many other environmental concerns as well, including genetic contamination of the environment. For example, StarLink is a variety of GM corn used for animal feed and was not approved for human consumption. However, once any crop is released into the environment, genetic drift occurs. StarLink has been found in hundreds of foods. We may have the power to recall the tortillas, but we don't have the power to get rid of them or recall GMOs!

Organic farmers are particularly concerned. If there are genetically modified crops growing in their area, or a truck carrying GMO grain drives past their organic farm, pollen is going to wind up in their field. It also gets there by way of the birds, butterflies, bees, and the wind. Then, not only is the crop no longer organic, but also if that seed is harvested the next season, you stand in violation of the patent owner's rights and you will have to pay for it. There are several cases where organic farmers have been sued for unwittingly growing crops as a result of genetic drift – crops that of course they didn't even want.

Another large concern is that genetically modified crops will continue to force small farmers out of business. Monsanto, for example, has created (with funding from the government) their "technology protection system" which renders seeds sterile. (Critics call it terminator technology or suicide seeds.) Saving seeds from season to season is how farmers have been able to continue growing food over the years. This new technology forces farmers to buy seed each year from a major corporation, taking farming away from the farmers.

Many consumer advocates oppose all patents on plants, animals and humans, and on their genes, suggesting that life should not be a commodity.

Genetic modification also limits biodiversity, another substantial threat to ecological sustainability.

Also, genetic engineering is far from precise. For example, one common way to introduce artificial genes into a plant or animal is to blast genes into DNA with a gene gun. Scientists coat tiny shards of gold or tungsten with the foreign genes and fire it into a dish of cells, hoping that at least some of the foreign genes will end up in the right place. They don't understand how the DNA shot into a cell actually gets incorporated into the cell's DNA, nor can they control the process. They just shoot the DNA into the cell using trial and error until they are satisfied with the results. This process always causes mutations, mutations which can alter the functioning of the organism. However, the mutations can't be adequately tested for, given the complexity of living organisms. The mutations may not have a noticeable immediate effect, and may not be realized until it is too late.

In fact, this has already occurred. Scientists genetically engineered bacteria to make tryptophan, a popular supplement sold as a sleep aid. The bacteria effectively made the tryptophan, but also created a toxin which was not discovered in the research lab. The tryptophan was put on the market. The result? Fifteen hundred Americans permanently disabled and 37 dead.

Also of concern is the current use of antibiotic-resistant genes to mark cells that have taken up foreign genes. The presence of antibiotic-resistance genes in foods could have two harmful effects. First, it is possible that eating these foods could reduce the effectiveness of antibiotics to fight disease when these antibiotics are taken with a meal. The antibiotic-resistance genes produce enzymes that can degrade antibiotics. If a food with an antibiotic-resistance gene is eaten along with an antibiotic, it could destroy the antibiotic in the stomach.

Second, the resistance genes could be transferred to human or animal pathogens, making them impervious to antibiotics and aggravating the already serious health problem of antibiotic-resistant disease organisms. While the transfer of genetic material from plants to bacteria is unlikely, the possibility may exist.

When the European Union evaluated the research regarding the possible health and environmental risks, they chose to take a "precautionary" approach, restricting imports on GM crops and food made from them. The United States promptly sued them, and the World Trade Association recently ruled in the U.S.'s favor, stating that the EU breached international rules. The ramifications of this remain to be seen, but there is speculation that the EU may choose to pay fines rather than accept GM goods.

Proponents of genetically engineered food claim that few of the concerns about genetic modification are conclusive. This may be true. In fact, perhaps most concerning is what we don't know. GMOs have not been adequately tested and the long-term effects have not been evaluated. There is already plenty of preliminary research to suggest reason for concern[412] and we're the guinea pigs in this ongoing experiment.

Interestingly, no one – not the FDA nor the biotech industry – has declared GMO foods to be safe. Instead, both proclaim that they are not proven to be unsafe. That doesn't help me sleep better at night.

And let's be honest here. If the goals of genetic engineering were to feed the hungry or improve nutrition, we would be developing seeds that accomplished that directly, such as making seeds cheap and without restrictive licensing, making seeds that could grow on substandard soil, making crops that feed people not animals ... Few of these are currently available as GMOs and few, if any, are in development.

Don't let the proponents of GMOs fool you when they discuss genetic modification as a simple improvement on the selective breeding that farmers have long conducted. Selective breeding works within the context of evolution, nudging a crop or animal in a desired direction. But once you tamper with genes outside nature's usual checks and balances, you run far greater risk, perhaps threatening nature itself.

Indeed, I could choose to tell the story behind virtually any genetically modified seed to support this point. Consider a commonly used seed in which a bacterium called Bacillus thuringensis (Bt) is spliced into a corn plant. Bt is a pesticide that causes caterpillars' stomachs to explode, but doesn't appear to directly harm humans, birds or bees. It's a naturally occurring germ and has been commonly used by farmers. In the context of natural laws, when it is applied directly to corn plants it's fairly effective at destroying a specific pest and not causing untoward damage beyond that.

But genetic engineering pushed the limits of its effectiveness. With the Bt gene spliced into the corn, each of the corn's cells became equipped to kill caterpillars. The problem arises when the Bt corn sheds its pollen and the wind dusts the pollen on the trees and bushes. When the butterflies munch on the plants, they meet the same fatal fate as the caterpillars: exploding stomachs. Monarch butterfly populations are dwindling fast. And other butterflies are becoming increasingly endangered as well.

Another problem is also arising: While the massive exposure to Bt is killing many predators, there are a few that have mutated a resistance. These super-resistant pests are growing in number and Bt is losing its effectiveness.

The challenges of genetic modification are profound. Engineered genes just don't play by the usual rules of nature that develop over the course of evolution. This type of gene manipulation could easily work from the inside to destroy habitat or some of the links on the food chain – both of which threaten our survival.

One more example should hammer this point home. GMO salmon have been developed that grow significantly faster and larger than ordinary salmon. What happens when these transgenic salmon escape from fish farms (which inevitably happens) and mate with or compete with wild stock for food and spawning sites? Odds are it's a recipe for havoc in the wild, and extinction for salmon as we know it.

The Food and Drug Administration has decided that consumers don't need to know whether foods have been genetically modified. No labeling is required, limiting the consumer's ability to make informed choices. Unless the manufacturer informs you that the product is GMO-free (or certified organic), you just don't know. Consumer advocates are fighting hard to make labeling mandatory, which is strongly opposed by the biotech industry. In the absence of federal protection, several counties have declared themselves GMO-free zones.

However, you have eaten genetically modified foods. Thus far, genetic engineering on a large scale has been largely limited to three basic food crops: soybeans, corn, and canola, all of which are common in processed foods. In fact, approximately 70 percent of processed foods in U.S. grocery stores contain GMO ingredients, including virtually all breads, sodas, and beers. Other foods include Hawaiian papayas, some varieties of summer squash, and milk and dairy products derived from cows injected with a genetically engineered hormone.

Cloned Animals

Another biotech experiment may soon find its way to our dinner tables: meat and milk from cloned animals.

When "Dolly," a much-celebrated sheep, was cloned in 1997, she aroused worldwide interest and concern. Science magazine even named her the breakthrough of 1997. The cloning technology involved fusing the genetic material of a cell from one sheep into an egg from another sheep. After the egg was fertilized in a laboratory, it was then implanted into the uterus of a third sheep, which gave birth to Dolly. Dolly lived until the age of 6 (about half the expected lifespan), when she was euthanized after developing arthritis and lung disease.

So far, I'm not aware of any evidence that eating food derived from cloned animals is unsafe, but it also doesn't appear that sufficient research has been conducted to feel confident. Ian Wilmut, one of the scientists responsible for cloning Dolly, acknowledges that even slight imbalances in a clone's hormones, fat, or proteins can render its meat or milk unsafe[413]. And the National Academy of Sciences warns us that no method exists to determine subtle health problems in clones[414].

But food safety is just one small issue that cloning raises. Cloning will move us more towards uniformity. Already, because of pressure from the industrialization of food products, one breed of farm animal disappears every month[415]. This trend deeply worries the United Nations Food and Agriculture Organization (FAO) which sees these disappearances as "the biggest global threat to farm animal diversity"[415].

Biodiversity is our insurance against nature's inconsistency. With too much uniformity, we lose our ability to confront natural catastrophes such as global warming and the emergence of new disease. Biodiversity allows risk to be spread out so that we can retain some species when others are wiped out by a particular circumstance.

Additionally, cloning poses animal welfare concerns. There is a high failure rate (90 percent), resulting in deformities and premature deaths to large numbers of clones and surrogate mothers[416].

Small ranchers are quite concerned. As they are less likely to be able to afford the new technology, many anticipate increased corporate control of our food supply. Attempts to patent cloned offspring add to this apprehension.

Despite these concerns, the Food and Drug Administration (FDA) has announced plans to lift a moratorium on selling meat and milk products from cloned animals. The FDA has also indicated that it won't require labeling.

Action Tips...

Food Irradiation
- Most foods are already government-approved for irradiation.

- Labels only have to appear on whole foods. (Since many irradiated foods are sold to restaurants or are a component of processed foods, they are frequently not labeled by the time they reach the consumer).
- If the radura symbol appears, you know the food was irradiated. However, the absence of a radura does not mean that the food was not irradiated, unless you are buying it directly from the manufacturer.
- If you choose to avoid irradiated foods, your best bet is to choose organic products, as organic foods cannot be irradiated.

Genetic Modification

- Labeling of GMO foods is not required, so you may not know for sure whether a food contains GMOs. However, you can purchase foods that specifically say GMO-free. Also, you can choose organic foods, as organic foods cannot be genetically modified.
- The Greenpeace True Shopping List has a long list of name brand items, telling you whether or not GMOs are present: http://www.truefoodnow.org/.

Cloned Animals

- Food from cloned animals is not currently sold, but the FDA has announced that it will soon be legal, and that no labeling will be required.

Get Informed...

Organic Consumer's Association has a great section called "**food irradiation** information for students," at http://www.organicconsumers.org/irrad/ForStudents.cfm#FactSheets. Also, Public Citizen and the Center for Food Safety did a good analysis which can be found at: http://www.citizen.org/documents/HiddenHarm_-_PDF.pdf.

Jeffrey Smith's book, *Seeds of Deception*, is an excellent resource on **GMOs**, and his website also provides good information: http://www.seedsofdeception.com/. You can also sign up for his free e-mail alerts.

Andrew Kimbrell also came out with an excellent primer called *Your Right to Know*.

The Center for Food Safety also has on-line information about food irradiation, genetic modification and cloned animals: http://www.centerforfoodsafety.org/, and a particularly good fact sheet on cloned animals: http://www.centerforfoodsafety.org/pubs/fact%20sheet.pdf.

John Robbins' book *The Food Revolution* also covers irradiation and genetic modification.

Agriculture and Sustainability

Agriculture – and the need to eat - connects us with the world. How we produce our food has a dramatic effect on the health and well-being of the earth and its peoples.

In the past, farmers served as stewards of the land, protecting and nurturing it for future generations. Animal agriculture and plant agriculture were closely interwoven, and farm animals played an integral role in supporting plant agriculture and nourishing our land and peoples. They ate weeds and crop wastes, pulled plows, and their manure fertilized the soil. And of course they were also slaughtered, allowing the waste products they ate to be recycled into food for humans.

Much has changed in recent times. At the beginning of the century, over 39 percent of Americans lived on farms; less than 2 percent do today[417]. Farms no longer resemble the pictures portrayed in storybooks: the majority of our food comes from large agribusiness, not family farmers with a personal commitment to the products they grow.

Today, most plant products are grown with harmful chemicals that harm workers and damage the soil and other natural resources, presenting problems that limit the viability of their future growth. Most animals raised for food spend much of their lives on huge factory feedlots in such overwhelming numbers that they now pose much more threat to our survival than support. World meat production *quadrupled* in the fifty years between 1940 and 1990, such that we now have *triple* the number of livestock compared to humans[418]; put in other terms, farm animals now comprise four times the weight of humans[419].

This has very profound ecological and social consequences. The current impact of agriculture on the planet is disturbing, and the topics discussed in this book, particularly this section, carry an emotional punch. If we want a viable future, we cannot continue on our current path.

In 2005, the Secretary General of the Food and Agriculture Organization (FAO) of the United Nations delivered a report on the state of the ecosystems of the earth, based on the work of over 1,500 scientists. He hypothesized that if we continue to live the way we do, humans will possibly be extinct in 300 years. What was most shocking about this report was what he named as the single greatest element responsible for this destruction: agriculture (the production of food).

The word "**sustainability**" refers to making choices now to save the world for future generations. In order to allow for everyone on this planet to eat while simultaneously protecting the world for generations to come, we cannot sustain our current eating habits.

Sustainable agriculture doesn't harm the ecosystem. Sustainable farmers don't use harmful pesticides and chemical fertilizers, and crops are rotated to ensure that nutrients in the soil get replenished. Sustainable farmers raise only as many animals as the land is capable of handling. Waste products are returned to fertilize the soil. Some types of organic agriculture are examples of sustainable practices.

Conversely, unsustainable agriculture pollutes the air, water and land. Factory farming of animals is an example of an unsustainable practice. A factory farm may have huge numbers of animals (predominantly fish, cows, pigs, chicken and turkeys) confined in a small space. Given their concentration in small places, their wastes exceed ranchers' ability to make use of them, polluting the environment. They also require an enormous amount of limited resources, such as land, water and fossil fuels. Additionally, the animals are fed antibiotics, pesticide-laden plants and other chemicals, which further damage the environment and endanger the health of the wildlife and humans that eat them.

In 1992, more than 1,600 senior scientists from 71 countries, including half of all living Nobel Prize winners, signed a document entitled "World Scientists' Warning to Humanity."[420] The following is an excerpt from the introduction:

> Human beings and the natural world are on a collision course. Human
> activities inflict harsh and often irreversible damage to the environment

and on critical resources. If not unchecked, many of our current practices put at serious risk the future that we wish for human society and the plant and animal kingdoms, and may so alter the living world that it will be unable to sustain life in the manner that we know. Fundamental changes are urgent if we are to avoid the collision our present course will bring about...

Further in the document, they warn us:

We the undersigned, senior members of the world's scientific community, hereby warn all humanity of what lies ahead. A great change in our stewardship for the Earth and life on it is required, if vast misery is to be avoided and our global home is not to be irretrievably mutilated.

Why did so many well-respected scientists feel compelled to make such a dramatic statement, repeating their plea at an international summit five years later[421]? Why is the Food and Agriculture Organization of the United Nations sounding such a serious alarm? You don't need to be a Nobel Laureate to understand the issues that provoke this concern, and this section will help to clarify agricultural sustainability.

Soil, Forests and Land

Fertile **soil** is amazing stuff, teeming with life which is necessary to sustain humans. A mere teaspoon can contain 5 billion bacteria, 20 million fungi, and 1 million protests[422]. This amounts to a lot more microbes in a teaspoon than humans on the entire planet[422]! These microbes are vital to our existence as they help recycle our wastes into rich organic matter and comprise the base of our food chain. Topsoil is particularly valuable; it is loaded with nutrient-rich organic materials and its consistency helps to regulate how much water the soil can absorb.

Thanks to the soil, most rainfall hitting our planet is trapped and absorbed, watering plants and replenishing aquifers, rivers, lakes and streams. If the soil didn't catch this water, it would run off the land into the oceans, and the continents would be barren.

Conventional farming methods have been devastating to the soil: its valuable nutrients are being depleted and topsoil is eroding about 17 times faster than it can be replenished[422]. The fertilizers[423] and pesticides[424] that are applied to growing crops have played a large role in this devastation, as have the heavy metals that are added to fertilizers[423] and livestock feed[425]. Many of these chemicals upset the balance by killing both pests and beneficial soil organisms. They can also be toxic to insects, birds and other pollinators that are necessary for fertilization.

Healthy soil is porous: air accounts for about half its volume, providing channels for water to flow, pathways for roots and space for organisms to move around. Animal grazing has also been devastating to the soil; when animals graze in large numbers they trample the plants and compact the soil, depleting the oxygen and making it harder for plants to grow. Also, since the compacted soil does not absorb water as well, heavy rains carry away topsoil[426]. One scientist puts this into practical perspective, stating that every hamburger causes the loss of five times its weight in topsoil[427].

It can take hundreds of thousands of years for an inch of fertile topsoil to form, although careless farming can deplete it in just a few growing seasons. To ensure our continued existence, we need to protect and nurture our soil.

Plants, trees and forests are also integral to human survival. Humans have a symbiotic relationship with plants and trees. We breathe in oxygen and then exhale carbon dioxide as a waste product. Plants and trees do the opposite, thus maintaining oxygen for the survival of humans and other animals and clearing the excess carbon dioxide (the most pervasive of the greenhouse gasses).

They also recycle or purify our water, and their roots prevent soil erosion, especially along riverbanks, helping to keep them from flooding.

And of course, our forests serve as home for wildlife. Additionally, tree wood can be used for fuel or as building material. Also important, our forests are a source of beauty.

Land, of course, is in limited supply. Growing crops for animals requires enormous amounts of space. According to the USDA Economic Research Service and Agricultural Research Service, it takes sixteen pounds of grain to produce a pound of beef[428]. In other words, by cycling our grain through cattle, we end up with only six percent as much food available to feed humans! (Much of the food energy that animals take in is converted to energy for movement or growing and maintaining body parts that are not consumed; only a small component is converted into edible weight gain.)

The Cattlemen's Beef Association disputes this number, stating that it only takes 4.5 pounds of grain to produce a pound of beef[429]. Regardless of which figure is more accurate, the point remains that plant foods are a much more efficient use of limited land resources.

Cattle typically roam on open land for the early part of their lives, grazing on weeds and grasses. About 40 percent of the land area in the United States is currently used for livestock grazing[430]. The U.S. Department of the Interior reports that in the Western United States, cattle have left about ten percent of the land desertified (barren), and about two-thirds substantially degraded[426]. Just about the only area that isn't grazed in the western U.S. are places that can't be, such as inaccessible areas, dense forests, dry deserts, sand dunes or developed areas.

In fact, today virtually all of the potentially productive soil on this planet is being exploited by agriculture; what is unused is typically too wet, too dry, or lacking in nutrients[431].

Given the limited availability of additional United States' land, Americans depend on other countries to grow crops and raise cattle to support our meat consumption. As a result, the world's forests are also currently being depleted at a very fast rate, particularly tropical rainforests[432]. Cattle ranchers cut down the trees, burn the forest, and then plant grass. Then they bring in cows to feed on the grass. When the cows are grown, they are slaughtered and turned into beef.

Scientists calculate that to produce every quarter pound fast food hamburger, fifty-five square feet of rainforest must be cleared[433]. (That's about the size of a small kitchen.) Since most of the nutrients in the rainforest are in the plants, when the trees are cleared, nutrients are lost and the soil becomes eroded and no longer available for re-use. The number one factor in tropical rainforest destruction is cattle grazing[434], leading one scientist to describe it as the "hamburgerization of the rainforest[432]."

Clearing forests to produce beef also destroys the homes of forest animals. The U.S. Congress General Accounting Office names it as the leading cause of species endangerment and extinction in the United States[435, 436].

Species extinction is a big concern these days, with species disappearing from our planet at a rate unseen since the days of the dinosaurs. Loss of species is not just a moral issue, but one to be concerned about from the selfish perspective of our own health. About one quarter of the pharmaceuticals used in the United States contain plant ingredients – or at least ingredients that were first discovered in plants[437]. We wouldn't even have common aspirin if it weren't for plants. When we lose our plant diversity, we may also be losing a potential medicine to treat AIDS, atherosclerosis or cancer.

Elimination of enough species may eventually cause the web of interdependency to come crashing down; we just don't know what will happen if we continue our current practices. Cute pandas or majestic sharks engage our sympathies, but their protection isn't enough; the ugly and less popular animals at the bottom of our food chain are essential to our survival at the top of that food chain – and need equal protection.

Rainforests have been called the "lungs of the Earth" because they filter our air by absorbing carbon dioxide while emitting the oxygen we need to breathe – yet another reason we should be doing our best to preserve them.

The higher we eat on the food chain, the greater the environmental damage. To put this in perspective, the Union of Concerned Scientists calculates that red meat causes 20 times as much impact on land use as pasta, and that meat and poultry consumption accounts for a quarter of threats to natural ecosystems and wildlife[430, 438, 439†]. Other researchers compared a meat-based diet to a soy-based diet, and reported that meat production took 6-17 times as much land[440].

Water

Contrary to common perception, water is a limited resource. It is easy to think of water in endless supply, especially those of us that live close to the ocean. But most people don't realize that the salt water from our oceans is not viable as a drinking source or to support agriculture. More than 97 percent of the earth's water is salty. Desalinization (removing the salt) is time-consuming and cost-prohibitive.

Of the remaining 3 percent which is sufficiently salt-free to drink or use for agriculture, almost all of it is locked away in glaciers or ice, or too deep underground for us to access. In fact, only about .0001 percent of fresh water is accessible. To help put this into perspective, if all the earth's water fit into a gallon (3.8 liters) bottle, the fresh water available for human use would equal just over a tablespoon (15 milliliters).

Where do we get the water that we use? Of course, rain delivers some to us, which we capture in reservoirs. However, we are currently using water at a faster rate than is replenished by rain. We therefore require a supplementary source of water, and aquifers serve this purpose.

Aquifers are underground storehouses of water that were formed when ice from the Ice Age melted. We don't have massive quantities of ice anymore and as the aquifers get used, they don't get replenished. (A small amount of rainwater drains into aquifers, but this amount is inconsequential when compared to pumping rates.)

This is resulting in the draining of our aquifers, and at a particularly alarming rate. If this trend continues, experts predict that by the year 2025, one-third of the world will face severe water scarcity, with devastating consequences for the environment, food production, human health, the world economy, and peace[441].

Access to water is a big factor in establishing and preserving agricultural regions. The Ogallala Aquifer makes agriculture in the Midwest viable and provides an example of a diminishing water resource. One of the world's largest aquifers, it stretches under eight states, supplying water needs from the Dakotas to Texas. It is currently pumped much more quickly than natural rates of replenishment, and will probably be depleted within a generation. (Ann Veneman, the former Secretary of Agriculture, speaking in front of the United Nations in 2001, cautioned that the aquifer could be dried up within 30-40 years[442].)

Adverse effects are already evident. For example, one-quarter of the Texas share of the Ogallala aquifer had been depleted by the early 1990s. Due to the limited water supply, more than a third of the land that had been irrigated in the 1970s has lost its water and become unable to grow food[443].

---

† The Union of Concerned Scientists analyzed two environmental studies, one conducted by the Environmental Protection Agency, the other by the California Risk Project, to quantify the effects of eating meat versus eating pasta. This symbol will denote conclusions drawn from their analysis.

Once depleted, farmers will have no other dependable water supply and agriculture in the area is destined to fail. Without adequate water, the region will eventually become inhospitable for human habitation as well.

Similar scenarios can be expected for Lybia's use of the Nubian Aquifer and pumping of aquifers in the Middle East. The situation is so dire that Egypt has threatened to go to war to protect its water supplies[441]. President Gaddafi of Libya warns that "the next Middle East war would be over dwindling water supplies."[441]

It is time to plug the drain! Water is a limited resource and we need to increase our efforts at conservation.

Of course, water conservation has already entered the public awareness, and many of us are actively contributing. Perhaps you use a low-flow toilet or shower and try to be conscientious when washing dishes or your car, or brushing your teeth. While these efforts are valuable and to be encouraged, few of us recognize that we can have an even more dramatic impact if we consider water conservation while making food choices. Since agriculture is the single largest user (and waster) of water, changes in our agricultural practices can have a large impact on sustainability. To give you a sense of the disparity, we use about 1,430 gallons per person in the United States. Only 100 gallons of that is household use per person.

Foods differ in their water usage. Here's one estimate, made by the Soil and Water specialists at the University of California Agricultural Extension in conjunction with livestock farm advisors[444]:

1 pound of lettuce	23 gallons
1 pound of tomatoes	23 gallons
1 pound of potatoes	23 gallons
1 pound of wheat	25 gallons
1 pound of chicken	815 gallons
1 pound of pork	1,630 gallons
1 pound of beef	5,214 gallons

Others present a more conservative view of water usage for Californian beef. For example, the Water Education Foundation estimates it to be half as much: 2,464 gallons[445]. (Part of the discrepancy is due to the fact that meat produced in different climates and terrains requires different amounts of water.)

As John Robbins points out, **you can save more water by not eating a pound of beef than you would by not showering for a year**[443k]! (If you use the Water Education Foundations' estimate, this would change from a year to six months, which still makes a dramatic statement.)

To put this in a different perspective, the International Water Management Institute calculates that meat-eaters consume the equivalent of about 5,000 liters of water a day compared to the 1,000-2,000 liters used by people on predominantly vegetarian diets in developing countries[446]. Other researchers compared a meat-based diet to a soy-based diet and reported that the meat-based diet required 4.4 to 26 times the water[440].

Water conservation is not our only concern, but water pollution is also mounting. A large contributor to water pollution is the manure generated by factory farms[447]. While manure is not a waste when formed in small quantities, the massive amounts that are generated by our huge factory farms overwhelm our ability to safely recycle the manure[418]. The waste is contaminated with antibiotics and other veterinary drugs that pose additional threats to environmental and human health[447, 448].

When factory farm buildings are cleaned, they are typically flushed with water that is distributed to holes in the ground called lagoons, huge cesspools of dilute urine and manure. Given the vast

---

[k] This comparison is based on a daily seven minute shower, with a shower head flow rate of 2 gallons per minute.

quantities of waste that are produced, lagoons grow large and often spill or routinely leak. Livestock waste enters the soil and water, polluting rivers and oceans and sickening wildlife and people.

In June of 1995, for example, a lagoon in North Carolina broke, releasing 25 million gallons of waste[449]. Ten million fish were killed in the New River, and 364,000 acres of coastal wetlands had to be closed to shell fishing[284, 450]. (Did you read about this in the papers? I didn't! Was the company made to take responsibility for clean up? No – this is business as usual.)

This example was of course an unusually large and devastating event. However, lagoon spillage and its accompanying damage, while not usually of this magnitude, is a common occurrence. A report by the American Society of Agricultural Engineers estimates that half of existing lagoons are leaking badly enough to contaminate ground water[451].

Government regulation of lagoon waste is inadequate at best. The Clean Water Act prohibits factory farms from discharging any traceable animal waste into nearby waterways, and requires them to obtain permits that offer exemptions under certain circumstances, such as when there's runoff after a storm. Sounds good so far, doesn't it? But a loophole[452] renders the law meaningless when it comes to regulating fecal discharge. The factory farms themselves get to determine what constitutes a polluting discharge and whether a permit is needed at all[453].

Livestock are producing copious amounts of waste: twenty tons of livestock manure are produced for every household in this country[430]. To view it in another perspective, the Environmental Protection Agency (EPA) reports that the waste produced per day by one dairy cow is equal to that of 20-40 people[454]. The EPA further reports that animal wastes pollute waterways more than the total of all other industrial sources, accounting for 20 percent of all water pollution[455].

And when the Union of Concerned Scientists compared the cost of producing a pound of red meat to a pound of pasta, they calculated that red meat causes 17 times as much water pollution†.

Humans can't survive without water, but you would never know from how we have been treating our oceans and other waters. Like plants, oceans absorb carbon dioxide and provide oxygen for us. They also are the source of most of the water we drink (evaporation from oceans forms the clouds, which in turn drop rain and snow that fill fresh-water sources).

Yet our oceans are dying as a result of pollution. As an example, there is now a "dead zone" in the Gulf of Mexico covering over 8,000 square miles from Louisiana through Texas[456]. "Dead-zone" means what it sounds like: it can't support aquatic life. The main reason is agriculture, due to the fertilizers, pesticides and animal wastes that seep into the water[456]. These compounds feed large algae growths that rob the water of oxygen and make it uninhabitable for other sea life.

Fishing for Trouble

Seafood poses different environmental considerations than plant or animal agriculture. From 1950-1990, oceanic fish catch jumped from 19 to 89 million tons. Since 1990, there has been no growth in catch. Why? Overfishing[457]! (Overfishing refers to taking fish out of the water before they reproduce to sustain a healthy population.)

According to a Food and Agriculture Organization (FAO) estimate, about 70 percent of marine fisheries are so heavily exploited that they are on the verge of depletion (34 percent) or have already been pushed over the edge (25 percent)[458]. A startling 90 percent of the world's large predatory fish, including tuna, swordfish, cod, halibut, shark and flounder, have disappeared in the past 50 years[457].

The situation is dire: in fact, it is predicted that world seafood stocks may collapse in our lifetimes (2048) if we don't significantly reduce consumption levels[459]. Even the United Nations, in their report ominously titled "In Dead Water," echoes the dire predictions of scientists[460].

Unless we act soon, our kids may just experience a world without seafood. Study after study shows that overfishing, aquaculture, and climate change threaten to do the fish in.

Trawling, the most widely used method for catching fish, has been particularly damaging, capturing not only the targeted fish species but killing numerous other species, such as dolphins, sharks, sea turtles and sea birds. Trawling involves pulling a net behind one or more boats, and catching everything in its path. One-quarter of the world's annual catch is thrown back into the sea, typically dead or dying[461, 462]. (Bottom trawling is often compared to clear-cutting forests in its environmental impact[463].)

If you thought the situation with the disappearing rainforest was bad, think about this: the coral reefs of the Indian and Pacific oceans are vanishing twice as quickly[464]. Home to 75 percent of the world's coral reefs, these oceans have lost nearly 600 square miles of reef each year since the late 1960s. Also, coral cover - a measure of ocean-floor coverage that reflects reef health - has shrunk from an average of 50 percent to about 20 percent in 2003.

The United Nations report isn't all doom and gloom however. The report does say that fisheries could recover if countries reduced global carbon emissions and shipping pollution and stopped overfishing and damaging fishing practices such as bottom trawling.

Aquaculture (fish farming) is now the fastest growing food production activity[458, 465]. Unfortunately, it has not helped the overfishing problem since it takes 2 pounds of wild fish to produce 1 pound of farmed fish. In fact, fish farming is now a major contributor to depleting wild fish[466].

Another difficulty posed by fish farming is that diseases and parasites thrive in the over-crowded pens[466]. To counteract this, chemicals and antibiotics are applied to kill bacteria, herbicides to prevent growth of vegetation, and other drugs to treat the diseases and parasites[466]. An additional challenge includes fish escaping; they then spread disease to wild stocks, and breed with them, contributing to extinction of wild varieties[466].

There are some fish farms that are dedicated to sustainable practices, and these will typically be noted at the point of sale.

Shrimp farming has been particularly damaging. In Thailand, Ecuador and several other tropical nations, coastal forests of mangroves have been cut down and replaced with shrimp farms. The mangroves were an important habitat for fish, and this has resulted in reduced fish for the local people. Mangroves also filter water and protect the coast against waves. Waste products build up over time and the farmers have to move on. That means no more shrimp farms - and no mangrove forest.

Farmed oysters, clams and mussels are often raised in more sustainable ways. They filter plankton out of the water for their food, which means that they don't need extra feed and they are also improving water quality. Since oysters, clams and mussels must come from non-polluted water when farmed for human consumption, these farms often get involved in keeping coastal waters clean.

Water: A Human Right or Human Need?

Water is no longer a gift of nature, but is also quickly becoming a profit center. A few multinational corporations have already taken ownership of this precious resource, with devastating results. Bechtel Corporation, for example, bought the water rights to the town of Cochabamba, which is in Bolivia, the poorest country in South America. Two months after taking over the water system, they hit water users with enormous price increases – increases which many people just could not afford.

A popular uprising by desperate citizens broke out (called the "Water War"), leaving one boy dead and more than a hundred injured. For the people, this war was about survival, not political ideology. Bechtel finally withdrew and the uprising subsided. Bechtel has now filed a complaint against Bolivia with the World Court, asking for $25 million as compensation for its lost opportunity to profit.

Many people believe that access to water is a basic human right and should not be privatized. This is a highly contentious issue being fought in courts in the U.S. as well as abroad.

Fuel

Cheap oil and gas fuel much of our lives in modern America. All the luxuries – and even what we consider necessities – depend on fossil fuels: air conditioning, central heating, cars, airplanes, electric lighting, cheap clothing, movies, supermarkets, surgery, you name it. We are so entrenched in our dependency that we have not faced a fact of nature: fossil fuels exist in finite, non-renewable supplies. Once depleted, they are gone forever. Seems a little short-sighted to build our lives on such an ephemeral resource, doesn't it? Conservation is essential (as is developing replacements).

What does this have to do with agriculture? We are eating a lot of oil. No, I'm not talking about olive oil or corn oil, but about crude oil derived from fossil fuels. Producing, manufacturing and transporting any kind of food require energy.

Until the last century, all of the food available on this planet was derived from the sun, a renewable resource, but much has changed since. In fact, 17 percent of all fossil fuel used in the U.S. is currently used for food production[467]. We use fossil fuels to power heavy farming machinery, to refrigerate foods during transportation, in various capacities to process foods and to produce packaging materials, to manufacture fertilizers and pesticides, and of course, to transport the food and related materials.

Conventional agriculture is remarkably inefficient in fuel usage. It takes an astonishing amount of fossil fuel calories to produce our food calories: some scientists estimate that it takes as many as ten fossil fuel calories for each food calorie produced.

To put that in perspective, it takes about 20,000 fossil fuel kilocalories to produce the 2,000 kilocalories of food energy that the average person eats per day. In more familiar units, the average four person family consumes almost 34,000 kilowatt-hours (kWh) of energy, or more than 930 gallons of gasoline. Compare that to their average household consumption of electricity: about 10,800 kWh, or 1,070 gallons of gasoline. In other words, we use as much energy to grow our food as we do to power our homes! Once again, the message is clear: if you care about energy conservation, your food choices are an extremely effective tool for change.

Not all forms of agriculture drain fossil fuels to the same extent. For example, "...(f)eed (for livestock) takes so much energy to grow that it might as well be a petroleum byproduct," writes Worldwatch Institute in their analysis[468]. Their argument is supported by extensive research conducted at the Fort Keogh Livestock and Range Reserve Laboratory, demonstrating the high dependency of the beef industry on fossil fuels[469]. Check out the following data which was compiled by John Robbins from the sources cited[443]:

Amount of fossil fuel needed to produce 1 kilocalorie of protein from:
- soybeans: 2 kilocalories[428, 470, 471];
- corn or wheat: 3 kilocalories[428, 470, 471];
- beef: 54 kilocalories[428, 470, 471].

Amount of greenhouse warming carbon gas released by driving a typical American car, in one day: 3 kilograms[468];
Amount released by burning enough Costa Rican rainforest to produce beef for one hamburger: 75 kilograms[468].

Robbins points out that people consuming protein from soybeans are, in effect, using only 4 percent as much energy – and producing only 4 percent as much carbon dioxide – as people eating meat[443]. While many people are conscientiously driving less to save on gas, I wonder how many realize that they could save 25 times the amount of energy by eating one less hamburger than they would by not driving their car for a day[443, 468]!

Others calculate that meat production results in meat-eaters using 6 to 20 times the fossil fuels compared to those consuming a soy-based diet[440]. While the disparity in these different estimates indicates that it is very difficult to quantify, it is certainly evident that eating lower on the food chain can dramatically reduce our fossil fuel usage.

David Pimental estimates that if all humanity ate the way Americans do, we would exhaust all known fossil fuel resources in just seven years[472]. (Critics challenge Pimental's figures. But their estimates don't change the picture much: they claim he's off by as much as 30 percent. Okay. Ten years instead of seven.)

What is particularly alarming about our fossil fuel dependency is that resources are not spread equitably throughout the world. Resource wars have already begun.

Global Warming

Sunlight reflects down, warming the land, water and air. In turn, the warmed up land, water and air give off heat, which rises into the atmosphere. The earth is like a giant greenhouse, and atmospheric gases act like a greenhouse's glass walls, keeping heat contained, and maintaining the earth's warm climate. This heat trap keeps our world at fairly stable, predictable temperatures – well, at least it did for most of our history. For the past century or so, the earth is warming up more than usual – and this is what is referred to as global warming.

Global warming is a hot topic these days. It is no longer theory, but an established scientific consensus. (Scientific organizations that recognize it as a serious problem include: the United Nations' Intergovernmental Panel on Climate Change (IPCC), the National Academy of Sciences, the Environmental Protection Agency, the National Oceanic and Atmospheric Administration, the Goddard Institute of the National Aeronautic and Space Association, the Union of Concerned Scientists...) Scientists warn we may soon cross a threshold of no return; in fact, some believe it could already be too late. Clearly, there is an urgency to reversing – or at least leveling - global warming now.

If the earth gets hotter, the following would be expected to occur:

Because heating water makes it expand, water levels will rise, causing coastal cities to flood.

Regions that currently receive frequent rain and snowfall may become hotter and drier. Lakes and rivers will dry up and forest fires will occur more frequently. Droughts will make growing food more difficult. Less water will be available for drinking and showers.

Plants and animals unable to take the heat will go extinct.

Hurricanes, tornadoes and other weather conditions caused by changes in heat and water evaporation will occur more frequently and be more intense.

Diseases will spread more easily because warmer temperatures increase the geographic range that disease-carrying animals, insects and microorganisms - as well as the germs and viruses they carry - can survive.

Unfortunately, this is not merely a forecast for the future: all of these are already occurring, as the Earth gets hotter at an unprecedented rate. The severity of Hurricane Katrina was not an accident. It was a smaller storm when it crossed Florida, and roared to full life when it encountered the abnormally hot water of the Gulf of Mexico. A month earlier, hurricane experts showed that tropical storms are now lasting half again as long and producing winds 50 percent more powerful than just a few decades earlier[473]. The only plausible explanation: the higher temperatures on which these storms thrive. Preventable human actions – like global warming – turn natural hazards into humanitarian nightmares.

Waves are already washing over islands in the South Pacific, coastal cities and low-lying countries are encountering severe flooding, polar ice caps and glaciers are melting, polar bears and other species are threatened with extinction, crop failures are mounting, diseases are spreading more easily.

Of course, there are many human activities that contribute to global warming that you may already be familiar with: among the biggies, for example, are generating electricity, powering cars, trucks and planes, deforestation, smoking, militarism. (The U.S. military is the world's biggest consumer of oil and the world's biggest polluter.) What many people do not know, however, is that the production of meat has a significant effect. Let's take a look at why.

The main gases that cause the greenhouse effect are water vapor, carbon dioxide, methane and nitrous oxide. Carbon dioxide, in particular, has been increasing dramatically. Whenever energy is derived from coal, oil or gas, carbon dioxide is released, and the massive amounts of fuel used in agriculture is having a decided impact on global warming.

The greenhouse gas that plays the next largest role in climate change is methane, followed by nitrous oxide. Methane is actually much more potent a greenhouse gas than carbon dioxide (perhaps 24 times as potent), though it is found in much smaller quantities[474]. Levels of atmospheric methane have also been rising quickly, now almost triple the concentration at the start of the century. Methane is produced by a number of sources, such as coal mining and landfills, but what's the number one source worldwide? Animal agriculture. Strange as it may seem, these high levels of methane can be blamed in large part on cows burping.

Part of the problem is that we have vast quantities of cattle, and the other difficulty is that we are feeding them a diet unsuited to their physiology. This diet results in excessive eructation (burping) and flatulence (gas), and each releases a little methane gas. One cow releases up to 400 quarts of methane daily; in the United States, this accounts for over 3.8 million metric tons annually. Manure lagoons used to store untreated farm animal waste also release high quantities of methane and nitrous oxide. (Manure lagoons are already a target of environmentalists' for their role as the number one source of water pollution in the U.S.)

And of course the clear-cutting of forests for cattle grazing and to grow feed for cattle also generates more greenhouse gasses.

In fact, a United Nations report blames livestock for 18% of all greenhouse gases[475]. This alarming figure takes into account clear-cutting forests for grazing, the petroleum used to produce fertilizers, the fuel needed to produce and transport meat, and the gases created by manure and flatulence. (Livestock also produces more than 100 other polluting gases, including more than two-thirds of the world's emissions of ammonia, one of the main causes of acid rain.)

For all of these reasons, the most effective way to reduce global warming is to reduce our consumption of foods from animals. "The impact is so significant that it needs to be addressed with urgency," concludes the United Nations[475].

Another U.N. reports highlights the dangers posed by nitrogen fertilizer in conventional (non-organic) agriculture.[476] This has a potent effect on global warming – in addition to damaging ecosystems, polluting water, and harming the health of humans and wildlife.

There are two ways to slow global warming: the first is to produce less greenhouse-warming gases, and the other is to reduce what is already there by pulling it out of the air and storing it somewhere else, such as in the soil. Some types of farming - and shopping - can do both.

Organic agriculture helps tame global warming as growing food organically emits less carbon dioxide than non-organic methods. Conventional agriculture uses large amounts of nitrogen fertilizer[427] – a fossil fuel - which accounts for as much as a third of agriculture's carbon dioxide emissions. Organic farms, on the other hand, do not use synthetic nitrogen, relying instead on crop wastes and manure as fertilizer. Recycling this organic matter provides another advantage as it can increase the amount of carbon stored in the ground.

Food Miles

Growing food, however, addresses only part of the issue. Getting it to the table also emits carbon dioxide. The average meal in the United States typically travels 1,500 miles before landing on the dinner plate. The food industry is the largest user of freight transportation in the country. Buying more locally grown food reduces those miles, keeping more carbon out of the sky.

Because industrial agriculture has grown so large and centralized, food is now shipped extraordinarily long distances before it reaches consumers. Ironically, wonderful apples are grown 20 miles from my house, yet the local supermarket stocks apples grown 2,000 miles away.

And I was surprised to learn that my local fishmonger was selling fish that had traveled 8,000 miles after its death. It was caught on the west coast of North America, shipped to Asia to be processed (skinned and filleted), then shipped back to North America to be eaten. All because the (subsidized) cost of oil makes shipping cheap enough to access the cheaper labor in Asia.

Once I was sitting in a café in Hawaii and I got curious about the sugar packets on the counter. They were the familiar packets I've seen all across the country, produced by C&H Sugar, which operates a refinery near my home in California. Turns out the sugarcane is grown in Maui, just a few miles from the café I was sitting in. But the food miles involved in getting that sugar to me are extraordinary. The sugarcane was picked and then shipped to the refinery in California, where it was refined into white sugar. It was then shipped to New York, where it was packaged into the little packets, and then distributed around the country, including the café I was sitting in in Hawaii.

Eating food that is locally grown and distributed can therefore also dramatically reduce fossil fuel usage.

In fact, buying locally grown food is likely to be even more beneficial from an environmental perspective than buying organic[477]. A diet composed of some meat, grains, vegetables, and fruit from conventional sources can entail four times the energy and four times the greenhouse gas emissions compared to that same diet from domestic sources[478].

The United States is the largest single source of greenhouse gas emissions, accounting for 22 percent of total world emissions (though we are only 5 percent of the population). We have refused to participate in international conventions to limit greenhouse gas emissions, such as the widely respected Kyoto Accord endorsed by most countries. Saving the planet will require that the United States join with the world community, rather than continuing to undermine its efforts.

No doubt New Orleans will be rebuilt. But if hurricanes like Katrina increase from being unusual, once-in-a-lifetime events to once-in-a-decade-or-two, as some scientists predict, can we continue to rebuild and recover? Global warming means that the future will be filled with this kind of horror and devastation. We can't continue to be shortsighted about our future. The questions plaguing agriculture are not just about how we feed ourselves, but whether we survive at all.

Biodiversity

Biodiversity is also critical to our survival. You're unlike your sister, even less like your mail carrier, and every kernel of corn holds a slightly different destiny. Some corn seeds will grow into tall plants, other short, some will yield sweet corn and others starchy. In a good growing year, all or most will thrive, but in a bad year high winds might take down the taller stalks.

Since all plants are vulnerable in different ways, having diversity means that a single biological event can't wipe out your entire crop. Suppose, for example, that a bug loved a particular type of potato. If that bug found the potato, it would eat and destroy it, and then move on to the next potato. If the next potato was of a different type that was less appealing to the bug, the devastation would be limited. These are simple stories that demonstrate the importance of biodiversity. In simple terms, biodiversity is nature's insurance policy.

This was evident when a million Irish people died in the infamous Irish Potato Famine in 1845. The Irish had relied on a single variety of potato, and a fungus was able to destroy the entire potato crop.

Unfortunately, in an important departure from tradition, the crops we now grow in the United States are remarkably similar genetically. Conventional agriculture is dominated by a few large agriculture companies that sell relatively few varieties of seeds.

Not only that, but monoculture prevails among large industrial farms, meaning that they plant row after row of identical plants. This makes caring for your plants easy, until a certain disease or pest comes in. If one plant is vulnerable, all are vulnerable.

Biodiversity is also critical because of the vast interdependency all creatures share. If humanity, being at the top of the food chain, disappeared, much of the rest of life would benefit. Forests would return, atmospheric gases would stabilize, pollution in the oceans would recover, allowing fish to thrive again, the list goes on. In contrast, if ants, near the foundation of the food chain, were to disappear, the results would be disastrous. Ants aerate the soil and help dead creatures to decompose, making the soil more nutrient-dense, which in turn feeds everything else that grows from the soil. It would likely result in the collapse of some ecosystems.

And since industry's focus is predominantly on hardiness as a measure of successful harvest (as opposed to taste or nutritional content, for example), the more tasty varieties are disappearing. What we gain in durability, we often sacrifice in flavor.

A hundred years ago, you could roam the earth and find about 7,000 varieties of apples; about 85 percent of them have since become extinct[479]. And almost all of our milk comes from one breed of cows, and most of our eggs from a single strain of hens[480].

Many of us believe that we have extensive choice in the supermarket, but this choice is illusory. For example, check out the cereal options. Though there are hundreds to choose from, every cereal contains the same basic ingredients, grown from the same few varieties of staple grains. The grains that are hardiest and easiest to turn into cereal are made in major quantities, and variations of those grains, and other types of grains, are disappearing. Slight twists in flavoring, packaging or marketing differentiate the brands, making the chemists and marketers more actively involved in food production than the farmers.

Wheaties, made by General Mills, provides an example of how this gets played out. Wheaties had adequate sales, but GM wanted to do better. So they added 1.5 cents worth of vitamins and minerals, changed the flavoring chemicals slightly, called it Total cereal, and marketed it differently. Total was so successful that they are able to sell it for 65 cents more per box, and sales are greatly increased over Wheaties.

The truth is that our food choices are dwindling, and plant biodiversity is quickly decreasing, as a direct result of our growing practices. Because it is irreversible, it may be the most serious of ecological threats. There is a renewed call for "heirloom" varieties from environmentalists and concerned consumers. Heirloom crops are grown from seeds that have been passed down from one generation of farmers to the next, offering a variety of tastes, textures and other qualities, and preserving biodiversity.

Trash Ecology

The amount of waste generated through agriculture, particularly packaging, is also astounding. Increased trash means more garbage collection trucks wasting gas and spewing carbon into the atmosphere. Incinerating the trash releases toxic chemicals. And growing landfills take up more and more precious space, leaching hazardous chemicals and noxious odors.

Packaging comprises the largest (and most rapidly growing) part of our trash, fueled by take-out restaurants and convenience foods. Disposable products – like paper cups and plates, plastic utensils - also rank high.

Protecting us from Pollution?

The Environmental Protection Agency (EPA) is the regulatory agency predominantly responsible for generating and enforcing laws protecting natural resources and human health. Unfortunately, agriculture has been exempt from many of these laws, which were enacted in earlier times when farmers did minimal damage and it was deemed in the natural interests to promote agriculture[32]. For example, there is an exemption for "agricultural storm water," so that runoff from farm fields is exempt from water pollution laws, and an exemption from "fugitive dust" emission, meaning that agricultural dust is not considered a contaminant under the Clean Air Act[32]. This has essentially given agriculture a license to pollute at will, with any clean up that is accomplished frequently done at taxpayer expense.

The use of pesticides and herbicides is governed by the United States Department of Agriculture (USDA), which has been similarly lax in regulating the industry. As discussed in the food safety section, many legal pesticides and herbicides are known to be toxic.

Farmers and Agricultural Workers

Sustainable practices require that we respect the workers' health, safety and quality of life. Farm workers have extraordinarily high rates of illnesses, injuries and deaths, whether it is from exposure to toxic pesticides or the dust and gases emitted by concentrated manure. Unfortunately, they are viewed as disposable workers in today's workforce. Farm labor history is one shameful tale after another of adversity and exploitation.

Annual rates of work-related deaths among agricultural farm workers are two to four times greater than those for the general workforce[481]. Twenty-five to thirty percent of all factory farm workers report serious respiratory ailments[482], and 70 percent of all pig confinement workers suffer from some form or respiratory illness or irritation[483]. Working conditions at slaughterhouses are particularly hazardous. According to the U.S. Department of Labor, meatpacking is the most dangerous job in the United States; slaughterhouse workers are injured or ill three times more than the average factory worker[42].

Human Rights Watch investigated conditions in slaughterhouses and meatpacking plants[484]. Their analysis showed that workers risk losing their jobs when they exercise their rights to organize and bargain collectively to improve working conditions. Immigrant workers are particularly at risk as language difficulties often prevent them from knowing their rights and understanding specific hazards in their work. Undocumented workers risk deportation if they seek to organize and to improve conditions.

Animal Welfare

How we treat our fellow animals is another issue relevant to sustainability. Please refer to the chapter "Transforming Animals Into Food" for more discussion.

Cheap Food: Can We Really Afford It?

Hidden costs and huge subsidies contribute to making our food appear relatively cheap. Studies show that Europeans spend between 25 and 50 percent more of their income on food than Americans[485].

The cheapness of food is in part made possible by the externalization of ecological and social costs. We overlook the true costs when we only consider the price paid at the checkout stand. Agriculture's destructive effects on the environment and society, for example, are not paid up front. We pay through taxes for medical expenses, environmental clean up, or the social and economic impact of employing low paid workers in substandard conditions.

The cheapness of food is also made possible by tax-payer financed government subsidies (estimated at $143 billion over the last decade). Subsidizing food seems a noble cause to make it more accessible. Theoretically, if food is cheaper, people should not have to go hungry. So why do some object to making foods more affordable?

Part of the problem is who benefits from food subsidies, and what types of food we subsidize. According to a report by the Agricultural Policy Analysis Center, the farmers and the environment lose out, while major agribusiness thrives[486]. "Get big or get out" is the general message sent to farmers. The livestock and processed food industries, in particular, benefit greatly[486].

As one example, much public land is cheap or free to cattle grazing[487]. In 1994, the U.S. government paid $105 million to manage the land used for cattle grazing; they only received $29 million from ranchers in return[487]. This keeps expenses down for cattle ranchers, although the savings come from taxpayers' dollars. These subsidies and many others play a role in making meat cheap. Some estimate that if meat prices reflected their true costs, meat would be sold for between $35 and $200 a pound[443, 468]. Sugar (and processed food) subsidies are similarly disproportionately high[488]. The government does not seem to be prioritizing making more nutrient-dense unprocessed plant foods affordable.

Trade agreements have also hurt American farmers, while bolstering the profits of large agribusiness. Many agricultural products can be produced more cheaply in low-wage countries. It is simply less expensive to grow oranges and soybeans in Brazil than in Florida or Illinois.

The new trade deals such as the North American Free Trade Agreement (NAFTA) have reduced the political barriers to food imports, while technological improvements in refrigeration and irradiation have reduced the physical barriers to shipping food long distances without spoiling. When you follow the money you can see that American farmers struggle (and increasingly more are going out of business), while major processors and commodity brokers such as Cargill and Archer Daniel Midland, continue to post impressive profits; these companies just go where wages are cheapest.

The trade agreements are not supporting developing nations either; contracts go to internationally-held corporations, putting local farmers out of business. Desperate farmers sell their land and return to work their fields as low-paid farm workers, barely able to feed their families. Thousands of illegal Mexican immigrants are also crossing the border following NAFTA because cheap (subsidized) American corn has flooded the Mexican market. Farmers can't compete against U.S. corn on their soil, and many end up picking fruit on ours.

It is also a myth that the "efficiency" and size of agribusiness and factory farms makes food cheap for consumers. There are remarkable costs for all the middle-people, such as the costs involved in processing, packaging and preparation for the retail marketplace. Without the intermediary costs associated with the middle-people – if farmers could get fresh foods more directly to consumers – food would be far cheaper and healthier for consumers *and* more profitable for farmers. For example, a farmer that sells through a distributor may only be making about ten or fifteen cents per dollar of the sales price. However, by selling the product directly to the consumer, they may make eighty to ninety cents of that dollar. The food cost to the consumer is the same, but the return to the farmer is far higher.

The grocery store cost also doesn't reflect the damage to our health.

We just can't afford "cheap" food anymore!

Sustainable Agriculture

This has been a depressing story, hasn't it? But there is a flipside. You do have the power to change the direction of our future. You can make choices that are sustainable, and applying these practices *will* make a difference. If you are concerned about the planet, adopting socially and ecologically sound eating habits is one of the simplest and most powerful ways you can make change. Each time you eat and each time you spend money, you are casting a vote for the world you want.

Perhaps most important, you can choose to **buy locally grown products**, which helps minimize fuel consumption and pollution, and better supports the local economy. Farmers' markets are a fun way to shop, and give you a direct sense of where your food comes from.

Community-supported-agriculture (CSA) is another helpful and feel-good alternative. When you become a member of a CSA, you pay money which helps guarantee that the farm can produce food. In return, you get a delivery of whatever fresh seasonal produce is grown. You get top quality produce, and it is often well below retail prices. CSAs save you shopping time – and most also provide you with great recipes to accompany the produce, helping you to try new seasonal foods and in ways you may not be familiar.

Food cooperatives are another alternative in some areas. A food coop is a member-owned business that provides groceries and other products, usually at a discount. Joining usually requires you to pay some dues and/or volunteer your time. Many coops stock organic and/or locally grown foods.

My second recommendation tends to meet more resistance. Environmental science is forcing us to face a fact that those who like pork chops and ribs may not want to hear: our appetite for meat is a driving force behind the environmental damage that threatens our future. Virtually every major threat is included: soil erosion, deforestation, water scarcity and pollution, air pollution, global warming, species endangerment and loss of biodiversity, social justice… **Reducing consumption of animal products** is another very potent solution to our ecological crisis. When and if you do consume animal products, you can choose to get them from more sustainable sources.

You can also choose to **buy organic foods**. If a food is certified organic, that means that the growers did not use any synthetic pesticides, herbicides or fertilizers to grow crops or feed for animals; they did not use crops or feeds that were genetically modified, fertilized with sewage sludge, or irradiated; they did not feed animals the by-products of other animals; they gave animals access to the outdoors; and they were inspected to make sure they followed these rules. Products certified with a "USDA organic" label help to ensure sustainability (except when applied to seafood, which lacks strict legal standards).

Organic foods are clearly a healthier choice, although not primarily because of their direct effects on personal health. Their larger value comes from what they do for the land, air and water, for farm workers, for animals, and for other environmental and social factors. (Note that as helpful as organic labels may be, some small farmers may choose not to become "certified organic" due to the high costs associated with certification. Get to know your local farmers: some may have more sustainable practices without the label.)

There are also plenty of nutritional advantages to going organic. For example, it is well documented that organic foods have higher mineral content than their conventional counterparts. They also have higher antioxidant content: of the fifteen studies with quantitative comparisons, thirteen found higher antioxidant levels, on average 30 percent higher[489]. (Interestingly, organic plants are healthier because they are forced to defend themselves against pests and diseases, resulting in greater production of beneficial phytochemicals.)

Though organics are still only a small percentage of the food market, their sales are increasing dramatically, far outpacing increased sales of conventional agriculture. This has resulted in the emergence of "corporate organics," where the large agricultural giants are relegating small fields to organics, doing little different regarding other practices relevant to sustainability, such as fuel or water conservation or respecting workers' rights. While the organic label does protect you against synthetic pesticides, consider other factors in your choice: there is a huge difference in impact when you support your local organic farmer compared to Safeway Organics.

Nonetheless, the major chains are bringing organics more into the mainstream because they are able to keep prices down, partly because store brands don't require as much advertising.

Attempts to weaken the organic standards have been relentless, and on several occasions the USDA almost bowed to the pressure. At one point they were prepared to allow organic formers to use genetic modification, irradiation and sewage sludge, but backed down after receiving 275,000 outraged letters from consumers. In 2004, they were prepared to allow organic farmers to use pesticides that contained ingredients prohibited by the Environmental Protection Agency, but again backed down when faced with consumer pressure. That "corporate organics" have been so relentless about attacking the organic standards tells us that corporations are clearly resistant to sound stewardship, though they want to capitalize on the success of the organics. And the success of consumer resistance tells us that we do have power and we can make our voices heard.

"Fair trade" products are another ethical choice, supporting fair wages for foreign growers and helping to ensure that our purchases are not contributing to the exploitation of another country's workers. Many growers that are certified "fair trade" reinvest their revenues into strengthening their communities through building health clinics and schools, starting scholarship funds, building housing, and providing leadership training and other community development programs. Many are also committed to sustainable growing practices.

The Slow Food Movement provides a great model for implementing sustainable habits. Its goal is to link pleasure with awareness and responsibility. Slow Food summarizes its vision in the phrase "the right to taste," and fights to preserve the pleasure of food so it does not get lost in the homogenization of fast food. They are active in helping to protect agricultural biodiversity.

Increasingly more restaurants are also showing a commitment to sustainable practices. The phenomenal success of Chez Panisse in Berkeley, owned by Executive Chef Alice Waters, demonstrates that it is possible for restaurants with a commitment to sustainability to thrive, and that there is a strong market for sustainable (and delicious) foods.

Alice Waters has expanded her vision to another highly successful venture: the Edible Schoolyard at Martin Luther King, Jr. Middle School. There, middle school students help grow a sustainable organic garden and landscape. They are involved in all aspects of farming, in addition to preparing, serving and eating the food. These children are experiencing first-hand the connection between what they eat, where it comes from, and the pleasures of eating well.

The strategy is working: the kids report new-found appreciation for the wholesome foods and environment they create. Involving young kids in feeding themselves, from growing foods to eating them, as part of their educational experience, appears to be very effective in creating a new attitude and respect for food.

You can also support sustainability by being more conscientious around packaging and disposable materials. Minimize your use of these products. Carry your own washable dishes and utensils around with you: keep them in the office, bring them to potluck parties, provide your own coffee mug in cafes.

Confused about the choice between paper or plastic choice? How about neither? Using precious resources for a bag you will use for the few minutes it takes to get from store to car and then car to house is remarkably wasteful. Bring reusable canvas totes wherever you go. And perhaps you want to bike to the store?

You can be part of creating the future you want... and you will taste the difference.

Action Tips for ecological sustainability...

- Support locally grown food
  - ○ Shop at farmers' markets
  - ○ Participate in Community-Supported Agriculture (CSA)
  - ○ Support your local food coop
  - ○ Patronize restaurants committed to sustainable practices
- Eat lower on the food chain
  - ○ More grains, fruits, vegetables; fewer animal products
  - ○ Substitute poultry for beef or pork
  - ○ If you eat animal products, get them from sustainable sources
- Buy organic and sustainably grown products
- Seek out heirloom varieties
- Grow your own food
- Eat more fresh, unprocessed foods
- Reduce garbage by buying in bulk and minimally packaged goods
- Join a food cooperative
- Eliminate waste with creative recycling of leftovers
- Use fuel efficient cooking (pressure cookers, woks)
- Use nontoxic cleaning solutions

Get informed...

Check out these excellent books: John Robbins' *The Food Revolution*, Cynthia Barstow's *The Eco-Foods Guide*, E Magazine's *Green Living: The E Magazine Handbook for Living Lightly on the Earth*, Jane Goodall's *Harvest for Hope*, and Anna Lappe and Bryant Terry's *Grub: Ideas for an Urban Organic Kitchen*. All are inspirational books that will help you get up to speed on agricultural sustainability.

Also, check out www.sustainabletable.org.

Be sure to sign on at www.sustainableagriculture.net to stay on top of the latest public policy issues and how you can get involved.

Co-Op America can further educate you and also help you connect with businesses committed to sustainability: http://www.coopamerica.org.

The Union of Concerned Scientists is another excellent resource on this topic: www.ucsusa.org.

To find more sustainable food choices (both plant and animal), plug your zip code into the Eat Well Guide, at www.eatwellguide.org.

Another group that educates about sustainability is Small Planet: http://www.small-planet.org/.

To learn more about identifying sustainable practices on food labels, check out the Consumers Union Guide to Environmental Labels at www.eco-labels.org.

Art Sussman will help you understand the big picture of human interconnectedness with the land and other animals in *Dr. Art's Guide to Planet Earth*.

Michael Brower and Warren Leon of the Union of Concerned Scientists can help you figure out which lifestyle changes to prioritize to have the greatest environmental impact. Read their book, *The Consumer's Guide to Effective Environmental Choices*.

Want to learn more about shifting to a whole foods, plant-based diet? Check out this website: http://www.vegpledge.com/. Local organizations such as Bay Area Vegetarians (http://www.bayareaveg.org/) are also quite helpful.

The SmartSoul Path to Sustainability will help you to learn about what you can personally do to lead a more sustainable lifestyle. It can also help you to find a like-minded community of others. Visit them at http://www.smartsoul.com/ssp_index.html. Or you can take their short quiz to learn about your personal "ecological footprint": http://www.earthday.net/footprint/index.asp.

There are some local groups that support individuals in leading "whole foods" lifestyles. They also provide education and participate in political actions. All of the groups promote a vegetarian or vegan diet; there aren't any comparable groups for omnivores that I am aware of:

Bay Area Vegetarians: http://www.bayareaveg.org/

EarthSave! (Bay Area Chapter): http://bayarea.earthsave.org/

San Francisco Vegetarian Society: http://www.sfvs.org/

To find a farmers' market near you, search the listings at Local Harvest: http://www.localharvest.org/farmers-markets/.

To find out more about Community Supported Agriculture – a cheap, convenient and tasty way to ensure that you get health-enhancing food - check out http://www.nal.usda.gov/afsic/csa/. They have a database you can search to find farms local to your neighborhood.

Check out the Slow Foods Movement to help you find the pleasure in food: http://www.slowfood.com/.

World Hunger and Food Insecurity

Almost 800 million people suffer from chronic hunger, meaning that their daily caloric intake is insufficient for them to live active and healthy lives[490]. This includes one-quarter of all children. Six million children under the age of five die each year of complications related to insufficient food.

The problem is worsening: the number of hungry people in developing countries increased by 18 million in the second half of the 1990s alone.

Hunger and Food Insecurity in the United States

In many developing nations, hunger manifests as severe and visible malnutrition. In the United States, it is often less visible, in part because social service programs provide a safety net for many. Overt starvation seldom occurs here, though many do go hungry and are malnourished. This malnourishment can have harmful effects on learning, development, and physical and psychological health.

"Food insecurity" is a new phrase that has emerged to describe the widespread but less severe hunger problems typically encountered in developed nations. It refers to the lack of access to enough food to fully meet basic needs at all times.

The problem of hunger and food insecurity is also worsening in the United States. During 2006, requests for food assistance increased by 12 percent, with 76 percent of cities surveyed reporting an increasing need for food[491]. The USDA reports that in 2004, 11.9 percent of all U.S. households were "food insecure." Of the 13.5 million "food insecure" households, 4.4 million were classified as "hungry."

Do We Care?

The greatest tragedy in these numbers is that **hunger need not exist. It is about a lack of compassion, not a lack of food.** The real causes of hunger are poverty and inequality. Let's take a look at some of the associated myths[l][395].

First, food is not scarce. This is one of the most damaging and widely-held social justice myths. The problem plaguing agriculture is abundance and glut – not scarcity. There are enough calories produced to feed every human being with 3,810 calories per day[492], far more than the average person needs, if distributed equitably[m][493]. Even most countries where malnourishment is a serious problem have more than enough calories to feed their populace, though they may be net exporters of food.

Food surpluses rot by the sides of the road in India, while millions starve. There is so much food on the market that farmers – globally and in the U.S. - can't get paid enough for what they grow to make a living. Mountains of food are stockpiled or wasted. A study in United States estimates that nearly half of the food produced in this country is wasted before it even gets to our plate. Fields of vegetables are left to rot because they aren't pretty enough. There is nothing wrong with them, but they are not the identical size and shape to meet the needs of agribusiness. And it is not in the farmer's best economic interests to ship them where they might be better appreciated.

We should also remember that most of the grain and soy we produce goes to feeding factory farmed animals, which only return a fraction of these calories to us in meat. In the United States, seventy percent of the grain that is grown is fed to animals. In Latin America, Asia, and Africa there are huge amounts of land that are devoted to soybean production for export to Europe to feed cattle. If it

---

[l] This section is in large part drawn from *World Hunger: 12 Myths, 2nd Edition*, by Frances Moore Lappe, Joseph Collins, and Peter Rosset, with Luis Esparza.

[m] While the exact number of calories may be disputed, it is well established by organizations such as the United Nations Food and Agriculture Organization that we produce more than enough calories to feed everyone. The FAO database calculates that we produce 2,804 kilocalories per day.

were possible to redistribute that food, so that instead of feeding cattle we fed people, we could immediately end hunger.

Likewise, increasing population growth is not to blame. It may go hand in hand with hunger as they both result from inequities that deprive people of economic opportunities, but it does not explain hunger. While it is true that some densely populated countries like Bangladesh suffer from severe hunger, there are plenty of examples of similarly densely populated countries, like Nigeria or Bolivia, where abundant food resources coexist with hunger[395]. The Netherlands illustrates the flipside: while there is very little land per capita, there is also little hunger[395].

Another commonly accepted myth is that nature is to blame for many "hunger" deaths. It's not – nature challenges us, but it is human policies and attitudes that determine who gets to eat during hard times. Even when there have been huge famines in Africa and Asia, people starved because they didn't have any money to buy food, not because there wasn't any food. Plenty of food could be found in neighboring villages, provinces, or the next country. The people who were hungry were hungry because they were broke.

"Conflicts" and wars, of course, limit people's access to food and keep farmers away from their land. In Afghanistan in 2002, for example, farmers weren't able to get to their fields to plant crops, resulting in massive starvation. Many killed their livestock to survive, obviously a short-term solution which limits their future potential to grow food. The U.N. Food and Agricultural Organization reports that the 2004 violence in Greater Darfur in Sudan forced 1.2 million people from their fields, resulting in massive starvation.

Free trade is not the answer either. In most developing countries, exports are big business while hunger persists or worsens. U.S. government subsidies compound the problem since they lead to a surplus of food that costs less than it should. When this gets shipped abroad, it cripples the local farmers.

U.S. aid has usually worsened the problem. Emergency shipments of food often fail to reach those in need. And when the cheap grain is available for famine relief, it undermines local food production, resulting in the local farmers unable to sell their crops.

Check out the current situation in Malawi, a small country in southern Africa[494]. It's May, and corn is abundant. The country has been through a rough time, devastated by AIDS and by famines in 2002, 2003 and 2005. In the most recent famine, one-third of the people ran out of food, so one would think that the current abundance of corn would be reason to celebrate.

But a good harvest doesn't mean prosperity. The price of corn is so low that there isn't anywhere to sell it. Why? Because of U.S. government "aid." We're shipping tons of corn to Malawi as food aid. But our food aid comes with conditions: it has to be bought from American farmers and put in American ships to be transported to Malawi. So the country is flooded with more corn, and the Malawi farmers can't sell what they've got.

If the U.S. gave money instead of food, we could feed more than 2-1/2 times as many people. But then we couldn't offload our surplus. It seems like the primary beneficiaries of U.S. food aid policy are multinational agribusiness and shipping companies.

To make matters worse, a report by the U.S. Congress found that U.S. shipments are often contaminated or infested by insects by the time it gets to the country that needs it[494].

So think twice next time you hear of U.S. generosity. History shows us that our food aid volume increases when prices in the U.S. are depressed; buying farmers' surpluses is a way of subsidizing them – often at a steep cost to the countries we purport to help[494]. Even large charities are critical of U.S. policy: CARE, one of the world's biggest charities, walked away from some $45 million a year in federal financing, saying American food aid supports major American agribusiness firms and may hurt some of the very poor people it aims to help [495].

Also, when governments are controlled by wealthy beaurocrats with little concern for their country's poor, "food aid" just reinforces the status quo.

As corporate globalization expands, we find that the demands of the wealthy seriously and negatively impact the poor in developing countries. People in wealthier nations are consuming more and more of the food resources of poorer nations. We now have a global corporate structure where less developed countries are struggling with poverty and hunger while they deplete their land and resources to feed people in wealthier countries. And when we purchase food from other countries, the money goes to the multi-national corporations, not the local people.

Nor is biotechnology helping the world hunger crisis. Most pesticides that are used by developing countries are applied to export crops, playing little role in feeding the locals that are hungry. In the United States, many are used to improve cosmetic appearance as opposed to nutritional value. Also, genetically modified foods have not been proven to increase crop yields[396-399]. Research conducted at the University of Nebraska, and in Australia and Argentina, found significant drops in production associated with the switch to biotech crops on the order of 10 to 30 percent.

Personal stories about the experience of hunger following the transformation to biotechnology are heart-wrenching. Farming communities that were once self-sufficient – with farmers owning the land and replanting seeds for generations – now rely on costly inputs of fertilizers, pesticides and seeds. The land is being devastated, the water depleted – and small farms can't survive. Thousands of farmers in India have committed suicide by drinking the pesticides that destroyed their livelihood. According to government data, 17,103 farmers made this choice in 2003 alone, the most recent year that data is available[496].

There is no need for increased food production to feed the hungry. What we need is a more just way to distribute the food that we already produce. We have the knowledge, information, and resources to substantially end world hunger; what is lacking is the moral and political will to do so.

Our future

New threats to food security loom on the horizon, some effects already evident. The loss of biodiversity of plant and animal species, for example, is particularly alarming. Seventy-five percent of the genetic diversity of agricultural crops has been lost since the beginning of the last century. Food security depends on diversity in order to be able to adapt to different climates and growing conditions.

Many factors contribute to this loss of biodiversity, including wars, climate change, urbanization and habitat destruction, and large-scale farming techniques that rely on monoculture.

Large-scale farming techniques also contribute to food insecurity by increasing the likelihood of diseases, such as the avian flu, and misusing antibiotics, which weakens our ability to fight pathogens. They additionally increase our vulnerability to bioterrorism: it is a lot easier to introduce disease (whether malicious or unintended) into a huge operation than a smaller, more diverse farm.

The problem of world hunger will continue to worsen given that these root causes are increasing in severity.

The Solution: Food Democracy

Nobody, of course, chooses to be hungry. World hunger and food insecurity are imposed on individuals by a system lacking appropriate fairness and compassion. The vision for a more just world has been termed a "food democracy," a concept which acknowledges that we all deserve the right to sufficient, safe, nutritious food. Included in this, is that people are also deserving of fair access to land to grow food, and fair return on their labor for producing it. Additionally, the land requires our protection so that it is viable to produce food, now and in the future.

Action tips…

Huge institutional changes will be necessary to combat food insecurity. However, individuals also have great power to make a difference. Note that concerns raised in the ecology section go hand in hand with food insecurity, and reviewing the action tips in that section will be valuable. Here are some powerful suggestions that will help make a difference:

- Buy locally produced heirloom products.
- Support farmers with sustainable growing practices.
- Support fair trade products.
- Encourage stores and restaurants to do the same.
- Help spread the word!

Get informed…

A must read is *World Hunger: 12 Myths, 2nd Edition*, by Frances Moore Lappé, Joseph Collins, and Peter Rosset, with Luis Esparza. It will fill in many details for the short blurb provided above.

Follow that up by reading another powerful book, *Hope's Edge: The Next Diet for a Small Planet*, by Frances Moore Lappé and Anna Lappé, which chronicles social movements addressing the root causes of hunger and poverty.

Be sure to check out Food First (www.foodfirst.org) for more information and suggestions on how to get involved in world hunger issues.

The Small Planet Institute (http://www.smallplanetinstitute.org/) will also inspire you and give you the tools to help create a more just world.

Worldwatch Institute (http://www.worldwatch.org) is another great resource, providing, in their words, "independent research for an environmentally sustainable and socially just society."

Food Categories

Fruits and Vegetables

Eating plenty of fruits and vegetables is probably the single most important nutritional habit for good health. This is one area where you'll find consensus among nutrition professionals! Of course, nobody makes much of an effort to help you follow this advice. Given the low profit margins of produce, the produce companies do little to market them. When was the last time you saw a commercial for a carrot?

And the government doesn't subsidize the produce that we directly eat, particularly when compared to the enormous subsidies they put into the foods that end up as added sugars and fats in processed foods (corn, soybeans, sugarcane, beets) or as feed for animals. So I encourage you to get creative about finding ways to enjoy and prepare these nutritional powerhouses. Fruits and veggies can be delicious and easy to eat or prepare, even if nobody's broadcasting it.

Each type of fruit and vegetable carries its unique nutritional punch. Color and smell are often good clues to nutrient content, as the more intensely colored and smelling vegetables are often more nutrient-rich. Leafy green vegetables top the nutrient-density list (such as kale, collards, spinach, chard, romaine lettuce and other leaf lettuces), followed by the solid green vegetables (broccoli, brussels sprouts, artichokes, bok choy, cabbage, celery, cucumber, okra, peas, peppers, kohlrabi, string beans, zucchini). Be sure to get a variety of colors in your diet to maximize the variety of nutrients. The skin of fruits and vegetables is most concentrated with fiber and nutrients, so eat it if you find it palatable.

How fruits and vegetables are grown and processed affects their taste and nutritional quality. Left on their own, fruits and vegetables generally grow to a point of perfect ripeness where their flavor and nutrient density is maximized: you can't beat the taste and nutritional punch of an apricot, ripe and freshly harvested from the tree.

However, life doesn't end when you pick that apricot. Even after being harvested, it is still a living organism; its cells are still breathing (an apricot may not have lungs, but each cell is still consuming oxygen) and enzymes are still functioning. These life processes begin to slow down upon harvest, and some of the flavor chemicals and nutritional value are diminished, increasingly more over time. Best to get your produce as close to harvest as possible.

When fresh isn't really fresh

Fruits and vegetables typically travel a long route before their arrival in your local supermarket. For example, this is the common scenario for a supermarket with centralized distribution: farm, local warehouse, regional distribution center near local warehouse, regional distribution center at destination, local supermarket. There's a lot of jumping around, and on average, somewhere between 1,500 to 2000 miles are traversed.

In order to decrease the perishability of foods, food scientists have developed numerous techniques to slow the post-harvest ripening process, the most common of which is to control the atmospheric gases. For example, virtually all apples are stored and shipped in a controlled environment with less oxygen and more carbon dioxide than common air. Kept in this way, they may be sold as long as a year after being harvested. Carrots are also typically kept in cold storage for months before delivery to a supermarket. Pre-cut salads are stored in bags with nitrogen gas added to prevent the browning and deterioration that would typically occur. While these methods are effective at reducing perishability, particularly cosmetic value, they are unfortunately accompanied by a loss in taste and nutritive value.

Freshness is a larger concern for some vegetables, such as the ones that are grown above ground (broccoli, cauliflower, lettuce, etc.), as opposed to those that are grown below ground (such as carrots and potatoes), which keep longer. Within a day of picking, broccoli might lose about a third of its Vitamin C content. However, after that initial nutritional drop, the rate of decrease goes down dramatically. You probably can't do much about that initial day, so I wouldn't worry about it too much. Besides, most micronutrients are much more stable than Vitamin C. Flavor chemicals, on the other hand, tend to be even more fragile, providing good incentive to purchase freshly harvested produce.

Most fruits and vegetables naturally produce ethylene gas while on the vine or tree, which causes them to ripen. Many companies pick their produce well before it has fully ripened so that it won't perish before getting to the market or your table. Unfortunately, picking produce before it is fully ripened also means that flavor chemicals won't fully develop.

Manufacturers apply chemicals to slow the ripening process, and more chemicals to enhance ripening once it gets to the stores. (Ethylene, the chemical that the produce would have naturally released if let to ripen on its own, is the most common ripening chemical used.) Most bananas have been bred not to ripen on their own, but to instead wait until they reach the gassing facilities.

Root vegetables ripen more slowly, and only minimally deteriorate when carefully stored in commercial warehouses that control humidity and temperature.

Beauty is more than skin deep

Keeping up appearances is important for food manufacturers, but appearances can be deceiving. Sellers assume that consumers are looking for cosmetic perfection, and fruit and vegetables that aren't picture perfect aren't accepted for sale. The grading system is all about looks. As much as 20 percent of the harvest is left in the field to rot because of cosmetic imperfections.

These expectations dictate excessive use of pesticides to prevent the smallest spot, even though those spots typically don't affect the taste or quality. For example, 13 of the 16 sprays used on conventionally grown Nova Scotia apples are aimed at a fungus that leaves a slight scab on the outside of the peel, which is easily sliced off and doesn't affect taste or nutrition[497]. And the plump look of fruits and vegetables could be from excessive use of nitrogen fertilizers, which cause plants to shoot up quickly and suck up extra water.

To prevent dry skin and wrinkling that comes with age, some vegetables get a wax coating (often impregnated with fungicides) to seal in their water. Vegetables that are commonly waxed include cucumbers, sweet potatoes, white potatoes, squashes, tomatoes, peppers, beets and rutabagas. Sometimes the wax is visible on the surface (cucumbers, for example), but it isn't usually obvious on other vegetables. Though the Food and Drug Administration requires that retailers post signs identifying waxed produce, I've yet to see any that comply with this regulation.

I was a little uncomfortable when I first discovered that the same wax is used for polishing cars and furniture, but on further examination, it seems unlikely to harm you. However, note that it seals in pesticides and fungicides along with the water. Besides, it's a clear indication that the produce can't be very fresh.

Some fruits are dyed to give them a more appealing presentation: oranges from Florida, for example, are green when ripe on the tree, but dyed orange prior to sale.

Processed produce

Good to keep a healthy skepticism if the food is pre-packaged. It's interesting how we get deceived at times. Those convenient baby carrots? They're really just ordinary carrots cut and shaped to give the perception that they're out of the ordinary.

Bagged produce that has been washed and pre-cut does provide convenient, though costly, access to ready-to-eat vegetables. (But is it really so difficult to wash and cut your own?) They are typically washed in chlorinated water, a not so environmentally-friendly method of cleansing. Little of the chlorine residue remains on the produce, however, and I'm not so concerned about its direct effect on your health.

Buying frozen, dried or canned produce are alternative options when fresh isn't convenient. While they are likely to be less tasty and nutritious than fresh, they are still a good way to get important nutrients and tasty food.

Frozen vegetables are typically blanched in hot water to deactivate enzymes that play a role in the vegetable's deterioration. This cooking, of course, results in some nutrient loss. They are then flash-frozen to minimize further nutrient loss. While frozen, they are still deteriorating, although at a much slower pace than if they were left at warmer temperatures. The longer frozen vegetables are stored, the greater the nutrient loss. If the frozen packages are handled carelessly as they are shipped between warehouses and the supermarket, they may thaw and refreeze, and the tissues break down further, causing additional loss of nutrients (and taste).

Despite this nutrient loss, frozen vegetables are still nutritional powerhouses, just less so than fresh vegetables. And sometimes vegetables are picked at peak ripeness, flash frozen, and much more nutritious than the limp "fresh" vegetables that are out of season.

Drying is a good way to preserve fruits and vegetables because most bacteria can't grow in the absence of water. Sun drying used to be the method of choice, but is rarely practiced now. Instead, fruits and vegetables are typically dried quickly in a blast of hot air. Nutrient losses aren't too high, and the valuable fiber is retained. Light colored fruits are dipped in a solution of sulfur dioxide and other compounds to prevent browning. This is unlikely to have any effects other than cosmetic.

Canned fruits and vegetables are lowest on the quality rung. Food is sealed in a can and then cooked at a temperature so high that it is equivalent to boiling vegetables on a home stove for about two hours. Of course, the tissue is damaged, and nutrients and flavor are lost.

Canned vegetables are still nutritional powerhouses when compared to many other food groups; if circumstances dictate, go for the convenience of canned vegetables rather than missing out on your vegetables entirely. In the winter months when fresh food is in limited supply, canned products serve a particularly valuable purpose.

Manufacturers of canned fruit typically add sugar to the canning water; the syrup prevents the fluid from draining out of the fruit pieces, and helps the fruit retain its firmness. However, just because the fruit retains its firmness doesn't mean that that it also retains its nutritional value; although the fiber and some nutrients remain, the nutrition is still compromised. The added sugars in many of the canned fruits make them more like candy than fruit, but on occasion you can find them without added sugar.

Conventional vs. organic produce

Is organic produce more nutrient-dense than its conventional counterparts? Research shows this to be the case, although the degree is up for debate. Most research shows substantially higher mineral content, which makes sense given how damaging conventional agriculture is to the soil. However, the vitamin differences are less impressive (although present), and overall, the nutritional advantages may not have a measurable effect on health. There are plenty of more important reasons to choose organic than its superior nutrient content (taste ranking high on the list!).

How to preserve your produce

The biggest enemy is moisture loss: minimize this by storing most of your produce in your refrigerator's crisper, which is a drawer that helps to retain moisture.

Cooking

Heat destroys living tissue – and that's in fact one of the reasons we cook vegetables, to break their tissues and make them softer. Unfortunately, heat also destroys some vulnerable nutrients. Furthermore, when you cook in liquids, vitamins, minerals and phytochemicals can leach into the liquid.

Steaming vegetables is one of the best ways to cook them while limiting nutrient loss, in contrast to boiling, which will most likely result in the greatest nutrient loss. Be sure to use the cooking liquid in soups or sauces to get some benefit from the leached nutrients.

Summing Up

Fruits and vegetables are now accessible independent of geography, season or weather conditions – and in a variety of convenient forms. But these advantages come at a price. While we get convenience, we often sacrifice flavor and nutritional value. You can't beat locally grown, freshly harvested, and minimally processed produce! However, there are plenty of alternatives and compromises available.

Fruit and vegetable buying tips, for maximum nutrition and health:
- Choose intensely colored and strong smelling vegetables and fruits for maximum nutrient variety and density.
- Shop frequently and use fruits and vegetables as soon as possible.
- Check for crispness or firmness.
- Buy locally grown, freshly picked produce. (Support farmers' markets and Community Supported Agriculture.)

Preparation and cooking advice:
- Don't wash or cut your vegetables and fruit until you are ready to use them.
- To maximize the nutritional punch, don't peel most unwaxed fruits and vegetables.
- Minimize cooking time. Most vegetables should be barely tender. (Of course, potatoes need to be cooked until soft.)
- Use minimal cooking liquid (e.g. steam, microwave or pressure cook as opposed to boiling).
- Serve vegetables promptly.

Grains

In their whole form, grains (such as wheat, rice, oats, etc.) and flours made from those whole grains (found in some cereals, pastas, breads, etc.) contain abundant nutrients: they are high in fiber, slowly absorbed carbohydrates, micronutrients and phytochemicals, have a good proportion of protein, and are low in fat (containing no cholesterol and an insignificant amount of saturated fat).

The part of the plant that is made into flour is called the kernel. In earlier times, people milled the grain by grinding the whole kernel. Over time we shifted to refining grains, which involves removing the bran and germ, and leaving only the endosperm. Refining makes the grain faster cooking and less perishable, but at a high cost to nutrition (and taste). Ironically, we then add the bran and germ to cattle feed, giving livestock the healthier components and saving the less nutritious stuff for us.

In 1936, research found that many people were suffering from deficiencies of iron, thiamin, riboflavin and niacin, which they used to receive from bread, prior to refining. So what does our government do? Makes it mandatory to add these nutrients – but not any of the others - back to flour! (Later, folate was added.) Wonder if anyone considered just using the whole grain again?

Whole grain products are rich in nutrients (and taste) and help to protect against disease. Refined grains have lost many nutrients, including their fiber. While enrichment may slightly improve the nutrient value of refined grains, they are still a far call from the whole grains they were made from. Their sugar and starch is quickly absorbed, leading to potential metabolic disturbances – and they rarely retain the original fiber.

Refined flour provides little nutritional value and squeezes healthier food out of our diets. Ironically, poorer countries tend to do better in this regard than the wealthier ones. For example, the percentage of total dietary energy in most traditional diets worldwide historically accounted for by whole grains is 75-80 percent. By comparison, the percentage of total dietary energy in the standard American diet accounted for by whole grains is only 1 percent! Replacing refined grains with whole grains is an easy change most Americans can make to improve their nutrition.

However, I also want to remind you that the nutritional impact of foods needs to be viewed within the larger context of one's total diet. For example, traditional Chinese culture uses high quantities of refined white rice, however, the incidence of diabetes and insulin resistance in that country is relatively low. That's because the rice is eaten with large quantities of fresh vegetables, and the fiber from the vegetables can help to lower the GI of the white rice and provide other nutritional benefits.

Many Chinese restaurants in the United States, on the other hand, continue to use traditional white rice, but serve it with meat-based dishes. While the protein and fat in the meat will also serve to lower the GI somewhat, thus lowering the risk for diabetes and insulin resistance, it doesn't contain the added benefits that come with the fiber and phytochemicals found in vegetables. (It's ironic that as people become better off financially, they abandon more traditional plant-based, whole foods diets in favor of less nutrient-dense diets consisting of more processed foods, fat and meat.)

Know your flours

<u>Not So Nutritious</u>

White flour has been refined and bleached for whiteness/softness.

Unbleached flour has the same (poor) nutritive qualities as white flour, sans the bleach.

Wheat flour is any flour made from wheat (including white flour).

Stone ground refers to a milling practice. It is often conducted on refined grains (unless of course whole grain is specified).

Brown bread is refined and colored wheat flour, unless the word "whole" appears.

<u>The Good Stuff</u>

Sprouted grains are made from the whole grain, and are the most nutritious form of grain. The grains are soaked in water, and allowed to germinate. The enzyme activity helps to "pre-digest" some difficult to digest carbohydrates, and make them and some of the micronutrients more accessible for absorption.

Whole grain refers to a grain milled in its entirety, not refined.

Whole wheat flour is made from whole wheat kernels and is whole grain.

Know your rices

Brown rice is the whole form of rice, as are the more exotic red and black rices; white rice, on the other hand, is the less nutritious refined form.

Curious about corn?

Contrary to popular belief, corn is a grain, not a vegetable. A whole dried corn kernel has a skin which contains fiber and a nutrition-packed germ. Unfortunately, both are usually removed before the corn is ground to make cornmeal, polenta and grits. Look hard to find whole grain cornmeal, and be sure to refrigerate it as it goes rancid quickly.

Wonder about oats?

In their whole form, oats are usually called groats. Steel cut oats (a coarse cut) or rolled oats (flakes) are also whole grains, even if they are quick-cooking or instant, which are partially cooked versions of the "old-fashioned" rolled oats. The quick-cooking and instant oats have a significantly higher glycemic index than "old-fashioned" oats but retain many of the nutrients.

Don't fall for trick labels!

Manufacturers employ many deceptive practices on food labels. If the word "whole" doesn't appear in the ingredient list, it's not likely to be a whole grain (e.g. wheat flour, brown bread, stone ground, multi-grain). Just because a bread is dark colored and called wheat bread, doesn't mean it contains whole wheat. More likely, molasses or caramel has been added as a coloring agent, and wheat (not whole wheat) flour is the predominant ingredient.

Also, be wary when you see a non-whole grain on the ingredients list followed by a whole grain. Most likely the whole grain is in very limited quantity, but a touch has been added so the manufacturer can legally claim that the product contains whole grain.

For maximum nutrition, **look for the word "whole" in the ingredients list and make sure it's the first ingredient.** Ignore other marketing ploys, such as pronouncements about "whole wheat goodness" or "multi-grain" and stick to the more reputable information provided on the nutrition facts panel and the ingredients list. You can find whole grain breads, cereals, pastas, rice, snack foods, etc.

Don't like whole grains? Some suggestions: Make the change slowly. Try mixing brown rice with white rice. You might enjoy the added texture. Experiment with different types of grains.

Cereal Chicanery

Breakfast cereals are the most highly fortified food on the market. Most are made with refined flour and fortified with high doses of vitamins and minerals. Only the flavoring chemicals, colors and shapes distinguish them. Since they are cheap to make, there is a high profit margin, and they are heavily advertised. Americans have clearly absorbed the advertising message, as cereals have a reputation for being a nutritious breakfast or snack choice. Hats off to the marketers. In fact, most cereals are more like candied vitamin supplements disguised as cereal.

Use your judgment around even the whole grain cereals (particularly the cold ones). Just because a food is a whole grain, doesn't automatically make it nutrient-rich. Many whole grain cereals are so processed that they don't have a significant amount of fiber or other nutrients relative to their other contents. And whole wheat flour that is finely ground is absorbed into your bloodstream rapidly, making it less wholesome than coarsely ground whole grains.

Which is not to say that you can't find wholesome cereal choices. You can. Look for whole grains that are high in fiber and low in sugar. Check the ingredients list for evidence of less processing.

Or make your own. It's not difficult. Leftover brown rice or kamut - or any grain - from the night before? Mix it with a little honey and cinnamon and toast it in the toaster oven. Add toasted nuts and fresh or dried fruit. The same strategy also works for old-fashioned oats: toast them with a sweetener and spices of your choice, and then add some toasted nuts and dried fruit for a delicious homemade granola.

Legumes (Beans, Peas, Lentils and some Nuts)

Legumes are jam-packed with nutritional benefits. In addition to containing carbohydrate (starch and fiber) and ample vitamins, minerals and phytochemicals, they are also a great source of protein and healthy fats. They're near the top of the nutrient density list (following most vegetables) and are the most concentrated source of fiber. Many provide as much calcium as milk, minus the acidic amino acids that cause your body to excrete some of its calcium.

One particular legume is quite prevalent, lurking in your cupboards, your cereal, bread, pasta, chips, cheese, condiments, yogurt, sausages, ice cream – even M&M's and lattes. Know what I'm talking about? Soy!

No doubt you've heard a lot of positive stuff about foods made from soy products. Even the Food and Drug Administration sanctions them, citing their ability to fight cardiovascular disease[498]. Numerous studies document soy's beneficial effects on cholesterol and other cardiovascular disease. (The same results could probably be expected from any beans – but only soy has been so well-tested.)

Given its popularity, however, it's not surprising that soy is mired in controversy. You also may have read counter-claims suggesting that soy may actually endanger health. That's not so surprising. All foods can have benefits in one system and pose detriments to others. Here's the scoop.

Soybeans are rich in phytochemicals, such as isoflavones, and the only beans that are complete proteins (contain a full complement of essential amino acids). (Most beans are rich in phytochemicals, particularly flavonoids, though isoflavones are particular to soy.)

Isoflavones, like those found in soy, typically act like weak estrogens. (For this reason, they are called "phytoestrogens.") These have well-documented positive effects, such as working with soy protein to lower blood cholesterol levels, and perhaps also lower the risk for osteoporosis and hot flashes and other uncomfortable symptoms of menopause.

However, estrogens are also known to increase cancer risk in women, and soy's role in promoting cancer seems to be the backbone of the media sensationalism raising fears about soy. So far, this concern (and others) doesn't appear to be well grounded by research, which shows contradictory results.

Nor am I particularly worried about another hot topic in the media, soy's effects on infants and children. One study did find that the highly concentrated phytoestrogens in soy formula might weaken the immune systems of babies, but this risk is largely theoretical. There's no evidence to date that soy formula is unsafe, or that infants have been harmed by drinking it. Nor was I able to find any scientific evidence documenting the popular claim that high soy intake causes boys to develop breasts or otherwise affects their reproductive development.

Most likely, beyond the positive effects on lowering cholesterol, the benefits and risks of soy are probably too small to make much of a difference. That those who consume high quantities of soy have lower rates of cardiovascular disease, menopausal symptoms and other health problems may have more to do with the overall benefits of a diet relatively high in plant foods and low in animal foods.

I suspect that another issue that confuses the research literature is that the quality of soyfoods differ dramatically. The less processed (edamame, tofu, and some soymilks) and the fermented forms of soy (tempeh, miso, natto), more typically used in Asian countries, act quite different than the soy derivatives (soy protein isolate, texturized vegetable protein, hydrolyzed soy protein) used in more highly processed foods. That Americans get more of their soy in the highly processed form may explain why the deleterious effects are showing up in the American research literature.

Industry has discovered a way to profit from every part of the bean. Most vegetable oils are made from soy; soy lecithin is a common emulsifier; soy flour is the base of many baked products; and various forms of soy protein are added to everything from fast food burgers to protein powders to animal feed – even cardboard. Extensive processing produces excitotoxin byproducts such as glutamate (think MSG) and aspartate (part of aspartame), which further complicate the health picture.

Soy is a great imitator. By itself soy protein has little taste, but it is adept at absorbing other flavors. Soy products, such as soy burgers and soymilk, are popular and easily accessible. Texturized vegetable protein is the stuff used to fool people into thinking they're eating meat. It's made from soy protein bundled with flavors, dyes, additives, and hydrolyzed vegetable protein, flavored and textured to resemble animal products like pork, beef, fish or duck. By the time it gets to that form, I doubt it maintains many of the characteristics found in the original soybean.

Meat, Poultry, Fish/Shellfish, and Eggs

Meat and Poultry

Meat and poultry are the central focus of meals for many North Americans. We eat dramatic amounts: though we only make up 7 percent of the world's population, we eat one-third of the world's meat supply.

The role of meat in our diet has come under great scrutiny, bringing up a wide range of sustainability concerns that affect personal, environmental and community health – and challenge our moral values. As a result, the meat in our diet is a highly emotional issue.

I teaching nutrition to culinary arts students, and it's been interesting to see how resistant students and the chefs on faculty have been to discussing these concerns. Meat is such a central part of many people's diets that we just don't want to think too much about anything that might threaten our enjoyment of it. Nonetheless, as difficult as it may be to acknowledge, it is well accepted by nutritionists, health care practitioners and environmentalists – indeed, anyone who studies meat - that Americans on the whole would benefit from reduced consumption.

Meat and poultry contain ample amounts of vitamin B12 (not easily found in vegan diets) and are also good sources of selenium, zinc, iron, phosphorous and B vitamins, placing them mid-range on the overall nutrient density scale.

Meat is also a concentrated source of protein, although given our over-consumption of protein, this doesn't appear to be a benefit. (It is not surprising that most Americans over-consume protein as meat plays such a central role in the American diet. There are seven grams of protein in a single ounce of meat, so eight ounces of meat (a half pound) alone supplies more than the Recommended Dietary Allowance for an average-sized person.)

If you choose to eat meat and poultry, moderation is recommended; small servings provide significant amount of nutrients.

The nutritional quality of meat depends in part on the conditions under which the animals were raised as well as how the food was processed.

Most animals (over 95 percent) are raised in crowded conditions on large factory farms. Disease rates are high, and animals are typically given antibiotics (which serves both as a protective measure to minimize disease and as a growth enhancer) and other chemicals to speed growth, which leaves less time for flavor chemicals to develop. They are fed a diet which predominates in grain, although their digestive tracts are not suited to properly digest the grain. Tight confinement results in little movement; as a result, their muscles stagnate and more fat develops.

Organic animals, in contrast, are free to roam, eat a diet more suited to their physiology, are only given medicines when sick, and are not given any growth hormones. For optimum quality, go organic. (Many claim that organic tastes better as well.)

How does the nutritional content of the different cuts of meat vary? Any time you cut something, you expose more surface area, making it susceptible to deterioration (oxidation). Un-cut products, like whole chickens and turkeys, are therefore more nutritious than cut products, and larger cuts, like steak, are more nutritious than hamburger meat. Grinding breaks the cell structure, causing loss of vitamins and minerals, allowing the essential fatty acids to oxidize, and exposing the foods to more bacteria. Freezing also causes the cell membranes to deteriorate, resulting in similar problems. (Note that it is legal to label items as "fresh" even though they were previously frozen; this is common at many deli counters.)

It's becoming less likely that the meat you buy in the supermarket is just meat and more common for animal foods to be injected with water, salt and chemicals in an effort to make up for the loss of taste that results from current breeding practices. (Check the label to see if your product has been "enhanced.")

Sausages, hot dogs, and deli meats are typically last on the quality list as they are often mixed with extra fat, emulsifiers, flavors, and other chemicals - which are generally cheaper than the meat. Also, they are usually made from meat that may be less appealing and can't be otherwise sold (cow lips and cheeks, , pig snouts and stomachs, etc.). Contrary to legend, they do not contain animal eyeballs, hooves or genitals.

Low-fat processed meats tend to be particularly low in nutritional quality. The main way meat is manipulated to lower the fat content is by adding water. In order to do that, it is necessary to add water-absorbing substances, like carageenan and food starch, which have a bitter taste. This typically results in more flavoring chemicals. In the end, these highly processed meats bear little resemblance to the original product they were derived from, and hold little nutritional value.

Fish and Shellfish

Seafood can be high in nutrient density, containing a good amount of vitamins and minerals in addition to protein. Their low saturated fat content gives them a distinct nutritional advantage over other animal foods. Cold-water fish contain an abundance of omega-3 fatty acids, a boon for your heart and brain.

But the great health benefits of seafood are possibly over-shadowed by their health drawback: the massive pollution of our waters. Fish absorb the toxins, making some quite toxic for us to eat. (See the food safety section.) This poses quite a dilemma: fish have excellent nutritional value, but their nutrients may be delivered in a toxic package. You are well advised to educate yourself on the different varieties of fish and their varying degree of toxin content – and to follow recommendations for moderating the fish you eat. And of course, fishing poses environmental concerns, addressed in the Ecology section. The appendix provides some information to help you make informed choices.

There's a challenge in getting seafood to our plate, particularly if we want the nutrients intact. Once dead, fish are quickly subject to deterioration. And bruising - almost inevitable when catching fish in large commercial batches - quickens the deterioration process. By the time the fish gets to you, there's not much quality time left: be sure to eat it quickly.

Top rank for nutrient-density is fresh, wild fish. Farmed fish suffer similar difficulties as other factory farmed animals: packed in confined spaces, they are prone to disease and receive antibiotics and swim in water with large doses of herbicides. Farmed fish are typically more contaminated than wild fish[352]. Additionally, they are fed less nutritious foods than their wild counterparts find, resulting in less omega-3s for you.

Lowest quality is the restructured seafoods, like the fake crabmeat, lobster, shrimp, etc., which is labeled "imitation" or "artificial." It is sold in that form, and also frequently found in seafood salads and soups. The fish is washed repeatedly until it loses all flavor and color, cornstarch, binders, flavors and sugar are added, and then it is shaped, painted and frozen. Almost all of the nutritive value has been washed out.

Fish retailers are required to inform you whether a fish is farmed or wild, and its country of origin. (Processed seafood, such as fish sticks, sushi, and canned products, is exempt.) Strangely, wild fish are labeled according to the country of origin of the fishing boat, not the location caught. This undermines the intent of the law. You may know that the northern coast of Europe is highly polluted, for example, but if the fish is harvested in the U.S., you would never know its true origin.

Given how difficult it is to get fresh fish to consumers quickly enough, much is immediately frozen and then thawed when it gets to market. For some reason, it is legal to then label the fish "fresh," so you may have some trouble distinguishing if your fish is really fresh.

Use your senses when buying fish. It should not have an odor, and its eyes should be clear and bright. The skin should be a vivid color – although it is easy to be fooled by the dyes that are now commonly added to the feed pellets fed to farmed fish. All farmed salmon, for example, contain added color. Rules are that added colors need to be disclosed, but I've rarely seen retailers comply.

Is the dye dangerous? It's not clear. Canthaxanthin has been found to accumulate in the retina of the eye, and its health consequences haven't been adequately examined. The European Commission's Health and Consumer Protection Agency has recommended reduced use of this dye, but U.S. agencies have been silent.

Some wild fish also get cosmetically altered. For example, wild tuna tends to brown, and seafood companies spray them with carbon monoxide to prevent this. This is unlikely to be harmful, but it can deceive you into thinking the fish is fresher than it really is. The European Union, Japan and Canada ban this practice.

While the term "organic" is usually a helpful term, holding manufacturers to high standards, it is relatively meaningless when applied to seafood. This is because the USDA's rules for the National Organic Program don't mention seafood. Without defined standards, producers can't be certified or use the USDA Organic Seal. However, many sellers use the term "organic" and define the standards for themselves. These standards are rarely described on the product, so you don't know what practices were followed, nor how they were monitored. I'd advise you to ask your fishmonger these questions before paying the higher prices of "organic" seafood. It may be good stuff, but the word "organic" alone - at least when applied to seafood - doesn't ensure that.

Eggs

Eggs get about 40 percent of their energy from protein (the white portion) and the other 60 percent from fat (the yolk). They have more cholesterol than any other single food - a large egg contains about 215 mgs, and the government's recommendation are for less than 300 mgs in a day - and much of their fatty acids are saturated. They also contain a moderate dose of micronutrients, including selenium, choline, and Vitamin E.

Given their high cholesterol content and the well-known association between diets high in cholesterol and heart disease, egg trade groups have worked aggressively to minimize cholesterol being seen as a health problem, and have funded several research studies designed to prove that eating eggs doesn't raise blood cholesterol levels. Remember those catchy ads, with the eggs breaking out of jail, implying that new news shows that their cholesterol is not problematic?

They are also hard at work trying to convince us of the great nutritional advantages. I remember a flyer put out by the Egg Nutrition Center, bragging that eggs have nutrients, satisfy hunger, make convenient snacks, taste good, and don't cost too much. All possibly true. But you could make the same claims about many other foods, like beans, fruits or vegetables, sans the cholesterol and saturated fat problem. Is that really the best they could do? So don't get suckered in. Eggs are not a super-food. Nor will they kill you, particularly if eaten in moderation.

You can get eggs laid by hens who were fed supplemental omega-3 fats, resulting in a higher omega-3 content in the eggs. Will these eggs be more nutritious? Sure. Most Americans are deficient in omega-3s. Worth the price? Hardly – you can get at least a month's supply of fish oil or flax for the cost differential of a dozen of eggs!

The color of the eggshell doesn't matter; the nutritional contents are the same. The grading system (AA, A or B) refers only to cosmetics and says nothing about nutritional differences.

Dairy

Milk

Many dairy products carry a decent nutritional punch, particularly the less processed ones (like milk), and the lower fat versions. However, as discussed in the nutrition politics section, dairy products are not the ideal foods they are espoused to be, and don't deliver on all the tenets they're promoted for. Their reputation as a super-food can mostly be attributed to super marketing.

Milk from any species is designed to make infants of that species grow. Though milk is clearly the perfect food for baby cows, it's value for humans is less well established. Let's take a closer look.

Fresh milk is a suspension of fat droplets in watery whey. Left to its own devices, the fat would naturally separate from the whey. Milk is first processed to fully separate the cream from the whey, and the cream is then added back in the right proportions to make the 1 percent, 2 percent, or full-fat milk. Since the sugar, protein, minerals and most vitamins dissolve in the watery part of the milk, removing the fat poses little detriment to the other nutrients. The fat-soluble vitamins A and D are reduced, but these are later supplemented.

The next step is homogenization, which mechanically mixes the milk together and breaks the fat globules into small enough pieces that they stay evenly suspended in the whey. The leftover cream is used to make butter, cheeses, and other products.

The milk is then pasteurized, which means that it is brought up to a high temperature to kill some of the bacteria. Heat damages the taste, so the temperature that is used is a compromise: high enough to kill most of the bacteria, but low enough to preserve much of the taste. (Ultra-pasteurization scalds milk under pressure at a very high temperature for a very short time.)

Raw milk enthusiasts prefer the taste of raw milk. They also get additional benefits, such as some healthy bacteria that are otherwise killed during pasteurization. Some of these bacteria make lactase, making raw milk much more palatable to lactose-intolerant individuals. And since some vitamins (but no minerals) are damaged during processing, raw milkers get additional nutrients, although the damage to the more important vitamins is to a relatively small degree. On the flip side, homogenization and pasteurization make milk safer and extend the shelf life. My advice to raw enthusiasts is to make sure you trust your source and that conditions are sanitary. There have been very few instances of problems with raw milk, but potential bacterial problems – which are typically solved by pasteurization - could be lethal. In most states it's illegal to sell raw milk, based upon government concerns about food safety (which may be exaggerated).

One negative to milk is that whole milk is high in saturated fat and cholesterol; as dairy foods make up about a third of the saturated fat that people consume and a fifth of their cholesterol, dairy plays a large role in many people's excessive saturated fat consumption. However, if eaten in moderate quantities as part of a diet that is overall low in saturated fat and cholesterol, this need not be problematic. And concerns about dairy's fat content are easily minimized or eliminated by choosing lower-fat or non-fat versions, though these have slightly reduced vitamin content.

There are a lot of great micronutrients in dairy products, including calcium, Vitamin B12, riboflavin, phosphorous, magnesium, potassium, zinc and supplemented Vitamins A and D.

Just don't bank on the common wisdom that suggests that dairy will strengthen bones and stave off osteoporosis. There is little research to support that[29]. (And there are plenty of other ways to get your calcium: most vegetables are loaded with it – and give other dramatic benefits as well. Besides, most experts agree that decreasing calcium loss plays a much more potent role in bone strength than increasing calcium consumption, making running around the block a more effective bone strengthening technique.)

Though the evidence isn't conclusive, research shows an association between milk consumption and several types of cancer, particularly ovarian, breast and prostate cancer. Milk has also been criticized for containing high levels of environmental toxins, such as dioxins and ammonium perchlorate, a component of rocket fuel. Perchlorate can harm the thyroid gland and disrupt the development of motor skills in children, as well as their intelligence.

Be sure to see the carbohydrates section for a discussion of milk's association with type 1 diabetes in genetically susceptible children.

The dairy industry promotes dairy as a weight loss aid. Despite the hype they have conjured, there is more evidence to support the opposite. Yes, there was one research study (funded by the National Dairy Council) that documented that when 32 people dropped their calories, those that ate a lot of dairy lost more weight than the others. But larger studies which attempted to replicate the results found no difference between the high-dairy and low-dairy subjects[499] and there are no studies which examine whether any weight change is maintained on a long-term basis, a fatal flaw endemic to almost all weight loss plans. Besides, there is plenty of other evidence to support that eating a more plant-based diet results in greater stimulation to your internal weight regulation system.

Another issue to consider is the growth hormones given to dairy cows in order to boost milk production. Most commercial cows are injected with rBGH (also called rBST), which refers to recombinant bovine somatotrophin growth hormone. Many people are concerned about its consequences.

Labels on milks produced by dairies that don't inject their cows with growth hormones are bound to generate confusion. In order to claim "no hormones added," they are required by law to also include a disclaimer: "The FDA has found no significant difference from milk derived from rBST treated cows and those not treated." If it doesn't matter, why make the claim?

Confusing statements like this can be simply explained by one word: politics. The thriving hormone-free industry threatens conventional dairies. The company that makes the growth hormone (Monsanto) put enormous financial resources behind lobbying the FDA. First, they made sure that when their rBST injections are given to cows, the dairies don't have to acknowledge this on their labels.

Then, when their competition starting advertising on their labels that the milk was made from cows not treated with hormones, Monsanto – along with the conventional dairies - grew concerned that this simple truth might lure consumers into thinking that the milk was actually different – or better – so their second campaign took the lobbying a step further, resulting in the above statement.

Does it matter? Other countries believe it does and have banned its use. Canada, for example, banned it, citing the increase in lameness, infertility and infections in cows. The European Union banned it, citing the stimulation of production of IGF-1 in cows, a growth factor connected to cancer. It is also banned in Australia and Japan. However, the U.S. Food and Drug Administration says it is harmless.

Here's the deal. All lactating cows (and humans) secrete hormones into their milk, although in such small quantities that the amounts don't seem to affect the cows or humans (infants or adults) that drink it. Cows make a natural form of BST (not recombinant) and this is found in their milk. At the time that the question of whether to require labeling of milk from rBST-treated cows came before the FDA, tests weren't sensitive enough to tell the difference between BST and rBST, and the FDA accepted Monsanto's argument that since there was no detectable difference, labeling needn't be required. Lab tests can now distinguish the two, and there are so far no proven differences in how they act. (This is not to say that they don't have different actions – we are still a long way from understanding the differences posed by genetic modification or being able to conduct the controlled research that would answer this question. See the Biotechnology section for more detail.)

Nonetheless, there are other issues that loom larger than the rBST itself that is found in milk. The first is the effects of the rBST on the cows. Cows just weren't designed to deliver so much milk, and the rBST injections result in infections, both at the injection site and in their udders (mastitis). This is not only painful for the cow, but results in high levels of pus in the milk that we drink. And the more infections they get, the more antibiotics are used, leading to increasing antibiotic-resistance. (See the Food Safety section for a discussion of antibiotics.)

It's also possible that the antibiotics may result in killing helpful bacteria in the digestive tracts of milk drinkers. (Although there are safeguards in place to keep the milk containing antibiotic residues out of our food supply, it is not clear that these safeguards are sufficient.)

The last issue has to do with the hormone IGF-1. IGF stands for insulin-like-growth factor, and IGF-1 is found in both cows and humans. In humans, it is strongly linked to increased risk for breast[21] and prostate cancer[22-24]. IGF-1 is a protein hormone, and typically most proteins are destroyed by stomach acid or intestinal enzymes during normal digestion. However, there have been several studies documenting that IGF-1 levels are boosted in people that drink milk; although inconclusive, this might explain the research showing an association between drinking milk and these types of cancer. Furthermore, women who consume dairy are five times more likely to have twins than vegan women, a fact which could again be explained by the higher IGF levels[500].

Consuming any dairy products increases blood levels of IGF-1 in humans, and consuming milk from cows that have been injected with synthetic growth hormone can have a correspondingly larger effect. In fact, Steinman, the author of the study showing the association between dairy consumption and increased likelihood of twins, attributes rBGH as the significant factor[501].

If you are concerned about hormone-treated cows, some dairies raise cows without giving them hormones, and their milk is often labeled rBGH-free. In the absence of a notice saying the product is rBGH or rBST-free, assume the cows were treated with hormones.

And remember issues related to lactose intolerance, discussed in the digestive disorders section. (Lactose is a carbohydrate found in milk, and some people don't make sufficient quantities of the enzyme lactase to digest it properly, resulting in stomach problems when lactose is consumed.)

So what's the take-home message about milk? There is a wide diversity of opinion among experts. But here's my take. Milk is certainly not an essential component of a healthy diet. Given the lack of evidence of extensive benefits and with so many unanswered questions and possible risks, there is no reason to go out of your way to drink it. Excellent alternatives exist – such as soy milk, almond milk, and rice milk, which carry no risks and many benefits.

At the same time, when considered from the perspective of personal health, while I have concerns, I'm not sufficiently convinced of the dangers of dairy to counsel against consuming it in moderation, if you enjoy it. (However, I would suggest it be avoided by children and young adults with a known susceptibility to type 1 diabetes.)

Many other products are made from milk, such as yogurts, cheeses and ice creams. Be sure to check nutrition labels when purchasing these milk products. Note that many highly processed dairy products, like sweetened yogurts, contain high levels of added sugar and are often low in nutrient density. Dairy-free alternatives to milk-based yogurts, cheeses, and ice cream can also be found.

Cheese

Earlier I mentioned that dairy is the leading source of saturated fat in American diets. Much of this can be attributed to cheese. (Meat is the second highest source of saturated fat, followed by milk.)

Most cheese is made by adding rennet, a curdling agent, to milk, along with bacteria that feed on the nutrients in milk and produce an acid by-product. The usual source of rennet is the stomach of slaughtered newly-born calves. Vegetarian cheeses are manufactured using rennet from either fungal or bacterial sources.

After the bacteria have done their work, the carbohydrates are gone (except for a small amount that remain when cottage cheese is made), the proteins are coagulated and dispersed among the fat, and the fat is loaded with flavor.

Most cheeses are predominately fat, with little protein. If you compare a one ounce serving of the different cheeses, you'll find a range of calories: the harder cheeses like parmesan contain a lot more (fat) calories than the softer ones like mozzarella. This can be attributed to differences in the water content.

Given the high saturated fat content of cheese, it is not possible to eat significant quantities of cheese and stay within the recommended healthy guidelines. An ounce of cheese (the equivalent of about a slice or a one inch cube) contains about 6 grams of saturated fat, which is ¼ of an average person's Daily Value for saturated fat.

Cheese is best eaten in small amounts as an accompaniment to other foods rather than slathered thick on your pizza. (One serving of Pizza Hut's PZone® Classic pizza – half a pie – gives you 11 grams of saturated fat, half the government's recommended daily allotment. And how many people really stop at half the pie?)

Yogurt and Other Fermented Dairy Products

Like cheese, plain yogurt is made by adding bacteria to milk. When the bacteria digest the nutrients in milk, they produce substances that curdle and flavor it. The bacteria digest much of the lactose, making yogurt more tolerable than milk to many who are lactose-intolerant.

The bacteria are quite healthy for you. Although research is inconclusive, they are likely to do a pretty good job of strengthening your immune system. (See discussion of probiotics in the digestion section for more information.) But this means they need to be alive: be sure to check the label for the "Live and Active Cultures" seal as some yogurts are so highly processed that the bacteria are destroyed. The seal is given to frozen yogurts at the time they were made, and I'm not sure that the bacteria will survive the freezing, so I'd be less apt to trust that any frozen yogurt has a significant amount of active cultures.

Sweetened yogurts are often more similar nutritionally to candy than milk. Be sure to check labels for sugar content and other additives.

Many other products are made by fermenting milk, including kefirs, buttermilk, sour cream, etc. These don't pose any additional nutritional issues beyond those covered. Labels can keep you informed about the specifics.

Beverages

Fruit Juices and Drinks

Juicing a fruit exposes the nutrients to air, which of course facilitates nutrient loss. Most of the nutrients - except the fiber - are retained in freshly squeezed juice, but the longer the time lag between juicing and drinking, the lower the nutritional value. In the case of many fruits, like citrus fruits, the pulp contains much of the fiber, making the "homestyle" juices much more nutritious.

Mixed juices can often be deceptive. The featured juice is rarely in high quantity, and the product's main ingredient is probably the cheaper apple or grape juice that is blended. (White grape juice is a tip-off to low quality.) Labels occasionally provide you with the percentage breakdown, but probably only when it is favorable. Remember that the order of the ingredients tells you which juices are in higher quantity.

Sparkling juices are typically a mix of carbonated water and juice (but check the ingredients to be sure), and can be a good way to get a sweet drink with a little less sugar.

To make juice concentrate, manufacturers heat the juice to evaporate the water. As a result, nutritional value plummets. Fruit juice concentrates are basically fruit-flavored sugar (and typically require additional flavor chemicals). Even the USDA Guidelines describe "fruit concentrate" as a euphemism for sugar. Premium juices that have never been concentrated deliver much more nutritional value.

To make juices "lighter" or with lower sugar content, manufacturers typically add water. No great chemical feat here.

Anything called a drink, blend, or punch probably features sugar and water and is unlikely to contain much actual juice. As far as nutrition is concerned, put them in the same category as soda.

Read labels carefully to avoid getting duped. The term "100 percent" may be meaningless if it is not followed by the word "juice." For example, I've seen "100 percent lemonade" composed of 3 percent lemon juice (and of course tons of refined sugar). The ingredients list can confirm for you if it is in fact all juice.

Soda

Soda is among the most heavily marketed products. They are especially cheap to make. Water is practically free, corn syrup costs only pennies per bottle (thanks to government subsidies), and flavor chemicals are used in such tiny amounts that their cost is insignificant. Since the main costs are in packaging, labor, advertising and marketing, the cost differential between making a small soda and a larger one are negligible. So bigger sizes are priced as bargains.

Soda is the prototype of an empty calorie food. No, it's not the cause of all evils, as it is frequently espoused to be. It won't rot your digestive tract nor make you diabetic. Nor will it give you any benefit. If you enjoy it, best to do so in moderation.

And of course, the bigger the container, the higher the calories. Those 64-ounce Big Gulps? 800 kilocalories – devoid of any nutritional value beyond their energy. Big gulp, indeed. I can almost feel the insulin surge!

"Vitamin Waters"

Bottled water is pricy enough, but manufacturers can make even more money if they pack in some vitamins and sell it as a health drink. If you feel the need to supplement, you won't get any advantages to choosing a drink over a much cheaper multi-vitamin/mineral pill.

One difficulty in making these waters is that vitamins taste awful. (Try dissolving a vitamin pill in water if you want to test this.) So manufacturers inevitably add sugar or an artificial sweetener.

The one thing vitamin waters typically have going for them is pretty bottles.

"Sports Drinks"

Athletes sweat and it is no doubt helpful to replenish body water. Water does this best. When the sweating is extreme, it may be helpful to also replenish some of the electrolytes that get lost in your sweat (sweat is salty), and a little sprinkle of salt will easily accomplish this. If you need to fuel yourself, calories are what you need – and there is nothing magical about the ones found in sports drinks.

In other words, if you like the taste of sports drinks, go for it. Just don't get deluded into thinking you're getting something special that you can't easily get elsewhere (and cheaper) – through water, sugar and salt.

Coffee and Tea Drinks and Smoothies

How you frame your marketing plays a large role in its success. A PDA would have gone nowhere if it were marketed as a little computer. But call it a glorified personal assistant and suddenly it is incredibly powerful. Starbucks wouldn't have people lining up if they called their frappucinos milkshakes. Yet their nutritional profile is not all that much different from the milkshakes sold at Baskin Robbins. Best to consider them desserts and enjoy them in that capacity.

And sure, Jamba Juice uses plenty of juice in their drinks, making some of their smoothies quite nutrient-dense. But don't confuse them with eating fruit. In the form of a smoothie, it's easy to take in large numbers of calories without it registering to the degree it would in the fruit's original form. For example, you are unlikely to eat 3 pints of strawberries without considering it an indulgence – yet that's precisely the energy equivalent of an "original" size Strawberry Whirl, an "all fruit smoothie." And some of their smoothies weigh in even more heavily on the calorie scale: most of the "Jamba Classics" tip the scales at just less than 500 kilocalories – making this one drink equivalent to 25 percent of the average person's daily energy intake.

Added Fats

When assessing the health impact of the fats that are added to foods, you need to consider not only the source of the fat, but how it was manufactured.

Most of our salad and cooking oils come from plant sources, a fact which is mostly driven by economics. Plant fats are much cheaper. Not long ago, people preferred cooking with butter and other animal fats, such as lard and tallow. To make the switch, manufacturers had to sell us on the idea that plant fats are healthier. That claim plays a larger role in how people perceive fats and how they are marketed. Many margarines, for example, boast that they are made from pure vegetable oil or are "a rich source of poly-unsaturated acids."

While it may be good advice that in their less refined forms, plant fats are likely to be a healthier option than animal fats, the tables may get turned as plant fats go through the manufacturing process.

But you are well educated enough not to be duped by the deceptive labeling. You know by now that just because something is made from vegetable oil, doesn't mean it's health-enhancing. When vegetable oils are hydrogenated, they are a much worse choice than animal fats. And of course "cholesterol-free" doesn't tell you anything exciting either; it's not a difficult claim since plants never contain cholesterol.

Another important issue to consider is the degree of oxidation. Let's take a closer look at vegetable oils, so we can compare the different terms. All vegetable oils are processed, which of course affects their nutritional profile. Vegetable oils begin in a seed, which is stored energy for the germinating seed. The oil is well protected, as it is packed in fiber and stored with powerful antioxidants, such as Vitamin E. Some seeds are edible – like pumpkin, sunflower and flax – and in this form, are at their most nutritious.

Extracting the oil from plants can be a pretty harsh process, and the result is that most commercially refined oils are considerably less nutritious. High temperature and exposure to air result in oxidized oils. The essential fatty acids are usually the first to be affected.

Most manufacturers use a solvent, usually hexane, to dissolve the oil. The solvent is then evaporated at a high temperature, but traces may remain. Whether the solvent itself affects your health is unknown, but it is clear that the high temperature oxidizes the oil. If the label doesn't tell you the extraction method, assume a solvent was used and that the product is heavily oxidized.

Solvent extraction isn't necessary and other extraction methods result in less damage. Before extracting the oil, the seeds are usually cooked until they are turned into a mash. This mash is then squeezed through a press. The more common method of pressing is called "expeller-pressed" which refers to using several tons of pressure to force the oil out of the seed, resulting in raising the temperature to about 185 to 200 degrees F. Expeller-pressing is a better alternative to solvent-extraction, although the initial cooking does introduce some oxidation.

Better yet, some manufacturers run cooling water through the expeller, called "cold-pressing," resulting in significantly less oxidation. Unfortunately, the term "cold-pressing" is not defined by law, and a cold-pressed oil may have been brought up to a high temperature or previously cooked. So while the odds are that an oil labeled "cold-pressed" is less oxidized than one that is expeller-pressed, there are no guarantees.

After extraction, the oil may be filtered and sold as "unrefined." It contains phytochemicals, Vitamin E, and some other nutritious components, and probably has a strong flavor and cloudy appearance. Manufacturers often further "refine" the oil, making it clearer and removing some of the odor and flavor – and further damaging its nutritional value.

How to make good choices? It's difficult, given the lack of information typically provided on labels, along with the lack of consumer protections. Buying cold-pressed (preferably) and expeller-pressed oils that are "unrefined," while they will cost you more, are likely to be much healthier options than oils without these claims.

There are some special terms applied to olive oil. Extra-virgin olive oil refers to oil that comes from the first pressing of the olive – it has a stronger flavor and retains a lot more of the nutrients. It is always mechanically pressed (not solvent-pressed). "Virgin" is the next quality ranking and is typically a blend of extra-virgin and solvent-extracted oil. "Pure" olive oil is solvent-extracted and refined. Last on the quality list is "pomace" which is the leftovers extracted from substances from higher quality extractions, and "light," which is intensely refined to remove any remaining flavor and color.

Curious what is meant by the anonymous title "vegetable oil?" Manufacturers are apparently concerned that soybean oil has a bad reputation, so that's become a common euphemism for soybean oil.

Other buying and storage tips:
- Best to buy your oil in dark bottles that protect it from being oxidized by the light.
- Avoid oils in plastic bottles as the oil leaches harmful chemicals out of the plastic.
- Keep oils capped to minimize exposure to air.
- Store oils in cool, dark places – or refrigerate them.

And watch for deceptive labeling around the energy content. Regardless of whether an oil is virgin, light, or whether it comes from soybeans, corn or olives, all oil contains the same 9 kilocalories of energy per gram – or expressed in other terms, 120 kilocalories per tablespoon. Even the oil in spray cans contains 120 kilocalories per tablespoon. The labels may say that they are fat-free, but that is only because the serving size is so small. A quarter second spray gives you a quarter gram of fat, and anything less than a half a gram can be rounded off to zero. Some cans have less propellant and give you the same amount of fat in a half second spray.

Some oils (sold in spray cans and tubs) are mixed with water and various chemicals, which results in a lesser energy content than those that are 100 percent oil.

Artificial Sweeteners

In an effort to minimize sugar (and calories), many people turn to artificial sweeteners. These are also known as "non-nutritive sweeteners" because they give you a sweet taste but have no nutritive value. They are so intensely sweet that they can be used in very small quantities, and their energy value is so low that most can be rounded off to zero.

The Internet is saturated with horror stories about all of them, while the Food and Drug Administration proclaims their safety, and many health organizations, such as the American Diabetes Association, tout their benefits.

Who do you believe? Are they safe? The truth is there are no clear-cut answers.

It is impossible to conduct definitive research, particularly since the concerns are about long-term use. It would be nice if we could do a 30-year study comparing people who regularly used artificial sweeteners to those who didn't but otherwise led identical lifestyles, but that kind of data just doesn't exist.

Most of the safety tests are conducted on rodents that are given large amounts of artificial sweeteners to speed up the process and account for potential differences between rodent and human metabolism. Interpretation is never clear-cut. When a study does indicate increased cancer risk, supporters claim that the dosage was higher than humans would ordinarily receive, and when no risk is determined, detractors claim that because humans aren't rats, the research is inconclusive.

Further clouding the issue is that testing is typically done by the manufacturers, rarely by the government or independent laboratories.

I tried to sort through the research on the most popular artificial sweetener, aspartame. Aspartame is sold under the brand names Nutra-Sweet and Equal and you'll find it in products like Diet Coke, Diet Pepsi, Diet Snapple and Sugar Free Kool-Aid. Visit the website of the Calorie Control Council, which is a trade group for makers of artificial sweeteners, and you are reassured that "Aspartame is one of the most thoroughly studied food ingredients ever, with more than 200 scientific studies confirming its safety."[502]

But before I popped open my Diet Snapple, I started wading through the scientific literature and came across an interesting review. Dr. Ralph G. Walton analyzed the 166 articles about aspartame that were published in medical journals from 1980 to 1985[503]. All 74 studies that were financed by industry attested to aspartame's safety. On the other hand, 84 of the 92 independently funded articles identified adverse health effects. Coincidence? I don't think so. Not with those numbers.

There's been some really damning evidence against aspartame when consumed by animals at levels comparable to humans ingesting diet sodas[504, 505].

After further examining the literature, my theory is that there certainly isn't enough evidence on any of the artificial sweeteners to give me confidence that they are safe. And there are indications that suggest wariness is appropriate with every single one of them. On the other hand, though I don't like being a guinea pig, my concern isn't strong enough to drive me to purity.

Processed Foods

When appropriate, discussion of certain processed foods was weaved in to the food categories, but of course, not everything got covered. Use the knowledge you've gained throughout the book to make your own judgments about the other processed food options.

Food scientists have a tough job. They may be making a cookie in Ohio, truck it across the country, and then have it sit in various warehouses for weeks or months before shipping to a store and eventually getting into your hands. And of course, when you open the package, you're looking for perfection. Not an easy accomplishment when you consider that many foods have a natural tendency to separate, melt, precipitate, et cetera, especially after being bounced around.

I always start by reading the ingredients list. Are the ingredients recognizable as food? Many labels are probably more appropriately found in a chemistry lab than on something intend to nourish us. An obvious point to keep in mind is that if the taste or nutrients from real food itself were preserved, they wouldn't be much need for the stabilizers, emulsifiers, flavors, dyes, and other chemicals that get added. So a long list of unrecognizable chemicals is often enough to stop me. It's rare that chemists have been able to improve on nature.

The most common additives are "gums." Examples include gelatin, corn starch, carrageenan, xanthan gum, cellulose gum, locust bean gum, agar, and so on. Gums are used to thicken, emulsify, change the texture, or stabilize the food (prevent ice crystals from forming or sugar from precipitating). Will they hurt you? Unlikely; concerns have been raised that carrageenan may increase risk for ulcers[506], but the others seem harmless.

Even if it tastes good, processed food typically provides cheap thrills, lacking creativity and relying heavily on the same old sugar, fat and salt. As discussed in the Taste chapter, excessive consumption of these gets you hooked and less able to appreciate a diversity of other flavors. In the end, this means food in general is less pleasurable.

A diet high in processed foods also prevents you from getting a good diversity of nutrients. Supermarkets are packed with options, giving us the illusion that we have many foods to choose from. But the truth is that food technology relies pretty heavily on four crops to create the raw materials for most processed foods. Corn gives us corn flour, corn syrup, high fructose corn syrup, corn starch, and corn oil. Wheat gives us flour and modified food starch. Soy beans give us soy bean isolate, texturized vegetable protein, and soybean oil. And refined sugar is derived from beets or cane sugar. Rely heavily on processed foods and you will be limited in your range of nutrients.

Manufacturers know that you are more likely to buy a food if you think that it is good for you, so they routinely throw in cheap vitamins, minerals and other compounds, and then boast of the nutritional value on their label. Don't fall for it. Nature knows best. There are tons of health-enhancing phytochemicals in "real food" that haven't even been identified, let alone developed for fortification. And we just don't understand the synergy of the various micronutrients that we do fortify with to know if they really have the same benefits when found in "real" foods.

If you feel the need to supplement your diet with extra vitamins and minerals, consider buying your own supplement. Judge your food on merits other than its level of enrichment or fortification. Vitamin-supplemented junk food is still junk food.

Why do you choose the foods you do?

Well, you did it. Your introductory journey through nutrition is over. Now it's time to reflect on how you've changed, and come up with a game plan of how you intend to continue to incorporate your "food values" into your everyday life choices. First, complete the below survey.

It is important to me that the food I eat on a typical day:

Rank		not at all important	a little important	moderately important	very important
	Satisfies my physical hunger.				
	Appeals to my senses (tastes, smells and looks good)				
	Is nutritious and has a positive impact on my health.				
	Results in my having stable or good moods.				
	Gives me comfort or cheers me up.				
	Is environmentally friendly.				
	Is convenient to buy, eat or prepare.				
	Supports my religious values or reflects my culture.				
	Is inexpensive.				
	Will help me to lose, maintain, or gain weight.				
	Attracts approval/does not attract disapproval from others.				
	Is a respectful choice in terms of minimizing world hunger.				
	Doesn't contribute to animal cruelty.				
	Is shared with others socially.				
	Is organic.				
	Has not been genetically modified.				
	Has not been irradiated.				
	Is locally grown.				

Rank		not at all important	a little important	moderately important	very important
	Is low risk for contamination in ways not specified above (e.g. harmful bacteria, viruses, or prions)				
	Other:				

Compare your responses to the survey you completed in the initial chapter of the book. Now that you have more knowledge about the implications of your food choices, do you have different priorities when choosing foods?

I do hope that this book was able to help you reclaim the joy in food, and that "appeals to my senses" ranked high on your list. I also hope that you now have a better sense of your "food values" and what's important to you. And don't worry if your values come into conflict with your tastes. Long-term substantive change requires time, and it may take a while before these become more congruent.

Reclaiming the Pleasure in Eating

Understanding where our food comes from helps us to look at the world with entirely different vision. How we choose to feed ourselves may be the single most important factor in creating the kind of life we want for ourselves, the community we want to be surrounded by, and the planet we want to inhabit.

As I think about how to close this book, I am reminded of an experience I had recently, during a visit to a world-renowned museum which had powerful exhibits documenting the ecological devastation caused by modern industry, with a large section devoted to industrial agriculture. After appreciating the museum's exhibits, we visited the museum cafeteria with a heightened sensitivity to the critical role food choices play in community sustainability. The cafeteria was loud and crowded, the décor unimaginative and institutional, and there was an overpowering smell typical of fast-food. None of the food was freshly prepared or organic, and no attention had been put into its presentation or serving it with friendliness and respect. It felt much more akin to a gas station than a place where true nourishment was possible.

This experience was a clarion call that helped me to understand the disconnect that happens in our culture. Caring about ourselves and our world is not something that happens separate from our everyday lives. The museum was not "living" the values it was encouraging.

I want to encourage you to actively engage with our world. Food is a source of joy, and it connects us to our planet. The dominant culture disconnects food from pleasure, nourishment, and its source. There is little attention given to the quality of life of individuals, let alone respect for the world community. This is the incredible challenge - and opportunity - before us. We all, as individuals, have the resources to heal that connection. What we do each day does matter. Each time we eat and shop provides new opportunity to transform our world. This is an opportunity for pleasure, celebration and connection – and you can join in the fun.

Transforming the Planet starts in your body

The single most important thing you can do is start by making peace with the wonderful body you were given. You don't need to measure yourself against someone else's standards. Look at that beautiful body you have and say, "I'm okay just the way I am." Then take it further and say, "I'm gorgeous." Yes, guys, you can say it too. It's okay to admit being attractive is important to you too. How we feel about our bodies affects how we feel about ourselves. The more you care about yourself, the more you make choices that honor yourself. You take good care of things you like.

Don't underestimate the power of body-acceptance. Large industries depend on our self-hatred and the underlying belief that we need to adopt the cultural standards (and buy their products) in order to be acceptable. Increased body-acceptance means that we have less need for these material enhancements; this could topple large sectors of the beauty, fashion and diet industries, for example – and severely weaken all the other industries that promote their products based on your buy-in to a valued cultural image.

I'd also like to encourage you to extend that openness to others and to look through new eyes that value our incredible human diversity. Support your friends and family in rejecting the cultural standards and valuing their bodies, regardless of size.

Transforming the Planet includes self-acceptance

This vision of self-acceptance extends well beyond how we view our bodies. Other industries act in parallel, trying to convince us that the only path to happiness is the purchase of material goods. This results in never-ending consumption - including food - and an increasing sense of emptiness as each new purchase fails to deliver on its promise. Our consumptive habits not only make us feel bad about ourselves, but have taken a serious toll on the environment, depleting many of our earth's resources.

You don't have to buy-in. Self-acceptance – appreciating who you are rather than your accumulation of material goods - is a truly revolutionary act. Apply this to how you treat and view others by learning to see their unique personal qualities, giving less value to their consumptive and material expressions.

Transforming the Planet: enjoy your connection to food

Next, take care to create an environment that supports the pleasure of food. You can start by buying foods in ways that help you feel more connected to their source and in places that provide friendly human interaction. Prepare and share your food with people you like, and eat in enjoyable settings.

Eat mindfully: notice the feeling of food in your mouth, the flavor and texture, how it feels in your body, whether it satisfies your senses. Take care to get the foods you enjoy, and commit to eating truly delicious food. Food should satisfy you and make you feel good. Pay attention to how the food affects you after you eat, noticing whether you are comfortably full, if you have stable energy and mood. Allow this information to inform future choices.

Transforming the Planet: expanding your vision

When I first started to become educated on issues of sustainability, I felt consumed by guilt over eating. Imagine this. You are invited to dinner at a friend's house. She serves broiled salmon and a green papaya salad, artfully displayed on a bed of arugula, red cabbage and microgreens.

It is easy to get overwhelmed with questions: Is it okay to take an animal's life? Did it have a painful death? Was the salmon farmed or wild? Should I be concerned about its mercury content? Was it laced with antibiotics, pesticides, dye? Was it part of a community that is dying from over-fishing? Was it caught through trawling, which involved painfully and unnecessarily killing numerous other animals and plants? Did it come from a large commercial industry that displaced the livelihood of the local fisher-people? How did it get to me? Was it transported thousands of miles in trucks running on gasoline? And what about the vegetables...

Education comes with a price. You can no longer participate in the mass fantasy in which the massive amount of manure we dump is not polluting our waters, the excessive energy we consume is not changing the climate, the extensive fishing is not depleting our oceans, fossil fuels won't run out, your health and vitality are not being compromised... and that these are intricately connected to your daily food choices.

I believe that we all care, and that we all want to be responsible. Who wants to be cruel to animals, to pollute our environment? How do we resolve the dilemma of being drawn to foods that may not support our values, and engage in a social world where others may not have the same awareness or share our values?

My perspective is that I don't believe that eating should be dictated solely by politics or health concerns. Eating is about pleasure and celebration, and insisting that I – or anyone else – eat in a certain manner diminishes the joy in the experience. While it is true that I *mediate* my food choices based on concerns other than taste, I let pleasure be the ultimate guide.

As I became more educated about food, I was pleased to see that to some extent, my tastes naturally changed to better support my values. Locally produced, organic plant products just taste good to me. Also, I learned there were ways that I could actively engage in changing my tastes to further support this shift. Fortunately, "ecologically-sensitive" eating also meant that I got better-tasting food and food that was more supportive of good health.

In terms of how I allow my values to mediate my food choice, I start with the recognition that we can't be pure. This is the reality of the world we live in. Sometimes I need the convenience of a supermarket.

Also, I recognize that shame and guilt about food are not helpful. My guilt will not feed a starving person nor prevent global warming. On the other hand, if I leave the shame and guilt behind, eating is pleasurable and can help me feel connected to the larger community. Since it is my commitment to being a responsible citizen and bettering our community that underlies my commitment to sustainability, I honor that pleasure.

So that's where I put my focus in food – on pleasure and connection to community. Also, I value my time attending to nurturing my body. I take a quiet moment before eating to feel gratitude. How lucky I am to have food, let alone good food! I get acquainted with my food, and learn about its pedigree. I think about where it came from, how it connects me to my community. When possible, I shop, cook and eat with my family and friends. I buy much of my food directly from the growers, and even grow a little myself. I eat slowly, making sure to honor my body, and to savor and appreciate my food.

Your value system may change, but it will be hard to make or sustain changes for yourself if your culture doesn't change to support you. If your social world, for example, is built around the fast food meals you share with your friends and family, eating sustainably grown foods and practicing a "slow foods" lifestyle may require vast social changes. Educating your friends and family members and inviting them to join you in the journey will be valuable.

I also get involved in trying to spread the word beyond my immediate circle. The more people are aware, the more they are compelled to do something about it. (That's one of the main reasons I teach and write!) And I get involved socially and politically in trying to make change around food practices. Actually doing something about it also helps to appease the guilt that sometimes comes with awareness. Being able to make sustainable choices is a possibility for some, but it can't substitute for considering ways to address the larger issue of how to improve the way we produce, distribute and eat food collectively.

Concluding Words

If we choose to feed ourselves respectfully and sustainably, we feed ourselves with fresh, local food, and we become part of a larger community of individuals trying to live in a more harmonious and responsible way. And fortunately, sustainable choices are also quite delicious! Compare a freshly picked in-season heirloom tomato that was purchased at a farmer's market to the "tomatoes" available in supermarkets and you'll understand. Fruits and vegetables that are bred for taste, allowed to ripen in the field and brought directly to you – no long-distance shipping, no gassing to stimulate the ripening process, no sitting in storage for weeks – typically are the tastiest! So an inevitable outcome of choosing to eat more consciously is that I eat better-tasting food. Get moving on this path and you will find that it is self-perpetuating.

When I present this information, someone typically complains that it is easy for me – someone who works and earns a livable wage – to suggest this type of eating, but for many Americans it is an out-of-reach luxury. This is just not true! Everywhere in the United States there are farmers' markets where someone is selling freshly harvested food – and its tasty and inexpensive. Community-supported agriculture (CSA) provides another affordable opportunity. Check it out for yourself! There are cheaper options than fast food, processed food, or supermarket produce.

This is not to deny that some foods that are conscientiously grown and harvested are pricier, bringing on a difficult challenge of how to navigate the complicated path of money and morality, and how the answer might differ across economic class. There are no easy answers here, but I want to encourage you to challenge our culture's core values. Is there responsibility that comes packaged with the privilege of being at the top of the food chain? Are you driven to earn excessive amounts of money to support possessions and a fast paced lifestyle that doesn't deliver on its promised happiness?

You can't expect your local organic farmer to have Walmart prices, but at least you can support him or her in good conscience, knowing that you are contributing to a more sustainable, compassionate world. You may just find that you are more content and that you sleep better at night with a simpler lifestyle, lived closer to the land – where you prioritize spending your money on nourishment, your life is predicated on respect for the earth and its inhabitants, and your entertainment lies in your connection with nature and community.

Some people buy pricier organic food, viewing it as a charitable contribution – a way to support the health of the planet or people trying to do the right thing. Others see it as a kind of health insurance, figuring that down the line they may be saving in health care costs.

And as we all navigate our own value choices, it is important that we simultaneously make changes on a more systemic level, making access to safe, healthy, environmentally-friendly food a basic human right for all individuals, regardless of income. It is a crime that the affluent have better access to safer, more nutritious, sustainable foods.

As you become more knowledgeable about where your food comes from, you may start to notice a natural shift in the types of food that are appealing to you. One of the best ways to support this process is to simultaneously explore the joys of a sustainable, whole foods lifestyle. There are plenty of easy ways to buy (or grow) and prepare delicious food. Explore farmer's markets, different ethnic cuisines, try cookbooks or "whole foods" social clubs to get some ideas. Join others to get support (and go to potlucks to taste new foods and preparations).

Thinking too much about the consequences of our food choices is not what robs us of our enjoyment about foods, but rather putting too little attention into the joys of food and the ways it can connect us to friends, our community and our planet. There is no reason to feel hopeless over the many problems with our food. There is a large "sustainability movement" that is also occurring simultaneously, that puts the joy back in eating. Food is a celebration of nature, and a way to design a compassionate future.

Transforming the Planet: you have the power

The world can at times seem overwhelming and beyond our control. Many people feel helpless in the face of the magnitude of the problems that result from our current attitudes towards food. Even if they care, they fall into apathy. How can one person make a difference? Do individual actions really matter? I want to reassure you that you can make a difference, and all it takes is living the change that you wish for the world[a].

In the words of Margaret Mead, "Never doubt that a small group of thoughtful, committed citizens can change the world. Indeed, it is the only thing that ever has." History shows this to be true.

My personal observation confirms this. I have been truly inspired by my students at City College of San Francisco. Some are quietly making personal changes, such as buying from local farmers or discussing the issues with friends and family members. Others are more aggressively muckraking: changing options in vending machines, school cafeterias, local markets, restaurants, their children's schools; joining advocacy groups, writing elected officials, participating in political campaigns and community groups, educating others. The revolution is already happening, and there are endless opportunities to participate.

---

[a] This is a paraphrase from Mahatmas Ghandi's famous quote: "Be the change that you wish in the world."

There is no magical tactic that will turn the tide, only the persistence of committed individuals making conscientious choices. And it all starts with your daily food choices.

I hope this book will support you and inspire you to honor your body, respect the earth, and help make this a more compassionate world. My prescription to accomplish this is fun: Enjoy what you eat, expand your tastes to include a diverse range of locally grown, unprocessed plant foods, and let your body support you in choosing amounts and types of food.

May you always *Eat Well…For your Self and For the World*!

About the Author

Linda Bacon earned her doctorate in physiology (specializing in nutrition and weight regulation) from the University of California, Davis. She also holds graduate degrees in both psychology (specializing in eating disorders and body image) and exercise science (specializing in metabolism), and has professional experience as a researcher, clinical psychotherapist, exercise physiologist, and educator.

Currently, Dr. Bacon is a Nutrition Professor in the Biology Department at City College of San Francisco. She also works as an Associate Nutritionist with the University of California, Davis.

Author Disclosure

I have no current or previous financial relationship with any food manufacturing, diet or pharmaceutical company (except for those that may, without my knowledge, be part of mutual funds that I own through "socially responsible investing").

While writing this book, I have been employed as a Nutrition Professor by City College of San Francisco and also serve as an Associate Nutritionist at the University of California, Davis. My research has received grant funding from the National Science Foundation and the National Institutes of Health. I have collaborated with researchers at the Western Human Nutrition Research Center, which is a branch of the United States Department of Agriculture.

I maintain memberships in the following organizations which are relevant to my work:

- Association for Size Diversity and Health (ASDAH)
- Co-op America
- The Ecology Center
- National Association to Advance Fat Acceptance (NAAFA)
- National Resources Defense Council (NRDC)
- Slow Food USA
- Union of Concerned Scientists (UCS).

Appendix

<u>Nutrient Density</u>
(from most dense to least dense)

Nutrient density compares the amount of helpful nutrients that a food contains to its energy content. The below rankings consider phytochemicals, vitamins, minerals, fiber, and essential fats. Special consideration was given to the antioxidant activity of the micronutrients. It is a general list provided to give readers an overview rather than strict rules, and should be interpreted with caution.

Raw leafy greens
Solid green vegetables
Non-green, non-starchy vegetables
Beans/legumes
Fruits
Starchy vegetables
Whole grains
Raw nuts and seeds
Fish
Fat-free milk and milk products
Poultry
Eggs
Red meat
Full-fat milk and milk products
Cheese
Refined grains
Refined oils
Refined sweets

Calculating Energy Requirements

The Harris-Benedict Equations[507], developed nearly 100 years ago, are the most commonly used and accepted measures of energy expenditure. Any predictive equation will be inaccurate as there is too much that can't get accounted for by math alone, as well as a great deal of individual variability. This formula may effectively estimate the average energy needs of a large group of people, but is unlikely to be very effective at determining an individual's needs. (The National Research Council estimates that 70 percent of people fall within +/- 20 percent of the average[508].)

All equations tend to be more accurate when considering people who are closer to the mean in size, proportion of lean mass to fat mass, and activity level. Use this formula at your own risk!

What are your daily energy needs? There are three components to this: a) basal metabolic rate; b) activity demands; and c) thermic effect of food.

a) How much energy does your body need to stay alive? This is your basal metabolic rate (BMR). To calculate your BMR:

First calculate your weight in kilograms, if you don't know it in kilograms already. Since 1 kg = 2.2 pounds, divide your weight in pounds by 2.2 to get your weight in kilograms.

_____ / 2.2 = _____
Weight (in pounds)   Weight (in kilograms)

Next calculate your height in centimeters, if you don't know it already. Since 1 inch = 2.54 cm, multiply your height in inches by 2.54 to get your height in centimeters.

_____ x 2.54 = _____
Height (in inches)   Height (in centimeters)

Next use these numbers to complete one of the following two formulas:
Adult Males:
88.362 + (4.799 x _____) + (13.397 x _____) - (5.677 x _____)
                  Height (in cms)   Weight (in kgs)   Age
Adult Females:
447.593 + (3.098 x _____) + (9.247 x _____) - (4.330 x _____)
                   Height (in cms)   Weight (in kgs)   Age

The result of the formula is your basal metabolic rate (BMR): _____ kcals.

b) How much energy do you need for your daily activities? An easy way to estimate it is to multiply your BMR by an activity factor. Find your activity factor in the chart below. If you are not sure which category you fit in, see the bottom of the next page for more details.

Level of Activity	Male	Female
Sedentary	0.3	0.3
Lightly Active	0.6	0.5
Moderately Active	0.7	0.6
Very Active	1.1	0.9
Extremely Active	1.4	1.2

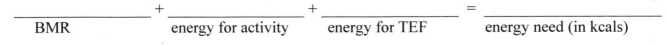

```
_____   x   _____   =   _____
     BMR               activity factor      energy needed for daily activities
```

c) How much energy do you spend metabolizing your food (called the thermic effect of food, or TEF)? One way to estimate is to add up the energy you need for your BMR and activity, and multiply these by 5% (which is the same as 0.05).

```
(_____   +   _____)   x 0.05   =   _____
   BMR (from a above)   energy for activity (from b)      energy for TEF
```

Now, you can calculate your energy need:

```
_____   +   _____   +   _____   =   _____
     BMR              energy for activity     energy for TEF       energy need (in kcals)
```

Estimating Energy Expenditure for Exercise

To simplify the estimation of your energy expenditure for exercise, choose one of the following five levels of activity: Sedentary, Lightly Active, Moderately Active, Very Active, and Extremely Active, defined below. If you fall between categories, choose a number for your activity factor that is between the two categories:

Sedentary: This is for you couch potatoes out there.

Lightly Active: Most students, office workers, and professionals; lawyers, doctors, shop workers, teachers, drivers, lab workers, playing a musical instrument, homemakers who use mechanical appliances, unemployed persons. This includes eight hours sleep and 16 hours of sitting or standing. Three of the 16 hours must include light activity (walking, laundry, golf, ping pong) and one hour must be moderate activity (tennis, dancing, walking briskly, aerobics, etc.).

Moderately Active: Most persons in light industry, electrical, carpentry and building trades (excluding heavy laborers), many farm workers, soldiers not in active service, commercial fishermen, people who work around the home without mechanical appliances. If you have an office or driving occupation (see Lightly Active category), you may have to average 1.5 to 2 hours of exercise per day (like jogging 5 to 6 miles/day) to be "Moderately Active."

Very Active: Full time athletes, unskilled laborers, some agricultural workers (especially peasant farming), forestry workers, army recruits and soldiers in active service, mine workers, steel workers. This level requires moderate intensity activity for most of the work day or exercise comparable to running 9 to 13 miles/day.

Extremely Active: Lumberjacks, blacksmiths, female construction workers, heavy manual digging, rickshaw pullers, and coal mining. Moderate to high level of physical activity for most of the work day or exercise comparable to running 14 to 17 miles/day.

Essential Fatty Acids

There are two families of essential fatty acids: the omega-3 family and omega-6 family. The omega-3 family comes from alpha-linolenic acid, and the omega-6 family comes from linoleic acid. We all create an enzyme that allows us to convert dietary alpha-linolenic acid to eiocosapentaenoic acid (EPA), which can then go on to form docosahexaenoic acid (DHA), and allows us to convert linoleic acid to a compound called arachidonic acid (AA).

EPA and DHA are fantastic stuff and have dramatic health benefits for your heart, your brain, and growth and development[509].

Some of the many benefits for your **heart** include:

- Reduces risk of strokes and heart attacks
- Thins blood
- Relaxes blood vessels (vasodilation)
- Lowers of blood pressure
- Reduces risk of blood clots in coronary arteries (thrombosis, anti-thrombotic properties)
- Protects against heartbeat abnormalities (arrhythmia, ventricular tachycardia, fibrillation)
- Protects against hardening of the arteries (atherosclerosis)
- Protects against plaque fat ruptures (which could lead to strokes and heart attacks)

Your **brain** also requires these to function optimally. (In fact, fathead, 60 percent of your brain is made out of fat – and you need a regular intake of fat to keep thinking clearly.) All of the following have been implicated in EPA/DHA deficiencies:

- Attention Deficit/Hyperactivity Disorder (ADHD)
- Dyslexia
- Depression and aggression
- Memory problems, Alzheimer disease and dementia

EPA and DHA are also essential for normal **growth and development**.

- They reduce inflammation and the risk of related disorders, such as:
  - Rheumatoid arthritis and other collagen vascular diseases such as lupus
  - Inflammatory skin disorders
  - Inflammatory bowel diseases

EPA and DHA are also the building blocks for the cells in your vital organs, and can guard against degenerative diseases such as:

- Degeneration of eyesight caused by macular degeneration
- Alzheimer disease
- Chronic kidney damage

Have I convinced you that they're good stuff?

The exact same enzyme that converts alpha-linolenic acid to DHA and EPA can also convert linoleic acid into a substance called arachidonic acid (AA), which is less helpful for our health. AA is involved in inflammation. In and of itself that isn't a bad thing; you need to have an inflammatory response as part of a healthy immune system. But there is danger in having too much of a good thing. Chronic inflammation upsets the delicate balance among all of our major systems: endocrine, central-nervous, digestive, and cardiovascular/respiratory, creating numerous health issues.

The enzyme prefers alpha-linolenic acid to linolenic acid – meaning it would rather make the EPA and DHA as opposed to the AA - but whether it gets the alpha-linolenic acid it wants depends on the ratio of linoleic acid (omega-6 fats) to alpha-linolenic acid (omega-3 fats) in your diet.

Recommended Ratio of Essential Fatty Acids

It has been estimated that thousands of years ago the diet of human hunter-gatherers consisted of approximately equal parts of omega-3 and omega-6 essential fatty acids[510]. Modern food processing has changed that dramatically. The food industry loves omega-6s because they are more stable (have a longer shelf life), so they generate more money. As a result, our ratio has risen dramatically and is out of balance for almost everyone. We make a lot more AA than we need, and not enough EPA and DHA. The current ratio in the American diet is estimated to be anywhere between 7:1 to 20:1.

While there is much debate about the optimal balance of omega-6 fats to omega-3 fats, many experts suggest a ratio of between 1:1 and 4:1.

Recommended Quantity of Essential Fatty Acids

Although there is also much debate on this issue, many experts advise consuming a minimum of 3% of energy from omega-6 fatty acids and 0.5% to 1% from omega-3 fatty acids; those who don't eat seafood should aim for the higher amount of omega-3 fatty acids since they don't get pre-formed EPA and DHA. If you consume 2000 kilocalories, this amounts to 60 kilocalories of omega-6 fats (6.7 g) and 20 kilocalories of omega-3 fats (2.2 g). Obtaining 6.7 g of omega-6s is almost impossible to avoid, even for those who consume diets very low in fat (10% fat). However, most Americans consume inadequate amounts of omega-3 fatty acids.

Sources of Omega-6 Fatty Acids

The primary source of omega-6 fatty acid in the diet is linoleic acid from the oils of seeds and grains. Corn, sunflower, and safflower oil are examples of where they are commonly found in our diets, and many processed foods are derived from these.

Sources of Omega-3 Fatty Acids

The primary source of omega-3 fats for Americans is fish. Fish eaters have it easy, because fish actually contains pre-formed EPA and DHA. That's why fish consumption has so many positive benefits and is so widely touted by health care professionals.

EPA and DHA are found primarily in oily cold-water fish such as tuna, salmon, and mackerel. Aside from seaweed, plant foods rarely contain EPA or DHA. However, alpha-linolenic acid (ALA), the precursor to EPA and DHA, is found primarily in dark green leafy vegetables, seeds, beans, and certain vegetable oils.

Note that saturated and trans fats have the potential to interfere with the metabolism of omega-3 fats, so for this reason, and many others, you may want to minimize them in your diet.

This next chart lists some of the more common plant foods that contain omega-3 fats. Since you want to shoot for about 2.2 grams per day, I listed the plant foods by the quantity that approximately provides this.

Food	Quantity	Grams of omega-3 fats
Flaxseed	1 tbsp	1.7 g
Flax oil	1 tsp	2.2 g
Walnuts	12 halves	2 g
Soybeans	1.5 c	2 g
Tofu	1.5 c	2 g

And here's the scoop on the omega-3 content of seafood.

Omega-3 Content of Fish and Shellfish (Amounts are in grams per 100g portion – which is 3.5 ounces uncooked, or approximately 3 ounces cooked) Source: USDA Nutrient Database for Standard Reference	Grams of Omega-3
Salmon, Atlantic, farmed, cooked, dry heat	1.8
Anchovy, European, canned in oil, drained	1.7
Sardine, Pacific, canned in tomato sauce, drained solid with bone	1.4
Herring, Atlantic, pickled	1.2
Mackerel, Atlantic, cooked, dry heat	1.0
Trout, rainbow, farmed, cooked, dry heat	1.0
Swordfish, cooked, dry heat	0.7
Tuna, white, canned in water, drained solids	0.7
Pollock, Atlantic, cooked, dry heat	0.5
Flatfish (flounder and sole species), cooked, dry heat	0.4
Halibut, Atlantic and Pacific, cooked, dry heat	0.4
Haddock, cooked, dry heat	0.2
Cod, Atlantic, cooked, dry heat	0.1
Mussel, blue, cooked, moist heat	0.7
Oyster, Eastern, wild, cooked, dry heat	0.5
Scallop, mixed species, cooked, dry heat	0.3
Clam, mixed species, cooked, moist heat	0.2
Shrimp, mixed species, cooked, moist heat	0.3

To look up information on other foods, check out the USDA Nutrient Composition Database yourself: http://www.nal.usda.gov/fnic/foodcomp/Data/index.html

Can you get omega-3 needs met through plant sources?

Vegetarians and vegans have no direct sources of EPA and DHA in their diets other than seaweed. EPA and DHA are not considered essential as the human body can convert alpha-linolenic acid into EPA and DHA, but even so, some of the body tissues of vegans have been found to contain less DHA and EPA than non-vegans. The consequences of this difference, if any, are not known.

Many factors affect the rate of conversion to EPA and DHA and one seems to be a high food intake of linoleic acid which is typical of vegan diets and may suppress the body's ability to convert alpha-linolenic acid to DHA. Vegans can achieve a better balance of PUFAs in their body tissues by using less linoleic acid-intensive oils such as sunflower, safflower and corn oils and more oils containing a higher proportion of alpha-linolenic acid such as canola oil, or soybean and walnut oils. This would encourage their tissues to make more DHA.

Research suggests that though the conversion is slow and incomplete, it is sufficient to meet most people's needs[511, 512].

Are you getting too many omega-6s?

An easy solution is to change your primary cooking oil. Use less corn oil, safflower oil, sunflower oil, cottonseed oil or "all-purpose vegetable oil." (It's okay to eat corn and sunflower seeds, as they don't give you concentrated amounts.) Instead, use mono-unsaturated oils, such as olive oil or canola oil. The former works better when you want the olive flavor, while canola oil is better when you are looking for a bland oil. Canola works particularly well for baking.

Getting enough omega-3s?

If you eat fish, you may be doing okay. Check out the chart at the end to see how you're doing. The American Heart Association recommends two servings of fatty fish per week. If you don't eat fish, odds are you're not getting enough from your diet.

Balancing your oils

The following table tells you about the balance of omega-6s and omega-3s in oils:

Oil	Omega-3 content	Omega-6 content	Ratio of Omega-6 to Omega-3
Flaxseed	53%	13%	1:4
Canola	9%	20%	2:1
Soy	7%	51%	7:1
Olive	1%	9%	9:1
Corn	1%	54%	54:1
Peanut	<1%	32%	32:1
Safflower	<1%	75%	75:1

You can see that flaxseed oil has four times the omega-3 content compared to omega-6 content, and therefore can do a good job of balancing out the omega-6s that we typically get in our diet. However, flaxseed goes rancid quickly and can't be used for cooking; it also imparts a strong taste and isn't always as practical for cold uses. Canola oil is also a good choice – particularly for cooking.

Supplementation

Given that it's hard to get the omega-3s you need from food, you may want to supplement. The two popular options are fish oils and flaxseed.

Fish oils work well, if you can tolerate the fishy smell. (And rest assured that tests show supplements to be low or free of mercury[513].)

The richest plant source of omega-3 fats is flaxseed. Flaxseed looks a bit like a sesame seed, but is a dark amber color. Best to take it in ground form as nature packages it in hard seeds which your body may not fully break down. Although there is some debate as to the best amount, 1-2 tablespoons a day is probably a good bet. You can buy it ground (called flaxseed meal), or grind the whole seeds yourself in a coffee or spice grinder. I think it tastes pretty good – kind of a nutty flavor. Some people like it sprinkled on cereals or mixed in yogurts or smoothies. It also works as a good egg replacer and is commonly used in recipes for foods like pancake batters and muffins.

Instead of ground flaxseed, you can also use flaxseed oil: 1-2 teaspoons is probably a good amount. Most people put it in salad dressings. Don't cook with flaxseed oil as it is easily oxidized. Many people prefer the ground form to the oil as it contains a lot of other beneficial nutrients, such as lignans, fiber and more antioxidants.

Special Notes on Vegetarianism and Veganism

Vegetarianism and veganism are becoming increasingly more popular and there are a host of compelling reasons to support these styles of eating, including animal welfare concerns (see the chapter on "Transforming Animals into Foods"), environmental and humanitarian concerns (see the chapter on "Agriculture and Sustainability"), and health (discussed throughout). Of course, some people enjoy vegan or vegetarian diets for the taste alone!

Many myths have been promoted about the viability of vegetarianism and veganism, some of which have also been discussed in the book. For example, the "Proteins" chapter discusses the myth that vegetarians get inadequate protein or amino acids and the "Micronutrients" chapter briefly confronts the myth that vegetarians get insufficient micronutrients.

Humans are designed to eat a varied diet, and eating a wide range of foods is necessary to ensure nutritional adequacy. A well-chosen vegetarian or vegan diet is abundant in a wide range of nutrients. In general, vegans tend to have a more nutrient-dense diet than vegetarians, and both vegans and vegetarians tend to have a more nutrient-dense diet than omnivores.

Regardless of whether you are a vegan, an omnivore, or somewhere in between, it is valuable to make sure that your varied nutrient needs are still being met, and this is intended to provide a little more depth to help those of you considering vegetarianism or veganism.

There are three micronutrients that tend to be low in the average vegan diet: calcium, iodine, and vitamin B_{12} [277].

The **calcium** needs of vegans in particular, and all individuals, remains a point of much discussion. Many factors affect calcium needs, including exercise levels and dietary protein content, both of which differ between the general population and vegans, making it very difficult to apply the research known about the calcium needs of the general population to vegans. Since there has been limited research specific to vegans, understanding this issue is particularly challenging. Vegetarians tend to eat a dairy-rich diet, making their calcium consumption similar to omnivores.

To meet calcium needs (and for a great nutritional punch in general), make it a point to include leafy green vegetables in your repertoire on a regular basis. Kale, collard, mustard and turnip greens are great sources of well-absorbable calcium. There are also a wide range of calcium-fortified foods commonly available, including tofu, soymilk, orange juice, baked beans, and molasses. You also don't want to overlook the contribution of other foods. While many beans and vegetables may not be rich sources of calcium, each supplies some, and a diet based on these nutritious foods adds up to sufficient quantities.

But if you're concerned about bone health, I have even more important advice: get moving! Weight-bearing exercise is likely to provide more benefit to developing and maintaining strong bones than dietary choices.

Changes in the food supply make **iodine** a difficult nutrient to find in unsupplemented foods. That's why it's commonly added to salt these days. If you stay away from processed foods (which typically have high salt content) and avoid the salt shaker, you are advised to either supplement iodine directly (75 to 150 mcg) or to add a small amount of iodized salt (1/4 tsp) to your diet.

Vitamin B_{12} tends to be *the* dietary issue for vegans (though not a concern for vegetarians). All Vitamin B_{12} comes from bacteria, and these bacteria live in the soil and in the intestines of animals. When they produce Vitamin B_{12}, it gets incorporated into their tissues, making animal foods such as meat, milk and eggs good sources of this nutrient. Bacteria on plants also produce Vitamin B_{12}, and historically plants were also a good source of Vitamin B_{12} for humans. Nowadays, however, cleaning foods eliminates much of the Vitamin B_{12} and plant foods are not a good source.

Fortunately, it is easy to meet Vitamin B_{12} needs on a vegan diet. Some foods are fortified with Vitamin B_{12}, such as certain brands of nutritional yeast and many breakfast cereals and meat analogs. Check labels. Supplements are also an easy option. If you choose to supplement, the recommended dosage is 10 mcg daily or 2,000 mcg weekly.

Vitamin B_{12} is readily stored on the human body and those that are new to veganism will have several months to consider whether they are getting sufficient amounts through fortified foods or whether they want to jump to supplementation.

Vegetarians and vegans tend to get more **iron** than omnivores, but I mention it here because it is a commonly discussed concern. The issue is not how much iron is in plant foods – there is plenty. The question is instead how much gets absorbed. Compounds found in many plant foods inhibit the absorption of iron. Also, the type of iron found in plant foods is less well-absorbed than some of the iron found in animal foods. That said, research indicates that vegans and vegetarians are no more likely to be iron-deficient than omnivores[172]. Most likely, the decreased absorbability is offset by the increased amount of iron typically found in a vegan diet.

Insufficient iron is the number one nutritional deficiency in the United States. It's helpful for people of all dietary styles - omnivore or vegan – to pay some attention to this nutrient and get sufficient amounts. Dried beans and leafy green vegetables are especially good sources.

WARNING: I do have two large concerns about vegetarianism and veganism for certain individuals. The first is that people sometimes take on these diets in the hope that they will result in weight loss. Indeed many professionals promote vegetarianism as a weight loss technique. Dr. John McDougall is perhaps the most famous example; McDougall frequently refers to the weight loss people experience while participating in his program.

If weight loss is your reasoning, you might as well go back to eating meat. There is no evidence to suggest that vegetarianism or veganism will help you to succeed at maintaining weight loss on a long-term basis, despite the widely accepted claims. (For more detail on this topic, see my other book, *Health at Every Size: The Suprising Truth About Your Weight*.) Indeed, when vegetarianism or veganism are undertaken for the purpose of weight loss, I suspect that they are more likely to provoke disordered eating, discomfort around food, and self-blame when weight loss is not achieved or maintained.

My second concern is that people with orthorexia and other eating disorders often subscribe to vegetarian or vegan diets, citing health reasons. When employed in this way, vegetarianism and veganism become dangerous, restrictive behavior.

Check out your motives for adopting these dietary styles. Health is much more broad-ranging than which nutrients you put into your body.

Resources

Vegan Outreach (www.veganoutreach.org) is a good starting point for learning about these dietary styles. Their pamphlets, "Why Vegan?" and "Vegetarian Living," are particularly popular and valuable and their website will help you link to much more information.

Also, check out this website: http://www.vegpledge.com/.

If a more traditional route is your style, you've got institutional support. "It is the position of the American Dietetic Association and Dietitians of Canada that appropriately planned vegetarian diets are healthful, nutritionally adequate and provide health benefits in the prevention and treatment of certain diseases."[172] Search the ADA's website for more information: www.eatright.org.

There are a lot of great books to be found – your best bet is to go to your local bookstore or library and scan the shelves for one that addresses your interests.

Environmental Working Group's
Guide to Pesticides in Produce

"The produce ranking was developed by analysts at the not-for-profit Environmental Working Group (EWG) based on the results of more than 100,000 tests for pesticides on produce collected by the U.S. Department of Agriculture and the U.S. Food and Drug Administration between 1992 and 2001." It is reproduced with permission from EWG (www.ewg.org).

Highest in Pesticides

These 12 popular fresh fruits and vegetables are consistently the most contaminated with pesticides — buy these organic.

- Apples
- Bell Peppers
- Celery
- Cherries
- Grapes (imported)
- Nectarines
- Peaches
- Pears
- Potatoes
- Red Raspberries
- Spinach
- Strawberries

Lowest in Pesticides

These 12 popular fresh fruits and vegetables consistently have the lowest levels of pesticides.

- Asparagus
- Avocados
- Bananas
- Broccoli
- Cauliflower
- Corn (sweet)
- Kiwi
- Mangos
- Onions
- Papaya
- Pineapples
- Peas (sweet)

Environmental Working Group's
Guide to Mercury Contamination in Fish

According to the Environmental Working Group, "Internal Food and Drug Administration (FDA) documents obtained by the Environmental Working Group (EWG) reveal that the agency is failing in its public health obligation to protect pregnant women and the developing fetus from the toxic effects of mercury." While their list is specifically directed towards pregnant women, high levels of mercury are dangerous to all of us. The following list is reproduced with permission from EWG (www.ewg.org).

Avoid
Shark
Swordfish
King mackerel
Tilefish
Tuna steaks
Canned tuna
Sea bass
Gulf Coast Oysters
Marlin
Halibut
Pike
Walleye
White croaker
Largemouth bass

Data From The 1970s Show High
Concentrations
(No Recent Data Available)
Porgy
Orange Roughy
Snapper
Lake Trout
Bluefish
Bonito
Rockfish

Eat No More Than One Serving From This List
Per Month
Mahi mahi
Blue mussel
Eastern oyster
Cod
Pollock
Great Lakes salmon
Gulf Coast blue crab
Channel catfish (wild)††
Lake whitefish

Lowest In Mercury
Blue crab (mid-Atlantic)
Croaker
Fish Sticks
Flounder (summer)
Haddock
Trout (farmed)
Salmon (wild Pacific)
Shrimp†

† Shrimp fishing and farming practices have raised serious environmental concerns.
†† Farmed catfish have low mercury levels but may contain PCBs in amounts of concern for pregnant women.

Co-op America's
Guide to Safe, Sustainable Seafood

Check out Co-op America at http://www.Co-opAmerica.org for great information on making ecologically-sensitive purchases. Their mission is to "harness economic power—the strength of consumers, investors, businesses, and the marketplace—to create a socially just and environmentally sustainable society." This seafood guide was drawn from an article that appeared in their Real Money newsletter, September/October 2005, which can also be found on their website at: http://www.coopamerica.org/pubs/realmoney/articles/seafood.cfm.
More in-depth information is provided in the article.

(T = High Toxin Levels, E = Environmental Issues)

Safe to Eat
Anchovies, Calamari, Clams, Crawfish, Dungeness crab, Fish sticks, Flounder (summer), Haddock, Hake, Herring, King crab, Lobster (spiny/rock), Mid-Atlantic blue crab, Northern shrimp (US-farmed), Oysters, Alaskan salmon (wild), Perch, White shrimp (US-farmed), Sardines, Bay scallops (farmed), Sole, Spot prawn, Stone crab, Tilapia, Whitefish

Caution (Limit to One Serving Per Month)
Blue mussel (T), Bluefish (T)*, Bonito (T)*, Channel (wild) catfish (T), Cod (except Atlantic) (T), Eastern oyster (T), Gulf Coast blue crab (T), Lake trout (T), Lake white fish (T), Mahi-mahi (T), Pollock (T), Porgy (T)*, Rockfish (T)*

Avoid
Catfish (farmed) (T), Caviar (wild) (E), Chilean sea bass/toothfish (E), Cod (Atlantic) (T, E), Grouper (E), Gulf Coast Oysters (T), Halibut (T, E), King mackerel (T), Largemouth bass (T), Marlin (T), Monkfish (E), Orange Roughy (T, E), Pike (T), Pacific rockfish/rock cod (E), Salmon (Great Lakes) (T), Salmon (Atlantic and most farmed) (T, E), Sea bass (T), Shark (T, E), Shrimp (wild, imported) (E), Snapper (T*, E), Sturgeon (wild) (E), Swordfish (T), Tilefish (T), Tuna (canned) (T), Tuna steaks (T, E), Walleye (T), White croaker (T)

*Based on data from 1977. No recent data available.
    Data from: FDA, EPA, Environmental Working Group, Monterey Bay Aquarium, Blue Oceans Institute, Environmental Defense.

Guide to Sustainable Food Label Terminology

Many food producers use specialty labels to attract consumers, and it's a challenge to read a food label and know what to trust. The most meaningful label is one that is certified to be "USDA Organic," which is described below. Except for the term "organic," none of the terms listed here is regulated or verified by the government. The below information was adapted from Sustainable Table, and more depth can be found on their website: http://www.sustainabletable.org.

100% vegetarian diet: As expected, this label means that animals are not fed any animal by-products.

Antibiotic-Free: This term is prohibited by the USDA, although I have seen it used. Know that it there is no legal definition.

Cage-Free: Birds are raised without cages. Does not indicate whether birds were raised outdoors or on pasture, if they had access to the outdoors, or if they were raised indoors in crowded conditions.

Electronic Pasteurization: Indicates the food has been irradiated.

Free-Range: The animal had some access to the outdoors on a daily basis (a door was at least left open). This term does not guarantee that the animal actually spent time outdoors.

GMO-free: Indicates the food was produced without genetic modification.

Grain-Fed: The animal was raised on a diet of grain. Does not guarantee that their diet was free of animal products. The grain may have been supplemented with animal by-products. (If you are concerned about Mad Cow Disease, animals raised on a "100% vegetarian diet" provide greater protection.)

Grain-Finished: Right before slaughter, the animal was fed only grain. (Some ranchers raise their animals on pasture, then switch them to grain shortly before slaughter to create a particular taste.)

Grass-Fed: Also known as "Pasture-raised," this indicates that animals graze on pasture and eat only grasses. The grasses are not supplemented with grain, animal by-products, hormones, and the animals were not given antibiotics to promote growth or prevent disease (although they may have been given antibiotics to treat disease).

Heritage: Indicates that the food was produced from a rare and endangered crop or breed of livestock. This helps preserve genetic diversity.

Hormone-free: This term is prohibited by the USDA, although I have seen it used. Know that there is no legal definition.

Made with organic ingredients: The product contains between 70 and 94% organic ingredients.

Natural: This term is meaningless except for minimal regulations applied to meat and poultry. "Natural" meat and poultry products can only be minimally processed and cannot contain artificial colors, artificial flavors, preservatives or other synthetic ingredients. (Note that "natural" meats and poultry are not necessarily sustainable or organic, and may contain hormones or antibiotics.)

No Antibiotics Administered: No antibiotics were given to the animal during its entire lifetime.

No Hormones Administered or **No Added Hormones**: No hormones were given to this animal. (Note that pigs and poultry cannot be given hormones by law, so the use of this term on labels is deceptive.)

Organic: This is a helpful, meaningful term to look for! To be labeled organic, a food must meet strict standards. The food cannot be grown with synthetic fertilizers, chemicals, sewage sludge, and cannot be genetically modified or irradiated. Organic meat and poultry must come from animals fed organic feed, and they cannot be treated with hormones or antibiotics. The animals must have access to the outdoors (although this doesn't necessarily mean that they go outdoors). (Note: "organic" as applied to seafood, on the other hand, is a meaningless term defined by the seller.)

Pasture or Pasture-Raised: Also known as "Grass-Fed," this indicates that animals graze on pasture and eat only grasses. The grasses are not supplemented with grain, animal by-products, hormones, and the animals were not given antibiotics to promote growth or prevent disease (although they may have been given antibiotics to treat disease).

Raised Without Added Hormones: See No Hormones Administered.

Raised Without Antibiotics: See No Antibiotics Administered.

Raised Without the Routine Use of Antibiotics: The animal did not receive antibiotics to promote growth or to prevent disease, but may have received them to treat illness.

rBGH-Free or **rBST-Free**: rBGH (recombinant bovine growth hormone), also known as rBST (recombinant bovine somatotropin), is a genetically engineered hormone that is injected into dairy cows to artificially increase their milk production. Milk with these labels is produced by cows that never received hormone injections.

Treated by Irradiation: The food was irradiated.

USDA certified organic: The product contains 95-100% organic ingredients. (See "organic.")

Guide to Egg Carton Labels and Animal Welfare

As there are no official standards or rules to enforce them, labels on egg cartons can be quite deceptive. Only four labels are backed by programs with official standards. For each of these labels, compliance is verified by independent auditors. The first three labels are well-respected by animal welfare advocates.

Certified Organic: the birds are fed an organic, vegetarian diet, without pesticides or antibiotics. They are uncaged inside barns or warehouses and have access to the outdoors. (Regulated through the USDA's National Organic Program.)

Certified Humane: The birds are uncaged, but may be kept indoors at all times. They must be able to nest, perch and dust bathe, and they meet requirements to minimize overcrowding. (Established by Humane Farm Animal Care.)

Free-Farmed: The birds are uncaged, but may be kept indoors at all times. They must be able to nest, perch and dust bathe, and they meet requirements to minimize overcrowding. (Established by the American Humane Association.)

This certification, created by egg manufacturers, is misleading:

Animal-Care Certified: Most egg producers comply with these standards and many proudly advertise that they do. Hens are confined in small cages (less than a sheet of paper) and can't perform natural behaviors, not even fully stretching their wings. (Established by the United Egg Producers.)

You may see these terms used as well, but no standards have been set, nor is compliance verified by independent auditors:

Free Range: This typically means that the hens are uncaged and have outdoor access. However, there are no standards regarding what the birds are fed, how crowded they are, the quality of the land, or frequency of outdoor access. (Note that the USDA has official standards for use of the term "free-range" as it applies to poultry products, but not for egg production.)

Cage Free or **Free Roaming**: Hens are uncaged, but typically don't have outdoor access. (The USDA has official standards for use of the term "free roaming" as it applies to some poultry products, but not for egg production.)

Vegetarian-Fed: Hens are fed a vegetarian diet; has no relevance to other animal welfare concerns.

Natural: No one is too sure what this means, but it has no relevance to animal welfare concerns.

Fertile: Hens lived with roosters, which means that they were most likely uncaged.

For more information, visit the Humane Society of the United States at http://www.hsus.org.

Guide to Food and Drink Packaging

Manufacturing certain types of food packaging materials releases toxic chemicals into the environment, such as benzene and dioxin, and some types leach chemicals as we use them or heat them. Reduced used of plastic, choosing plastic products carefully, and recycling are all important in protecting your own health as well as the earth.

Most plastics should have coded numbers, usually on the bottom. Of most concern to personal and planetary health are those labeled #3, #6, and #7, while #1, #2, #4, and #5 are better options.

Avoid these:

3 (Polyvinyl Chloride, also known as PVC):

PVCs are found in some cling wraps and bottles and are harmful on numerous levels. Their production releases highly polluting and carcinogenic compounds into the environment. They are often made with plasticizers such as phthalates which can leach out and have been shown to cause reproductive and developmental damage. And their incineration leads to the release of dioxins, also known to cause cancer, reproductive and developmental disorders, and immune dysfunction. They are not widely recyclable.

6 (Polystyrene):

Polystyrene is found in foam food trays, egg cartons, take-out cartons, coolers, and some plastic cutlery. The styrene can leach into foods and beverages and over a long-term basis cause cancer, and liver and nerve damage. On a short-term basis, it may have nervous system effects, including concentration difficulties, weakness and nausea. It is not widely recyclable. (They are also found in packing "peanuts" and some stores accept those for reuse.)

7 (Polycarbonates and others):

Number 7 refers to a wide variety of plastics that don't fit into another category. You can find them in plastic baby bottles, sport water bottles, and five-gallon water bottles, among many other items. They are made with bisphenol-A (BPA) which is an endocrine disruptor that can leach out. Rodent testing indicates that low doses alter brain chemistry and behavior, the immune system, and reproductive systems[514]. They are not widely recyclable.

Better choices include #1, #2, #4 and #5.

1 (Polyehtylene Terephthalate, also known as PETE or PET):

Used in clear bottles, and widely recyclable.

2 (High Density Polyethylene, also known as HDPE):

Used in colored and cloudy bottles, and tub containers such as those used for yogurt. Widely recyclable.

4 (Low Density Polyethylene, also known as LDPE):

Used in some cling wraps, garbage bags and food storage bags. Not widely recyclable.

5 (Polypropylene, also known as PP):

Used on butter/margarine tubs and some baby bottles and rigid containers. Not widely recyclable.

Here are some good general recommendations:

- Avoid using plastic containers or cling wraps in the microwave. Better microwave container options include glass or ceramic containers that are free of metallic paint.
- Minimize use of disposable plastic water bottles. If you do use them, don't use them for hot or warm liquids, and be sure to dispose of them when scratched or old.

And be sure to take special care with kids and during pregnancy as developing bodies are more susceptible to damage from toxins. Plastic baby bottles are of particular concern: avoid the polycarbonate bottles, which are generally rigid and have the number 7, and choose bottles of tempered glass or polyethylene and polypropylene (#1, #2, or #5). Use bottle nipples made of clear silicone rather than yellow rubber as the silicone is heat resistant (and hides less bacteria).

Bioplastics

Packaging made with bioplastics synthesized from corn, soy, sugar cane and other crops are increasingly being used by ecologically-sensitive consumers. They are made from renewable resources (rather than petroleum), and can degrade relatively quickly under the right conditions.

They are clearly a better alternative to the other plastics, but not concern-free. For example, since few people have access to composters which will help them degrade, they are likely to end up in landfills where they lack the light and heat necessary for degradation. Nonetheless, they provide a big advantage over synthetic plastics.

Tin Cans

Tin cans also pose safety concerns. Almost all have plastic liners, which on first consideration sound like a good idea. After all, when metal makes direct contact with food, it could affect the taste of the food and leach health-damaging heavy metals. But the problem with the protective liner is that it also leaches damaging compounds such as BPA. A safe, vegetable-based liner exists, but so far, Eden Organics, maker of canned beans, is the only company that uses it.

Why eat sustainable foods?

Sustainable agriculture allows us to grow food in a way that is socially and environmentally responsible, providing foods that are better for our bodies and the planet.

- Do it for the taste.
  - Savor a freshly harvested organic heirloom tomato from your local farmers' market. Next, munch on the conventionally-grown "tomato" purchased at your supermarket. You'll understand.

- Do it for your health.
  - Sustainably-grown food is more nutritious. Foods from sustainably-raised animals contain more omega-3 fats, higher vitamin content, less saturated fat, and fewer pathogens than those from conventionally raised animals. Sustainably-grown produce has higher phytochemical, vitamin and mineral content.

- Do it for the workers.
  - Farmworkers on conventional farms are exposed to toxic chemicals, rarely paid a livable wage, and highly exploited. Slaughterhouse work is considered the most dangerous job in the U.S. In contrast, when food is grown or raised sustainably, workers' health, safety and financial needs are respected.

- Do it for the environment.
  - Unsustainable practices pollute the soil, air and water, squander valuable natural resources, harm wildlife, and contribute to global warming. Sustainably-grown food preserves and nurtures resources.

- Do it for the animals.
  - In factory farms, animals are treated as commodities, not living, breathing, sentient beings. They are often crammed into small spaces with no access to sunlight or room to turn around, and subject to painful mutilation procedures such as debeaking, fire branding, or castration. Sustainable practices respect the animals and protect them from unnecessary suffering.

- Do it for your community.
  - The conventional food system is built on a foundation of impersonal, economic relationships. The legal mandate of corporations dictates the need to prioritize shareholder profits. Health and environmental concerns only play a role when in the corporation's financial interest. Sustainable farmers, on the other hand, are individuals who care about their land, their neighbors, and their customers. They help us stay connected to how our food is grown, and give us the opportunity to restore integrity to our relationships with each other and with the earth.

Flip to the next page for a guide on how to find sustainable foods.

Resources for Sustainable Eating

The **Eat Well Guide** (www.eatwellguide.org) is a directory of sustainably-grown or -raised meat, poultry, dairy and eggs. Plug in your zip code to find restaurants, farms and stores in your area.

Local Harvest (www.localharvest.com) can help you find local foods. They have an extensive listing of farms, farmers' markets, community supported agriculture, restaurants, and coops.

Eat Wild (www.Eatwild.com) lists pasture-based farms that supply grass-fed beef, lamb, goats, bison, poultry, pork and dairy products.

The **USDA Agricultural Marketing Service** (www.ams.usda.gov/farmersmarkets) includes a state-by-state listing of farmers' markets.

The **Biodynamic Farming and Gardening Association** (http://www.biodynamics.com/csa.html) has a listing of Community Supported Agriculture (CSA) by state.

The **USDA's Alternative Farming Systems Information Center** (http://www.nal.usda.gov/afsic/csa/) provides additional resources to help you find Community Supported Agriculture (CSA) near you.

Heritage Foods USA (www.heritagefoodsusa.com) contains a list of restaurants and stores that sell heritage foods. The foods they list are traceable, meaning they supply you with the details of where the food comes from and the way in which it was raised.

Excerpted from *Eat Well: For your Self, For the World*
(www.lulu.com/LindaBacon).
Eat Well provides much more extensive information on sustainable eating.

References

1. Hayflick, L., *The limited in vitro lifetime of human diploid cell strains.* Exp Cell Res, 1965. **37**: p. 614-36.
2. Sistrom, W., M. Griffiths, and R. Stanier, *The biology of a photo synthetic bacterium which lacks colored carotenoids.* Journal of Cellular and Comparative Physiology, 1956. **48**: p. 473-515.
3. Nestle, M., *Food politics. How the food industry influences nutrition and health.* 2002, Berkeley: University of California Press, Ltd.
4. Gallo, A., *Food advertising in the United States*, in *America's Eating Habits: Changes and Consequences*, E. Frazao, Editor. 1999, USDA: Washington, DC. p. 173-180.
5. Grassi, D., et al., *Short-term administration of dark chocolate is followed by a significant increase in insulin sensitivity and a decrease in blood pressure in healthy persons.* American Journal of Clinical Nutrition, 2005. **81**(3): p. 611-4.
6. Ambrosone, C., et al., *Breast cancer risk in premenopausal women Is inversely associated with consumption of broccoli, a source of isothiocyanates, but Is not modified by GST genotype.* Journal of Nutrition, 2004. **134**(5): p. 1134-1138.
7. Lesser, L., et al., *Relationship between Funding Source and Conclusion among Nutrition-Related Scientific Articles.* PLoS Med, 2007. **4**(1): p. 1-6.
8. Center for Science in the Public Interest, *Lifting the Veil of Secrecy. Corporate Support for Health and Environmental Professional Associations, Charities and Industry Front Groups.* 2003: Washington, D.C.
9. American Dietetic Association. *Home Page.* 2007 [cited 2007 February 1]; Available from: www.eatright.org.
10. American Dietetic Association. *Fact Sheet on Straight Facts on Beverage Choices.* 2004 [cited 2004 June 25].
11. Mello, M., B. Clarridge, and D. Studdert, *Academic Medical Centers' Standards for Clinical- Trial Agreements with Industry.* New England Journal of Medicine, 2005. **352**(21): p. 2202-2210.
12. Committee on Nutrition in Medical Education, *Nutrition education in U.S. medical schools.* 1985, National Academy of Sciences: Washington, D.C.
13. Zeisel, S. and C. Plaisted, *CD-ROMs for Nutrition Education.* Journal of American College of Nutrition, 1999. **18**: p. 287.
14. Fairfield, K., et al., *A prospective study of dietary lactose and ovarian cancer.* International Journal of Cancer, 2004. **110**: p. 271-.
15. Diabetes, 2000. **49**: p. 912-917.
16. Larsson, S., N. Orsini, and A. Wolk, *Milk, milk products and lactose intake and ovarian cancer risk: A meta-analysis of epidemiological studies.* International Journal of Cancer, 2005. **9999**(9999): p. NA.
17. Genkinger, J., et al., *Dairy Products and Ovarian Cancer: A Pooled Analysis of 12 Cohort Studies.* Cancer Epidemiol Biomarkers Prev, 2006. **15**: p. 364-372.
18. Akerblom, H.K. and M. Knip, *Putative environmental factors in Type 1 diabetes.* Diabetes Metabolism Review, 1998. **14**(1): p. 31-67.
19. Karjalainen, J., et al., *A bovine albumin peptide as a possible trigger of insulin-dependent diabetes mellitus.* New England Journal of Medicine, 1992. **327**(5): p. 302-7.
20. Scott, F.W., *Cow milk and insulin-dependent diabetes mellitus: is there a relationship?* American Journal of Clinical Nutrition, 1990. **51**(3): p. 489-91.
21. Hankinson, S. and e. al., *Circulating concentrations of insulin-like growth factor 1 and risk of breast cancer.* Lancet, 1998. **351**(9113): p. 1393-1396.
22. *Milk intake and bone mineral acquisition in adolescent girls.* British Medical Journal, 1997.
23. Chan, J. and e. al., *Plasma Insulin-Like Growth Factor-1 [IGF-1] and Prostate Cancer Risk: A Prospective Study.* Science, 1998. **279**: p. 563-6.
24. *Dietary changes favorably affect bone remodeling in older adults.* Journal of the American Dietetic Association, 1999.
25. Scrimshaw, N. and E. Murray, *The acceptability of milk and milk products in populations with a high prevalence of lactose intolerance.* American Journal of Clinical Nutrition, 1988. **48**: p. 1083-1085.
26. Kirk, A., et al., *Perchlorate in Milk.* Environmental Science and Technology, 2003. **37**(21): p. 4979 - 4981.
27. Environmental Protection Agency (EPA), *Perchlorate Environmental Contamination.* NCEA-1-0503, 2002.
28. New York Times Magazine. 1998.
29. Lanou, A., S. Berkow, and N. Barnard, *Calcium, Dairy Products, and Bone Health in Children and Young Adults: A Reevaluation of the Evidence.* Pediatrics, 2005. **115**(3): p. 736-743.
30. Weinsier, R. and C. Krumdieck, *Dairy foods and bone health: examination of the evidence.* American Journal of Clinical Nutrition, 2000. **72**: p. 681-9.
31. Feskanich, D., et al., *Milk, dietary calcium, and bone fractures in women: a 12-year prospective study.* American Journal of Public Health, 1997. **87**(6): p. 992-7.

32.   Midkiff, K., *The Meat You Eat. How Corporate Farming has Endangered America's Food Supply*. 2004, New York: St. Martin's Press.

33.   Mulkern, A., *When advocates become regulators*, in *Denver Post*. 2004.

34.   United States Department of Agriculture, *Major trends in the U.S. Food Supply, 1909-99*. FoodReview, 2000. **23**(1): p. 8-15.

35.   Putnam, J., J. Allshouse, and L. Kantor, *U.S. Per Capita Food Supply Trends: More Calories, Refined Carbohydrates, and Fats*. Food Review, 2002. **25**(3): p. 1-14.

36.   National Health And Nutrition Education Study (NHANES) I, NHANES II, and NHANES III.

37.   Rozin, P., et al., *Attitudes to food and the role of food in life in the U.S.A., Japan, Flemish Belgium and France: possible implications for the diet-health debate*. Appetite, 1999. **33**(2): p. 163-80.

38.   Drewnowski, A., et al., *Diet quality and dietary diversity in France: implications for the French paradox*. Journal of the American Dietetic Association, 1996. **96**(7): p. 663-9.

39.   Sandella, M. and P. Breslin, *Variability in a taste-receptor gene determines whether we taste toxins in food*. Current Biology, 2006. **16**(18): p. R792-R794.

40.   Rolls, E.T. and J.H. Rolls, *Olfactory sensory-specific satiety in humans*. Physiology and Behavior, 1997. **61**(3): p. 461-73.

41.   Nabhan, G.P., *Why Some Like It Hot: Food, Genes and Cultural Diversity*. 2004, Washington: Island Press.

42.   Schlosser, E., *Fast Food Nation*. 2001, New York: Houghton Mifflin Company.

43.   Rada, P., N.M. Avena, and B.G. Hoebel, *Daily bingeing on sugar repeatedly releases dopamine in the accumbens shell*. Neuroscience, 2005.

44.   Spangler, R., et al., *Opiate-like effects of sugar on gene expression in reward areas of the rat brain*. Brain Res Mol Brain Res, 2004. **124**(2): p. 134-42.

45.   Erlanson-Albertsson, C., *[Sugar triggers our reward-system. Sweets release opiates which stimulates the appetite for sucrose--insulin can depress it]*. Lakartidningen, 2005. **102**(21): p. 1620-2, 1625, 1627.

46.   Drewnowski, A., *Taste preferences and food intake*. Annual Review of Nutrition, 1997. **17**: p. 237-53.

47.   Drewnowski, A., et al., *Naloxone, an opiate blocker, reduces the consumption of sweet high-fat foods in obese and lean female binge eaters*. American Journal of Clinical Nutrition, 1995. **61**(6): p. 1206-12.

48.   Drewnowski, A., et al., *Taste responses and preferences for sweet high-fat foods: evidence for opioid involvement*. Physiology and Behavior, 1992. **51**(2): p. 371-9.

49.   Levine, A.S., C.M. Kotz, and B.A. Gosnell, *Sugars and fats: the neurobiology of preference*. J Nutr, 2003. **133**(3): p. 831S-834S.

50.   Levine, A.S., C.M. Kotz, and B.A. Gosnell, *Sugars and fats: the neurobiology of preference*. Journal of Nutrition, 2003. **133**(3): p. 831S-834S.

51.   Drewnowski, A. and A.S. Levine, *Sugar and fat--from genes to culture*. Journal of Nutrition, 2003. **133**(3): p. 829S-830S.

52.   Bertino, M. and F. Wehmer, *Dietary influences on the development of sucrose acceptability in rats*. Developmental Psychobiology, 1981. **14**(1): p. 19-28.

53.   Farm Animal Welfare Council. *5 Freedoms*. 2006 [cited 2006 July 15]; Available from: http://www.fawc.org.uk/freedoms.htm.

54.   Bouchard, C., et al., *Linkage between markers in the vicinity of the uncoupling protein 2 gene and resting metabolic rate in humans*. Human Molecular Genetics, 1997. **6**: p. 1887-9.

55.   Clapham, J., et al., *Mice overexpressing human uncoupling protein-3 in skeletal muscle are hyperphagic and lean*. Nature, 2000. **406**(6794): p. 415-9.

56.   Levine, J.A., *Nonexercise activity thermogenesis (NEAT): environment and biology*. American Journal of Physiology, Endocrinology and Metabolism, 2004. **286**(5): p. E675-85.

57.   Levine, J., N. Eberhardt, and M. Jensen, *Role of Nonexercise Activity Thermogenesis in Resistance to Fat Gain in Humans*. Science, 1999. **283**(5399): p. 212-4.

58.   Westerterp, K.R., *Diet induced thermogenesis*. Nutrition and Metabolism (London), 2004. **1**(1): p. 5.

59.   Acheson, K.J., et al., *Nutritional influences on lipogenesis and thermogenesis after a carbohydrate meal*. American Journal of Physiology, 1984. **246**(1 Pt 1): p. E62-70.

60.   Friedman, J.M., *Modern science versus the stigma of obesity*. Nature Medicine, 2004. **10**(6): p. 563-9.

61.   Cummings, J., *Constipation, dietary fiber adn the control of large bowel function*. Postgraduate Medical Journal, 1984. **60**: p. 811-819.

62.   Hallberg, L., et al., *Iron absorption from Southeast Asian diets. II. Role of various factors that might explain low absorption*. American Journal of Clinical Nutrition, 1977. **30**(4): p. 539-48.

63.   Greger, M., *Latest in Human Nutrition November 2003*. 2003.

64. Childs, P., *Dietary fat, dyspepsia, diarrhoea, and diabetes.* British Journal of Surgery, 1972. **59**(9): p. 669-95.

65. Holloway, R.H., et al., *Effect of intraduodenal fat on lower oesophageal sphincter function and gastro-oesophageal reflux.* Gut, 1997. **40**(4): p. 449-53.

66. Becker, D.J., et al., *A comparison of high and low fat meals on postprandial esophageal acid exposure.* American Journal of Gastroenterology, 1989. **84**(7): p. 782-6.

67. Van Deventer, G., et al., *Lower esophageal sphincter pressure, acid secretion, and blood gastrin after coffee consumption.* Digestive Diseases Sciences, 1992. **37**(4): p. 558-69.

68. Pehl, C., et al., *The effect of decaffeination of coffee on gastro-oesophageal reflux in patients with reflux disease.* Aliment Pharmacol Ther, 1997. **11**(3): p. 483-6.

69. Wendl, B., et al., *Effect of decaffeination of coffee or tea on gastro-oesophageal reflux.* Aliment Pharmacol Ther, 1994. **8**(3): p. 283-7.

70. Cohen, S. and G.H. Booth, Jr., *Gastric acid secretion and lower-esophageal-sphincter pressure in response to coffee and caffeine.* New England Journal of Medicine, 1975. **293**(18): p. 897-9.

71. Smit, C.F., et al., *Effect of cigarette smoking on gastropharyngeal and gastroesophageal reflux.* Ann Otol Rhinol Laryngol, 2001. **110**(2): p. 190-3.

72. Hogan, W.J., S.R. Viegas de Andrade, and D.H. Winship, *Ethanol-induced acute esophageal motor dysfunction.* Journal of Applied Physiology, 1972. **32**(6): p. 755-60.

73. Teyssen, S., et al., *Maleic acid and succinic acid in fermented alcoholic beverages are the stimulants of gastric acid secretion.* Journal of Clinical Investigation, 1999. **103**(5): p. 707-13.

74. Allen, M.L., et al., *The effect of raw onions on acid reflux and reflux symptoms.* American Journal of Gastroenterology, 1990. **85**(4): p. 377-80.

75. Murphy, D.W. and D.O. Castell, *Chocolate and heartburn: evidence of increased esophageal acid exposure after chocolate ingestion.* American Journal of Gastroenterology, 1988. **83**(6): p. 633-6.

76. Babka, J.C. and D.O. Castell, *On the genesis of heartburn. The effects of specific foods on the lower esophageal sphincter.* American journal of Digestive Disorders, 1973. **18**(5): p. 391-7.

77. Nebel, O.T., M.F. Fornes, and D.O. Castell, *Symptomatic gastroesophageal reflux: incidence and precipitating factors.* American journal of Digestive Disorders, 1976. **21**(11): p. 953-6.

78. Price, S.F., K.W. Smithson, and D.O. Castell, *Food sensitivity in reflux esophagitis.* Gastroenterology, 1978. **75**(2): p. 240-3.

79. Cranley, J.P., E. Achkar, and B. Fleshler, *Abnormal lower esophageal sphincter pressure responses in patients with orange juice-induced heartburn.* American Journal of Gastroenterology, 1986. **81**(2): p. 104-6.

80. Grigoleit, H.G. and P. Grigoleit, *Peppermint oil in irritable bowel syndrome.* Phytomedicine, 2005. **12**(8): p. 601-6.

81. *Position of the American Dietetic Association: Health implications of dietary fiber.* Journal of the American Dietetic Association, 1997. **97**: p. 1157-9.

82. Miller?, J.-B. and e. al?, American Journal of Clinical Nutrition, 2002: p. 5-56.

83. Ford, E., W. Giles, and W. Dietz, *Prevalence of the metabolic syndrome among US adults.* Journal of the American Medical Association, 2002. **287**: p. 356-9.

84. Mokdad, A., et al., *Diabetes trends in the U.S.: 1990-1998.* Diabetes Care, 2000. **23**(9): p. 1278-84.

85. Centers for Disease Control and Prevention, *National Diabetes Fact Sheet: General Information and National Estimates on Diabetes in the United States, 2000*: Atlanta, GA.

86. American Diabetes Association, *Type 2 diabetes in children and adolescents.* Diabetes Care, 2000. **23**: p. 381-89.

87. Ernsberger, P. and R.J. Koletsky, *Biomedical rationale for a wellness approach to obesity: An alternative to a focus on weight loss.* Journal of Social Issues, 1999. **55**(2): p. 221-260.

88. Bennett, P.H., *More about obesity and diabetes.* Diabetologia, 1986. **29**(10): p. 753-754.

89. Schwartz, M.W., et al., *Reduced insulin secretion: an independent predictor of body weight gain.* Journal of Clinical Endocrinology and Metabolism, 1995. **80**(5): p. 1571-6.

90. Longnecker, M. and J. Michalek, *Serum dioxin level in relation to diabetes mellitus among Air Force veterans with background levels of exposure.* Epidemiology, 2000. **11**(1): p. 44-8.

91. Cranmer, M., et al., *Exposure to 2,3,7,8-tetrachlorodibenzo-p-dioxin (TCDD) is associated with hyperinsulinemia and insulin resistance.* Toxicological Sciences, 2000. **56**(2): p. 431-6.

92. Rylander, L., A. Rignell-Hydbom, and L. Hagmar, *A cross-sectional study of the association between persistent organochlorine pollutants and diabetes.* Environmental Health, 2005. **4**: p. 28.

93. Lee, D., et al., *A strong dose-response relation between serum concentrations of persistent organic pollutants and diabetes: results from the National Health and Examination Survey 1999-2002.* Diabetes Care, 2006. **29**(7): p. 1638-44.

94. Kern, P.A., et al., *The effect of 2,3,7,8-tetrachlorodibenzo-p-dioxin (TCDD) on oxidative enzymes in adipocytes and liver.* Toxicology, 2002. **171**(2-3): p. 117-25.

95.   Kern, P.A., et al., *The stimulation of tumor necrosis factor and inhibition of glucose transport and lipoprotein lipase in adipose cells by 2,3,7,8-tetrachlorodibenzo-p-dioxin.* Metabolism, 2002. **51**(1): p. 65-8.

96.   Lee, D., et al., *A strong dose-response relation between serum concentrations of persistent organic pollutants and diabetes: results from the National Health and Examination Survey 1999-2002.* Diabetes Care, 2006. **29**(7): p. 1638-44.

97.   Gottlieb, M.S. and H.F. Root, *Diabetes mellitus in twins.* Diabetes, 1968. **17**(11): p. 693-704.

98.   Barnett, A.H., et al., *Diabetes in identical twins. A study of 200 pairs.* Diabetologia, 1981. **20**(2): p. 87-93.

99.   Kaprio, J., et al., *Concordance for type 1 (insulin-dependent) and type 2 (non-insulin-dependent) diabetes mellitus in a population-based cohort of twins in Finland.* Diabetologia, 1992. **35**(11): p. 1060-7.

100.   Perez-Bravo, F., et al., *Duration of breast feeding and bovine serum albumin antibody levels in type 1 diabetes: a case-control study.* Pediatr Diabetes, 2003. **4**(4): p. 157-61.

101.   Perez-Bravo, F., et al., *Genetic predisposition and environmental factors leading to the development of insulin-dependent diabetes mellitus in Chilean children.* Journal of Molecular Medicine, 1996. **74**(2): p. 105-9.

102.   Kostraba, J.N., et al., *Early exposure to cow's milk and solid foods in infancy, genetic predisposition, and risk of IDDM.* Diabetes, 1993. **42**(2): p. 288-95.

103.   Campbell, T., *The China Study. Startling implications for diet, weight loss and long-term health.* 2005, Dallas: Benbella Books.

104.   Dahl-Jorgensen, K., G. Joner, and K.F. Hanssen, *Relationship between cows' milk consumption and incidence of IDDM in childhood.* Diabetes Care, 1991. **14**(11): p. 1081-3.

105.   Virtanen, S.M., et al., *Cow's milk consumption, HLA-DQB1 genotype, and type 1 diabetes: a nested case-control study of siblings of children with diabetes. Childhood diabetes in Finland study group.* Diabetes, 2000. **49**(6): p. 912-7.

106.   Norris, J.M. and M. Pietropaolo, *Controversial topics series: milk proteins and diabetes.* Journal of Endocrinological Investigation, 1999. **22**(7): p. 568-80.

107.   Scott, F.W., *AAP recommendations on cow milk, soy, and early infant feeding.* Pediatrics, 1995. **96**(3 Pt 1): p. 515-7.

108.   Centers for Disease Control and Prevention, *National Diabetes Fact Sheet: General Information and National Estimates on Diabetes in the United States, 2000.* 2000: Atlanta, GA.

109.   Anderson, J., *Dietary fiber in nutrition management of diabetes,* in *Dietary fiber: Basic and Clinical Aspects,* V. Vahouney and V.a.D. Kritchevsky, Editors. 1986, Plenum Press: New York.

110.   Barnard, R.J., et al., *Response of non-insulin-dependent diabetic patients to an intensive program of diet and exercise.* Diabetes Care, 1982. **5**(4): p. 370-4.

111.   Barnard, R.J., et al., *Long-term use of a high-complex-carbohydrate, high-fiber, low-fat diet and exercise in the treatment of NIDDM patients.* Diabetes Care, 1983. **6**(3): p. 268-73.

112.   Knowler, W.C., et al., *Reduction in the incidence of type 2 diabetes with lifestyle intervention or metformin.* New England Journal of Medicine, 2002. **346**(6): p. 393-403.

113.   Tuomilehto, J., et al., *Prevention of type 2 diabetes mellitus by changes in lifestyle among subjects with impaired glucose tolerance.* New England Journal of Medicine, 2001. **344**(18): p. 1343-50.

114.   Brand, J.C., et al., *Plasma glucose and insulin responses to traditional Pima Indian meals.* American Journal of Clinical Nutrition, 1990. **51**(3): p. 416-20.

115.   Barnard, N., et al., *A Low-Fat Vegan Diet Improves Glycemic Control and Cardiovascular Risk Factors in a Randomized Clinical Trial in Individuals With Type 2 Diabetes.* Diabetes Care, 2006. **29**: p. 1777-1783.

116.   Hu, F., et al., *Diet, lifestyle and the risk of type 2 diabetes mellitus in women.* New England Journal of Medicine, 2001. **345**: p. 790-7.

117.   Willett, W.C., et al., *Reproducibility and validity of a semiquantitative food frequency questionnaire.* American Journal of Epidemiology, 1985. **122**(1): p. 51-65.

118.   Munger, R.G., et al., *Dietary assessment of older Iowa women with a food frequency questionnaire: nutrient intake, reproducibility, and comparison with 24-hour dietary recall interviews.* American Journal of Epidemiology, 1992. **136**(2): p. 192-200.

119.   Meyer, K.A., et al., *Carbohydrates, dietary fiber, and incident type 2 diabetes in older women.* American Journal of Clinical Nutrition, 2000. **71**(4): p. 921-30.

120.   Holt, S.H., J.C. Miller, and P. Petocz, *An insulin index of foods: the insulin demand generated by 1000-kJ portions of common foods.* American Journal of Clinical Nutrition, 1997. **66**(5): p. 1264-76.

121.   Bhathena, S. and M. Velasquez, *Beneficial role of dietary phytoestrogens in obesity and diabetes.* American Journal of Clinical Nutrition, 2002. **76**: p. 1191-1201.

122. Stephenson, T., et al., *Effect of soy protein-rich diet on renal function in young adults with insulin-dependent diabetes mellitus.* Clinical Nephrology, 2005. **64**(1): p. 1-11.

123. Marshall, J.A., et al., *Dietary fat predicts conversion from impaired glucose tolerance to NIDDM. The San Luis Valley Diabetes Study.* Diabetes Care, 1994. **17**(1): p. 50-6.

124. Feskens, E.J., et al., *Dietary factors determining diabetes and impaired glucose tolerance. A 20-year follow-up of the Finnish and Dutch cohorts of the Seven Countries Study.* Diabetes Care, 1995. **18**(8): p. 1104-12.

125. Manolio, T.A., et al., *Correlates of fasting insulin levels in young adults: the CARDIA study.* Journal of Clinical Epidemiology, 1991. **44**(6): p. 571-8.

126. Mayer, E.J., et al., *Usual dietary fat intake and insulin concentrations in healthy women twins.* Diabetes Care, 1993. **16**(11): p. 1459-69.

127. Marshall, J., D. Bessesen, and R. Hamman, *High saturated fat and low starch and fibre are associated with hyperinsulinemia in a non-diabetic population: the San Luis Valley Diabetes Study.* Diabetologia, 1997. **40**: p. 430-8.

128. Vitelli, L., A. Folsom, and E. Shahar, *Association of dietary composition with fasting serum insulin level: the ARIC Study.* Nutr Metab Cardiovasc Dis, 1996. **6**: p. 194-202.

129. van Dam, R., et al., *Dietary patterns and risk for type 2 diabetes in older Iowa women.* Annals of Internal Medicine, 2002. **136**: p. 201-9.

130. Meyer, K., et al., *Dietary fat and incidence of type 2 diabetes in older Iowa women.* Diabetes Care, 2001. **2001**(24): p. 1528-35.

131. Bessesen, D., *The role of carbohydrates in insulin resistance.* Journal of Nutrition, 2001. **131**(10): p. 2782S=2786S.

132. Kitagawa, T., et al., *Increased incidence of non-insulin dependent diabetes mellitus among Japanese schoolchildren correlates with an increased intake of animal protein and fat.* Clinical Pediatrics (Philadelphia), 1998. **37**(2): p. 111-5.

133. Llanos, G. and I. Libman, *Diabetes in the Americas.* Bull Pan Am Health Organ, 1994. **28**(4): p. 285-301.

134. Fraser, G.E., *Associations between diet and cancer, ischemic heart disease, and all-cause mortality in non-Hispanic white California Seventh-day Adventists.* American Journal of Clinical Nutrition, 1999. **70**(3 Suppl): p. 532S-538S.

135. Snowdon, D. and R. Phillips, *Does a vegetarian diet reduce the occurrence of diabetes?* American Journal of Public Health, 1985. **75**: p. 507-512.

136. Jenkins, D.J., et al., *Type 2 diabetes and the vegetarian diet.* American Journal of Clinical Nutrition, 2003. **78**(3 Suppl): p. 610S-616S.

137. Fraser, G., *Vegetarianism and obesity, hypertension, diabetes and arthritis,* in *Diet, Life Expectancy, and Chronic Disease.* 2003, Oxford University Press: Oxford, U.K. p. 129-148.

138. Nicholson, A.S., et al., *Toward improved management of NIDDM: A randomized, controlled, pilot intervention using a lowfat, vegetarian diet.* Preventive Medicine, 1999. **29**(2): p. 87-91.

139. Fox, M., *Vegan diet reverses diabetes symptoms, study finds,* in *Reuters.* 2006: Washington.

140. Ciliska, D., et al., *A review of weight loss interventions for obese people with non-insulin dependent diabetes mellitus.* Canadian Journal of Diabetes Care, 1995. **19**: p. 10-15.

141. Klein, S., et al., *Absence of an effect of liposuction on insulin action and risk factors for coronary heart disease.* New England Journal of Medicine, 2004. **350**(25): p. 2549-57.

142. Barnard, R., T. Jung, and S. Inkeles, *Diet and exercise in the treatment of NIDDM.* Diabetes Care, 1994. **17**: p. 1469-1472.

143. Barnard, R., et al., *Role of diet and exercise in the management of hyperinsulinemia and associated atherosclerotic risk factors.* American Journal of Cardiology, 1992. **69**: p. 440-444.

144. Boule, N.G., et al., *Effects of exercise on glycemic control and body mass in type 2 diabetes mellitus: a meta-analysis of controlled clinical trials.* Journal of the American Medical Association, 2001. **286**(10): p. 1218-27.

145. Lamarche, B., et al., *Is body fat loss a determinant factor in the improvement of carbohydrate and lipid metabolism following aerobic exercise training in obese women?* Metabolism, 1992. **41**: p. 1249-1256.

146. Gaesser, G., *Weight loss for the obese: panacea or pound-foolish?* Quest, 2004. **56**: p. 12-27.

147. Jenkins, D.J., et al., *Glycemic index: overview of implications in health and disease.* American Journal of Clinical Nutrition, 2002. **76**(1): p. 266S-73S.

148. Hu, F.B., J.E. Manson, and W.C. Willett, *Types of dietary fat and risk of coronary heart disease: a critical review.* Journal of the American College of Nutrition, 2001. **20**(1): p. 5-19.

149. Mozaffarian, D., et al., *Trans fatty acids and cardiovascular disease.* New England Journal of Medicine, 2006. **354**(15): p. 1601-13.

150. Black, P.H. and L.D. Garbutt, *Stress, inflammation and cardiovascular disease.* Journal of Psychosomatic Research, 2002. **52**(1): p. 1-23.

151. Descovich, G.C., et al., *Multicentre study of soybean protein diet for outpatient hyper-cholesterolaemic patients.* Lancet, 1980. **2**(8197): p. 709-12.

152. Carroll, K.K., *Hypercholesterolemia and atherosclerosis: effects of dietary protein.* Federal Proc, 1982. **41**(11): p. 2792-6.

153. Sirtori, C., G. Noseda, and G. Descovich, *Studies on the use of a soybean protein diet for the management of human lipoproteinemias,* in *Animal and vegetable proteins in lipid metabolism and atherosclerosis,* M. Gibney and D. Kritchevsky, Editors. 1983, Liss: New York. p. 135-148.

154. Sirtori, C.R., et al., *Cholesterol-lowering and HDL-raising properties of lecithinated soy proteins in type II hyperlipidemic patients.* Annals of Nutrition and Metabolism, 1985. **29**(6): p. 348-57.

155. Gaddi, A., et al., *Dietary treatment for familial hypercholesterolemia--differential effects of dietary soy protein according to the apolipoprotein E phenotypes.* American Journal of Clinical Nutrition, 1991. **53**(5): p. 1191-6.

156. Carroll, K., *Dietary proteins and amino acids - their effects on cholesterol metabolism,* in *Animal and Vegetable Proteins in Lipid Metabolism and Atherosclerosis,* M. Gibney and D. Kritchevsky, Editors. 1983, Alan R. Liss, Inc: New York.

157. Anderson, J.W., B.M. Johnstone, and M.E. Cook-Newell, *Meta-analysis of the effects of soy protein intake on serum lipids.* New England Journal of Medicine, 1995. **333**(5): p. 276-82.

158. Sirtori, C., G. Noseda, and G. Descovich, *Studies on the use of a soybean protein diet for the management of human hyperlipoproteinemias,* in *Current Topics in Nutrition and Disease, Volume 8: Animal and Vegetable Proteins in Lipid Metabolism and Atherosclerosis,* M.J. Gibney and D. Kritchevsky, Editors. 1983, Alan R. Liss, Inc.: New York. p. 19-49.

159. Terpstra, A., R. Hermus, and C. West, *Dietary protein and cholesterol metabolism in rabbits and rats.,* in *Current Topics in Nutrition and Disease, Volume 8: Animal and Vegetable Proteins in Lipid Metabolism and Atherosclerosis,* M.J. Gibney and D. Kritchevsky, Editors. 1983, Alan R. Liss, Inc.: New York. p. 19-49.

160. Kritchevsky, D., et al., *Atherogenicity of animal and vegetable protein. Influence of the lysine to arginine ratio.* Atherosclerosis, 1982. **41**(2-3): p. 429-31.

161. Unlu, N., et al., *Carotenoid Absorption from Salad and Salsa by Humans Is Enhanced by the Addition of Avocado or Avocado Oil.* Journal of Nutrition, 2005. **135**: p. 431-436.

162. Brown, M.J., et al., *Carotenoid bioavailability is higher from salads ingested with full-fat than with fat-reduced salad dressings as measured with electrochemical detection.* American Journal of Clinical Nutrition, 2004. **80**(2): p. 396-403.

163. Renaud, S. and M. de Lorgeril, *Wine, alcohol, platelets, and the French paradox for coronary heart disease.* Lancet, 1992. **339**(8808): p. 1523-6.

164. Hegsted, M., *Minimum protein requirements of adults.* American Journal of Clinical Nutrition, 1968. **21**: p. 3520.

165. Irwin, M., *A consensus of research on protein requirements of man.* Journal of Nutrition, 1975. **101**(385).

166. Scrimshaw, N., *An analysis of past and present recommended dietary allowances for protein in health and disease.* New England Journal of Medicine, 1976: p. 200.

167. Robbins, J., *May all be fed. Diet for a new world.* 1992, New York: Avon Books.

168. Reuben, D., *Everything you always wanted to know about nutrition.* 1978, New York: Avon Books.

169. Wright, J., et al., *Trends in intake of energy and macronutrients—United States, 1971-2000.* Journal of the American Medical Association, 2004. **291**: p. 1193-4.

170. Hardinge, M. and e. al., *Nutritional studies of vegetarians: Part I...* Journal of Clinical Nutrition, 1984. **2**(2): p. 84.

171. Hardinge, M. and e. al., *Nutritional studies of vegetarians, Part V, Proteins...* Journal of the American Dietetic Association, 1966. **48**(1): p. 27.

172. *Position of the American Dietetic Association and Dietitians of Canada: Vegetarian diets.* Journal of the American Dietetic Association, 2003. **103**(6): p. 748-65.

173. Skov, A., et al., *Changes in renal function during weight loss induced by high vs low-protein low-fat diets in overweight subjects.* International Journal of Obesity and Related Metabolic Disorders, 1999. **23**(11): p. 1170-7.

174. Kushi, L.H., E.B. Lenart, and W.C. Willett, *Health implications of Mediterranean diets in light of contemporary knowledge. 2. Meat, wine, fats, and oils.* American Journal of Clinical Nutrition, 1995. **61**(6 Suppl): p. 1416S-1427S.

175. Yang, C.X., et al., *Correlation between Food Consumption and Colorectal Cancer: An Ecological Analysis in Japan.* Asian Pacific Journal of Cancer Prevention, 2002. **3**(1): p. 77-83.

176. Holmes, M.D., et al., *Meat, fish and egg intake and risk of breast cancer.* International Journal of Cancer, 2003. **104**(2): p. 221-7.

177. Sieri, S., et al., *Fat and protein intake and subsequent breast cancer risk in postmenopausal women.* Nutrition and Cancer, 2002. **42**(1): p. 10-7.

178. O'Keefe, S.J., et al., *Rarity of colon cancer in Africans is associated with low animal product consumption, not fiber.* American Journal of Gastroenterology, 1999. **94**(5): p. 1373-80.

179. Campbell, T.C., B. Parpia, and J. Chen, *Diet, lifestyle, and the etiology of coronary artery disease: the Cornell China study.* American Journal of Cardiology, 1998. **82**(10B): p. 18T-21T.

180. Campbell, T.C. and C. Junshi, *Diet and chronic degenerative diseases: perspectives from China.* American Journal of Clinical Nutrition, 1994. **59**(5 Suppl): p. 1153S-1161S.

181. Messina, M. and V. Messina, *Soyfoods, soybean isoflavones, and bone health: a brief overview.* J Ren Nutr, 2000. **10**(2): p. 63-8.

182. Hu, J.F., et al., *Dietary intakes and urinary excretion of calcium and acids: a cross-sectional study of women in China.* American Journal of Clinical Nutrition, 1993. **58**(3): p. 398-406.

183. Song, Y., et al., *A prospective study of red meat consumption and type 2 diabetes in middle-aged and elderly women: the women's health study.* Diabetes Care, 2004. **27**(9): p. 2108-15.

184. Pennington, J., *Bowes and Church's Food Values of Portions Commonly Used.* Vol. 15th Edition. 1989, New York: HarperPerennial.

185. *Surgeon general to cops: Put down the donuts.* 2003 [cited 2004 August 18]; Available from: http://www.cnn.com/2003/HEALTH/02/28/obesity.police/index.html.

186. Mokdad, A.H., et al., *Actual causes of death in the United States, 2000.* Journal of the American Medical Association, 2004. **291**: p. 1238-45.

187. Flegal, K.M., et al., *Excess deaths associated with underweight, overweight, and obesity.* Journal of the American Medical Association, 2005. **293**(15): p. 1861-7.

188. Mokdad, A.H., et al., *The spread of the obesity epidemic in the United States, 1991-1998.* Journal of the American Medical Association, 2000. **282**(16): p. 1519-1522.

189. Mokdad, A., et al., *Correction: Actual Causes of Death in the United States, 2000.* Journal of the American Medical Association, 2005. **293**(93): p. 293.

190. American Dietetic Association, *Position of the American Dietetic Association: Weight management.* Journal of the American Dietetic Association, 1997. **97**: p. 71-4.

191. McGinnis, J.M. and W.H. Foege, *Actual causes of death in the United States.* Journal of the American Medical Association, 1993. **270**(2207-2212).

192. Manson, J. and G. Faich, *Phamacotherapy for obesity - do the benefits outweigh the risks?* New England Journal of Medicine, 1996. **335**: p. 659-60.

193. National Task Force on the Prevention and Treatment of Obesity, *Long-term pharmacotherapy in the management of obesity.* Journal of the American Medical Association, 1996. **276**: p. 1907-15.

194. McGinnis, J. and W. Foege, *The obesity problem [letter].* New England Journal of Medicine, 1998. **338**: p. 1157.

195. Flegal, K.M., et al., *Estimating deaths attributable to obesity in the United States.* American Journal of Public Health, 2004. **94**(9): p. 1486-9.

196. Waaler, H., *Height and Weight and Mortality: The Norwegian Experience.* Acta Medica Scandinavica. Supplemantum, 1984. **679**: p. 1-56.

197. Hirdes, J. and W. Forbes, *The Importance of Social Relationships, Socieoeconomic Status and Health Practices with Respect to Mortality in Healthy Ontario Males.* Journal of Clinical Epidemiology, 1992. **45**: p. 175-182.

198. Lotutu, P.A., et al., *Male pattern baldness and coronary heart disease.* Archives of Internal Medicine, 2000. **160**: p. 165-171.

199. Robison, J. and G. Kline, *Surviving "risk factor frenzy": The perils of incorrectly applying epidemiological research in health education and promotion.* International Quarterly of Community Health Education, 2002. **21**(1): p. 83-100.

200. Barlow, C.E., et al., *Physical fitness, mortality and obesity.* International Journal of Obesity, 1995. **19**(Suppl 4): p. S41-S44.

201. Lee, C.D., S.N. Blair, and A.S. Jackson, *Cardiorespiratory fitness, body composition, and all-cause and cardiovascular disease mortality in men.* American Journal of Clinical Nutrition, 1999. **69**(3): p. 373-380.

202. Farrell, S., et al., *The relation of body mass index, cardiorespiratory fitness, and all-cause mortality in women.* Obesity Research, 2002. **10**: p. 417-23.

203. Church, T.S., et al., *Exercise capacity and body composition as predictors of mortality among men with diabetes.* Diabetes Care, 2004. **27**(1): p. 83-8.

204. Blair, S.N. and S. Brodney, *Effects of physical inactivity and obesity on morbidity and mortality: current evidence and research issues.* Medicine and Science in Sports and Exercise, 1999. **31**(11 Suppl): p. S646-62.

205. Gulati, M., et al., *Exercise capacity and the risk of death in women: the St James Women Take Heart Project.* Circulation, 2003. **108**(13): p. 1554-9.

206. Kassirer, J.P. and M. Angell, *Losing weight - An ill-fated New Year's resolution.* New England Journal of Medicine, 1998. **338**(1): p. 52-54.

207. Fontaine, K.R., et al., *Body weight and health care among women in the general population.* Archives of Family Medicine, 1998. **7**(4): p. 381-4.

208. Olson, C.L., H.D. Schumaker, and B.P. Yawn, *Overweight women delay medical care.* Archives of Family Medicine, 1994. **3**(10): p. 888-92.

209. Fraser, L., *Losing it. False hopes and fat profits in the diet industry.* 1998.

210. McGinnis, J. and W. Foege, *The obesity problem [Letter].* New England Journal of Medicine, 1999. **338**: p. 1157.

211. McGill, H.J., *The Geographic Pathology of Atherosclerosis.* 1986, Baltimore: Williams and Wilkins.

212. Montenegro, M. and L. Solberg, *Obesity, body weight, body length, and atherosclerosis.* Laboratory Investigations, 1968. **18**: p. 134-143.

213. Gaesser, G., *Big Fat Lies: The Truth about Your Weight and Your Health.* 2002, Carlsbad: Gurze Books.

214. Patel, Y.C., D.A. Eggen, and J.P. Strong, *Obesity, smoking and atherosclerosis. A study of interassociations.* Atherosclerosis, 1980. **36**(4): p. 481-90.

215. Warnes, C.A. and W.C. Roberts, *The heart in massive (more than 300 pounds or 136 kilograms) obesity: analysis of 12 patients studied at necropsy.* American Journal of Cardiology, 1984. **54**(8): p. 1087-91.

216. Chambless, L.E., et al., *Risk factors for progression of common carotid atherosclerosis: the Atherosclerosis Risk in Communities Study, 1987-1998.* American Journal of Epidemiology, 2002. **155**(1): p. 38-47.

217. Salonen, R. and J.T. Salonen, *Progression of carotid atherosclerosis and its determinants: a population-based ultrasonography study.* Atherosclerosis, 1990. **81**(1): p. 33-40.

218. Applegate, W.B., J.P. Hughes, and R. Vander Zwaag, *Case-control study of coronary heart disease risk factors in the elderly.* Journal of Clinical Epidemiology, 1991. **44**(4-5): p. 409-15.

219. Gaesser, G., *Thinness and weight loss: Beneficial or detrimental to longevity.* Medicine and Science in Sports and Exercise, 1999. **31**(8): p. 1118-1128.

220. Williamson, D.F. and E.R. Pamuk, *The association between weight loss and increased longevity.* Annals of Internal Medicine, 1993. **119**: p. 737-43.

221. Gaesser, G., *Big Fat Lies.* 1996, New York: Fawcett Columbine.

222. Williamson, D.F., et al., *Prospective study of intentional weight loss and mortality in never-smoking overweight U.S. white women aged 40-64 years.* American Journal of Epidemiology, 1995. **141**: p. 1128-1141.

223. Yaari, S. and U. Goldbourt, *Voluntary and involuntary weight loss: associations with long term mortality in 9,228 middle-aged and elderly men.* American Journal of Epidemiology, 1998. **148**: p. 546-55.

224. Diehr, P., et al., *Body mass index and mortality in nonsmoking older adults: the Cardiovascular Health Study.* American Journal of Public Health, 1998. **88**: p. 623-9.

225. French, S.A., et al., *Prospective study of intentionality of weight loss and mortality in older women: The Iowa Women's Health Study.* American Journal of Epidemiology, 1999. **149**: p. 504-515.

226. Williamson, D.F., et al., *Prospective study of intentional weight loss and mortality in overweight white men aged 40-64 years.* American Journal of Epidemiology, 1999. **149**(6): p. 491-503.

227. Williamson, D., et al., *Intentional weight loss and mortality in overweight individuals with diabetes.* Diabetes Care, 2000. **23**: p. 1499-504.

228. Coakley, E.H., et al., *Predictors of weight change in men: Results from the Health Professionals Follow-Up Study.* International Journal of Obesity and Related Metabolic Disorders, 1998. **22**: p. 89-96.

229. Bild, D.E., et al., *Correlates and predictors of weight loss in young adults: The CARDIA study.* International Journal of Obesity and Related Metabolic Disorders, 1996. **20**(1): p. 47-55.

230. French, S.A., et al., *Predictors of weight change over two years among a population of working adults: The Healthy Worker Project.* International Journal of Obesity, 1994. **18**: p. 145-154.

231. Korkeila, M., et al., *Weight-loss attempts and risk of major weight gain.* American Journal of Clinical Nutrition, 1999. **70**: p. 965-973.

232. Stice, E., et al., *Naturalistic weight-reduction efforts prospectively predict growth in relative weight and onset of obesity among female adolescents.* Journal of Consulting and Clinical Psychology, 1999. **67**: p. 967-974.

233. Shunk, J.A. and L.L. Birch, *Girls at risk for overweight at age 5 are at risk for dietary restraint, disinhibited overeating, weight concerns, and greater weight gain from 5 to 9 years.* Journal of the American Dietetic Association, 2004. **104**(7): p. 1120-6.

234. Stice, E., K. Presnell, and H. Shaw, *Psychological and Behavioral Risk Factors for Obesity Onset in Adolescent Girls: A Prospective Study.* Journal of Consulting and Clinical Psychology, 2005. **73**(2): p. 195-202.

235. Miller, W.C., D.M. Koceja, and E.J. Hamilton, *A meta-analysis of the past 25 years of weight loss research using diet, exercise or diet plus exercise intervention.* International Journal of Obesity and Related Metabolic Disorders, 1997. **21**(10): p. 941-7.

236. Wilmore, J.H., et al., *Alterations in body weight and composition consequent to 20 wk of endurance training: the HERITAGE Family Study.* American Journal of Clinical Nutrition, 1999. **70**(3): p. 346-52.

237. Ballor, D.L. and R.E. Keesey, *A meta-analysis of the factors affecting exercise-induced changes in body mass, fat mass and fat-free mass in males and females.* International Journal of Obesity and Related Metabolic Disorders, 1991. **15**(11): p. 717-26.

238. Donnelly, J.E., et al., *Effects of a 16-month randomized controlled exercise trial on body weight and composition in young, overweight men and women: the Midwest Exercise Trial.* Archives of Internal Medicine, 2003. **163**(11): p. 1343-50.

239. Ernsberger, P. and R.J. Koletsky, *Weight cycling.* Journal of the American Medical Association, 1995. **273**(13): p. 998-9.

240. National Institutes of Health National Task Force on the Prevention and Treatment of Obesity, *Long-term pharmacotherapy in the management of obesity.* Journal of the American Medical Association, 1996. **276**(23): p. 1907-1915.

241. Ten-State Nutrition Survey 1968-1970, U.S. DHEW Publication No. (HSM) 72-8131.

242. Keesey, R., *A set-point theory of obesity.*, in *Handbook of eating disorders: Physiology, psychology, and treatment of obesity, anorexia, and bulimia*, K. Brownell and J. Foreyt, Editors. 1986, Basic Books: New York. p. 63-87.

243. Cohn, C. and D. Joseph, *Influence of body weight and body fat on appetite of normal lean and obese rats.* Yale Journal of Biological Medicine, 1962. **34**: p. 598-607.

244. Brooks, C., McC, and E. Lambert, *A study of the effect of limitation of food intake and the method of feeding on the rate of weight gain during hypothalamic obesity in the albino rat.* American Journal of Physiology, 1946. **147**: p. 695-707.

245. Keys, A., et al., *The biology of human starvation.* Vol. 1. 1950, Minneapolis: University of Minnesota Press.

246. Johnson, D. and E. Drenick, *Therapeutic fasting in morbid obesity. Long-term follow-up.* Archives of Internal Medicine, 1977. **137**: p. 1381-2.

247. Sims, E. and E. Horton, *Endocrine and metabolic adaptation to obesity and starvation.* American Journal of Clinical Nutrition, 1968. **21**: p. 1455-70.

248. Sims, E.A.H., *Studies in Human Hyperphagia*, in *Treatment and management of obesity*, G.B.J. Bethune, Editor. 1974, Harper and Rowe: New York.

249. Schwartz, M., *Brain pathways controlling food intake and body weight.* Experimental Biology and Medicine, 2001. **226**(11): p. 978-81.

250. Wooley, S. and O. Wooley, *Should obesity be treated at all?*, in *Eating and its disorders*, A.J. Stunkard and E.J. Stellar, Editors. 1984, Raven: New York.

251. Garrow, J., *Energy balance and obesity in man.* 1974, New York: Elsevier.

252. Braitman, L.E., E.V. Adlin, and J.L. Stanton, Jr., *Obesity and caloric intake: the National Health and Nutrition Examination Survey of 1971-1975 (HANES I).* Journal of Chronic Disease, 1985. **38**(9): p. 727-32.

253. Wooley, S., O.W. Wooley, and S. Dyrenforth, *Theoretical, practical and social issues in behavioral treatments of obesity.* Journal of Applied Behavior Analysis, 1979. **12**: p. 3-25.

254. Sims, E.A.H., *Experimental obesity in man.* Transactions of the Association of American Physicians, 1968. **81**: p. 153-170.

255. Edholm, O.G., et al., *Food intake and energy expenditure of army recruits.* British Journal of Nutrition, 1970. **24**: p. 1091-1107.

256. Spiegel, T.A., *Caloric regulation of food intake in man.* Journal of Comparative and Physiological Psychology, 1973. **84**: p. 24-37.

257. Bouchard, C., *Genetics of obesity: overview and research directions*, in *The Genetics of Obesity*, C. Bouchard, Editor. 1994, CRC Press: Boca Raton. p. 223-233.

258. Tambs, K., et al., *Genetic and environmental contributions to the variance of the body mass index in a Norwegian sample of first- and second-degree relatives.* American Journal of Human Biology, 1991. **3**: p. 257-267.

259. Bouchard, C., et al., *Inheritance of the amount and distribution of human body fat.* International Journal of Obesity, 1988. **12**: p. 205-215.

260. Maes, H., M. Neale, and L. Eaves, *Genetic and environmental factors in relative body weight and human adiposity.* Behavior Genetics, 1997. **27**: p. 325-51.

261. Rice, T., et al., *Familial clustering of abdominal visceral fat and total fat mass: the Quebec family study.* Obesity Research, 1996. **4**: p. 253-61.

262. Stunkard, A., et al., *An adoption study of human obesity.* New England Journal of Medicine, 1986. **314**: p. 193-8.

263.   Allison, D.B., et al., *The heritability of body mass index among an international sample of monozygotic twins reared apart.* International Journal of Obesity and Related Metabolic Disorders, 1996. **20**(6): p. 501-6.

264.   Stunkard, A., et al., *The body-mass index of twins who have been reared apart.* New England Journal of Medicine, 1990. **322**: p. 1483-7.

265.   Stunkard, A.J., T.T. Foch, and Z. Hrubec, *A twin study of human obesity.* Journal of the American Medical Association, 1986. **256**(1): p. 51-4.

266.   Williams, P., et al., *Concordant lipoprotein and weight responses to dietary fat change in identical twins with divergent exercise levels.* American Journal of Clinical Nutrition, 2005. **82**: p. 181-187.

267.   Ravussin, E., et al., *Effects of a traditional lifestyle on obesity in Pima Indians.* Diabetes Care, 1994. **17**: p. 1067-74.

268.   Bouchard, C., et al., *The response to long-term overfeeding in identical twins.* New England Journal of Medicine, 1990. **322**: p. 1477-1482.

269.   Poehlman, E.T., et al., *Heredity and changes in body composition and adipose tissue metabolism after short-term exercise-training.* European Journal of Applied Physiology, 1987. **56**(4): p. 398-402.

270.   al, B.e., FASEB, 1992: p. a:1647 (Abstr.).

271.   Bacon, L., et al., *Evaluating a "Non-diet" Wellness Intervention for Improvement of Metabolic Fitness, Psychological Well-Being and Eating and Activity Behaviors.* International Journal of Obesity, 2002. **26**(6): p. 854-865.

272.   Bacon, L., *Tales of mice and leptin: False promises and new hope in weight control.* Healthy Weight Journal, 2003. **17**(2): p. 24-7.

273.   Bacon, L., et al., *Size acceptance and intuitive eating improve health for obese, female chronic dieters.* Journal of the American Dietetic Association, 2005. **105**: p. 929-36.

274.   Fodor, J.G., et al., *Lifestyle modifications to prevent and control hypertension. 5. Recommendations on dietary salt. Canadian Hypertension Society, Canadian Coalition for High Blood Pressure Prevention and Control, Laboratory Centre for Disease Control at Health Canada, Heart and Stroke Foundation of Canada.* CMAJ, 1999. **160**(9 Suppl): p. S29-34.

275.   United States Department of Agriculture. *Report of the Dietary Guidelines Advisory Committee on the Dietary Guidelines for Americans.* 2005 [cited 2006 2/5/2006]; Available from: www.health.gov/dietaryguidelines/dga2005/report.

276.   United States Department of Agriculture, *Food and Nutrient Intakes by Individuals in the United States, by Region, 1994-96.*

277.   Waldmann, A., et al., *Dietary intakes and lifestyle factors of a vegan population in Germany: results from the German Vegan Study.* European Journal of Clinical Nutrition, 2003. **57**(8): p. 947-55.

278.   U.S. Preventive Services Task Force, *Routine vitamin supplementation to prevent cancer and cardiovascular disease: recommendations and rationale.* Annals of Internal Medicine, 2003. **139**(1): p. 51-5.

279.   Morris, C.D. and S. Carson, *Routine vitamin supplementation to prevent cardiovascular disease: a summary of the evidence for the U.S. Preventive Services Task Force.* Annals of Internal Medicine, 2003. **139**(1): p. 56-70.

280.   Bleys, J., et al., *Vitamin-mineral supplementation and the progression of atherosclerosis: a meta-analysis of randomized controlled trials.* American Journal of Clinical Nutrition, 2006. **84**: p. 880-7.

281.   Erdal, S. and S.N. Buchanan, *A quantitative look at fluorosis, fluoride exposure, and intake in children using a health risk assessment approach.* Environ Health Perspect, 2005. **113**(1): p. 111-7.

282.   Vinceti, M., et al., *A retrospective cohort study of trihalomethane exposure through drinking water and cancer mortality in northern Italy.* Science of the Total Environment, 2004. **330**(1-3): p. 47-53.

283.   Villanueva, C.M., et al., *Disinfection byproducts and bladder cancer: a pooled analysis.* Epidemiology, 2004. **15**(3): p. 357-67.

284.   National Resources Defense Council report, *Environmental and health consequences of animal factories.* 1998.

285.   National Resources Defense Council, *Bottled Water. Pure Drink or Pure Hype?* 1999.

286.   Lalumandier, J.A. and L.W. Ayers, *Fluoride and bacterial content of bottled water vs tap water.* Archives of Family Medicine, 2000. **9**(3): p. 246-50.

287.   Corporate Accountability International. *Think Outside the Bottle. Challenge Corporate Control of Our Water.* 2006 [cited 2006 11/21/06]; Available from: http://www.stopcorporateabuse.org/cms/page1353.cfm.

288.   U.S. Bureau of Census, *Table A-11: Infant and Child Mortality by Region, Country, and Sex: 2002.* 2002.

289.   *Bicycle seats and penile blood flow: does the type of saddle matter?* Journal of Urology, 1999.

290.   Klebanoff, M., et al., *Maternal serum paraxanthine, a caffeine metabolite, and the risk of spontaneous abortion.* New England Journal of Medicine, 1999. **341**(22): p. 1639-44.

291. Cnattingius, S., et al., *Caffeine intake and the risk of first-trimester spontaneous abortion.* New England Journal of Medicine, 2000. **343**(25): p. 1839-45.

292. Boorstin, D., *The Americans: The Democratic Experience.* 1973, New York: Random House.

293. Mead, P., et al., *Food-Related Illness and Death in the United States.* Emerging Infectious Diseases, 1999. **5**(5): p. 607-25.

294. Ames, I., *Foodborne pathogens: risks and consequences.* 1994, Council of Agricultural Science and Technology.

295. Greger, M., *Mad cow disease: Plague of the 21st century?* 2004, Massachusetts Institute of Technology.

296. Center for Science in the Public Interest. *Outbreak Alert! Closing the gaps in our federal food-safety net.* 2004 March 2004 [cited 2005 April 29]; Sixth:[Available from: http://www.cspinet.org/new/pdf/outbreakalert2004.pdf.

297. Nestor, F. and P. Lovera, *Hamburger hell: The flip side of the USDA's Salmonella testing program.*

298. Centers for Disease Control and Prevention. *Influenza: The Disease.* 2004 11/15/04 [cited 2005 3/29/05]; Available from: http://www.cdc.gov/flu/about/disease.htm.

299. U.S. Census Bureau, *Statistical Abstract of the United States: 2001-2005.* 2005.

300. DeWaal, C. and E. Dahl, *Dine at Your Own Risk. The Failure of Local Agencies to Adopt and Enforce National Food Safety Standards for Restaurants.* 1996, Center for Science in the Public Interest: Washington, D.C.

301. Food Safety and Inspection Service, U.S.D.o.A., *Pathogen Reduction and HACCP Systems...and Beyond: The New Regulatory Approach for Meat and Poultry Safety.* 1998: Washington, D.C.

302. Fox, N., *Spoiled: The dangerous truth about a food chain gone haywire.* 1997, New York: Basic Books/HarperCollins.

303. Schlosser, E., *Order the Fish,* in *Vanity Fair.* 2004. p. 210-257.

304. Center for Food Safety and Applied Nutrition/Office of Compliance, *FDA Report on the Occurrence of Foodborne Illness Risk Factors in Selected Institutional Foodservice, Restaurant, and Retail Food Store Facility Types (2004).* 2004: Washington, D.C.

305. United States Government Accounting Office, *FOOD SAFETY. Continued Vigilance Needed to Ensure Safety of School Meals.* 2002: Washington, D.C.

306. USDA/FSIS, *Nationwide young turkey microbiological baseline data collection program, August 1996–July 1997.* 1998, U.S. Dept. of Agriculture Food Safety and Inspection Service: Washington, D.C.

307. Food and Drug Administration, C.f.V.M., *HHS Response to House Report 106-157- Agriculture, Rural Development, Food and Drug Administration, and Related Agencies, Appropriations Bill, 2000. Human-Use Antibiotics in Livestock Production.* 2000: Washington, D.C.

308. Center for Science in the Public Interest, *News Release: How Hazardous is Your Turkey?* 1998.

309. Food Safety and Inspection Service, U.S.D.o.A., *Progress Report on Salmonella Testing of Raw Meat and Poultry Products.* 2000: Washington, D.C.

310. Center for Disease Control. *Salmonellosis.* 2004 [cited July 29, 2004]; Available from: http://www.cdc.gov/ncidod/dbmd/diseaseinfo/salmonellosis_g.htm#How%20common%20is%20salmonellosis.

311. U.S. Department of Agriculture, *Pathogen Reduction; Hazard Analysis and Critical Control Point (HACCP) Systems; Final Rule.* 1996: Washington, D.C.

312. Veneman, A. in *Food and Safety Summit and Expo.* 2003.

313. Behard, R. and M. Kramer, *Something smells fowl,* in *Time.* 1994. p. 42-5.

314. Rusin, P., P. Orosz-Coughlin, and C. Gerba, *Reduction of faecal coliform, coliform and heterotrophic plate count bacteria in the household kitchen and bathroom by disinfection with hypochlorite cleaners.* Journal of Applied Microbiology, 1998. **85**(5): p. 819-28.

315. Armstrong, G., J. Hollingsworth, and J. Morris, *Emerging foodborne pathogens: Escherichia coli 0157:H7 as a model of entry of a new pathogen into the food supply of the developed world.* Epidemiological Reviews, 1996. **18**: p. 29-51.

316. Avery, L.M., K. Killham, and D.L. Jones, *Survival of E. coli O157:H7 in organic wastes destined for land application.* Journal of Applied Microbiology, 2005. **98**(4): p. 814-22.

317. Hennessy, T.W., et al., *A national outbreak of Salmonella enteritidis infections from ice cream. The Investigation Team.* New England Journal of Medicine, 1996. **334**(20): p. 1281-6.

318. Gansheroff, L.J. and A.D. O'Brien, *Escherichia coli O157:H7 in beef cattle presented for slaughter in the U.S.: higher prevalence rates than previously estimated.* Proceedings of the National Academy of Sciences, 2000. **97**(7): p. 2959-61.

319. White, D.G., et al., *The isolation of antibiotic-resistant salmonella from retail ground meats.* New England Journal of Medicine, 2001. **345**(16): p. 1147-54.

320. Tollefson, L. and M.A. Miller, *Antibiotic use in food animals: controlling the human health impact.* Journal of AOAC International, 2000. **83**(2): p. 245-54.

321. National Institute of Allergy and Infectious Diseases, N.I.o.H., U.S. Department of Health and Human Services, *The Problem of Antibiotic Resistance*. 2004: Washington, D.C.

322. Union of Concerned Scientists, *Hogging it: Estimates of Antimicrobial abuse in livestock*. 2001.

323. Committee on Drug Use in Food Animals, P.o.A.H., Food Safety, and Public Health, National Research Council, *The Use of Drugs in Food Animals: Benefits and Risks*. 1999, Washington, D.C.: National Academy Press.

324. National Cattlemen's Beef Association, *Factsheet - January 2000*.

325. Scientific Committee on Veterinary Measures Relating to Public Health, *Assessment of potential risks to human health from hormone residues in bovine meat and meat products*. 1999, European Commission.

326. Brown, P. and R. Bradley, *1755 and all that: a historical primer of transmissible spongiform encephalopathy*. British Medical Journal, 1998. **317**(7174): p. 1688–1692.

327. Brown, P., et al., *Bovine Spongiform Encephalopathy and Variant Creutzfeldt-Jakob Disease: Background, Evolution, and Current Concerns*. Emerging Infectious Diseases, 2001. **7**(1): p. 6-16.

328. Greger, M. *Could Mad Cow Disease already be killing thousands of Americans every year?* 2004 1/7/04 [cited 2005 3/29/05]; Available from: http://organicconsumers.org/madcow/GregerCJDkills.cjm.

329. *Prion disease - spongiform encephalopathies unveiled*. The Lancet, 1990. **336**(8706): p. 21-2.

330. Neurology, 2000. **55**: p. 1075.

331. *European Commission Report on the assessment of the Geographical BSE-risk of the USA*. 2000. **July**.

332. USDA Food Safety and Inspection Service, *Current Thinking on Measures that Could be Implemented to Minimize Human Exposure to Materials that Could Potentially Contain the Bovine Spongiform Encephalopathy Agent*. 2002. **January**.

333. U.S. Department of Agriculture Animal and Plant Health Inspection Services, *Bovine Spongiform Encephalopathy*. 2001: Washington, D.C.

334. United States Department of Health and Human Services, F.a.D.A., *FDA Guidance for Industry 70: Small Entities Compliance Guide for Feeders of Ruminant Animals Without On-Farm Feed Mixing Operations*. 1998: Washington, D.C.

335. Greger, M., *U.S. Continues to Violate World Health Organization Guidelines for BSE*. 2004, Organic Consumers Association.

336. United States Government Accountability Office, *FDA's Management of the Feed Ban Has Improved, but Oversight Weaknesses Continue to Limit Program Effectiveness*. 2005: Washington, D.C.

337. Hunter, N., et al., *Transmission of prion diseases by blood transfusion*. Journal of General Virology, 2002: p. 83.

338. United States Department of Agriculture, A.a. and P.H.I.S.V. Services, *Dairy Herd Management Practices Focusing on Preweaned Heifers Veterinary Services*. 1993: Washington.

339. Cross, A.R., *Blood Donation Eligibility Guidelines: In-depth Discussion of Variant Cruetzfeld-Jacob Disease and Blood Donation*. 2002.

340. United States Government Accountability Office, *FDA's Management of the Feed Ban Has Improved, but Oversight Weaknesses Continue to Limit Program Effectiveness*. 2001: Washington, D.C.

341. United States General Accounting Office, *FOOD SAFETY. Controls Can Be Strengthened to Reduce the Risk of Disease Linked to Unsafe Animal Feed (GAO/RCED-00-255)*. 2000: Washington, D.C.

342. United States General Accounting Office, *Mad Cow Disease: Improvements in the Animal Feed Ban and other Regulatory Areas Would Strengthen U.S. Prevention Efforts (GAO-02-183)*. 2002: Washington, D.C.

343. KQED, *Mad Cow Disease in Canada*. 2003, KQED Forum hosted by Angie Coiro.

344. *Expert Warned that Mad Cow was Imminent*, in *New York Times*. 2004: New York.

345. Public Citizen, *Letter to the FDA and USDA Re: BSE*. 2001.

346. Brown, P., et al., *Iatrogenic Creutzfeldt-Jakob disease at the millennium*. Neurology, 2000. **55**(8): p. 1075-81.

347. Collinge, J., et al., *Kuru in the 21st century—an acquired human prion disease with very long incubation periods*. Lancet, 2006. **367**: p. 2068-2074.

348. *Prion disease--spongiform encephalopathies unveiled*. Lancet, 1990. **336**(8706): p. 21-2.

349. Harvard Center for Risk Analysis, *Evaluation of the Potential for Bovine Spongiform Encephalopathy in the United States: Executive Summary*. 2001, USDA/APHIS.

350. Harriss, R. and H. C, *Mercury-measuring and managing the risk*. Environment, 1987. **20**: p. 25.

351. Jacobson, J. and S. Jacobson, *Dose-Response in Perinatal Exposure to Polychlorinated Biphenyls (PCBs): The Michigan and North Carolina Cohort Studies*. Toxicology and Industrial Health, 1996. **May-August**: p. 435-445.

352. Easton, M.D., D. Luszniak, and G.E. Von der, *Preliminary examination of contaminant loadings in farmed salmon, wild salmon and commercial salmon feed*. Chemosphere, 2002. **46**(7): p. 1053-74.

353. Hawthorne, M., in *Chicago Tribune*. 2006.

354. Aspelin, A. and A. Grube, *Pesticides Industry Sales and Usage: 1996 and 1997 Market Estimates*, Environmental Protection Agency, Office of Pesticide Programs: Washington, D.C. p. 3.

355. Schafer, K., et al., *Chemical Trespass: Pesticides in our Bodies and Corporate Accountability*. 2004, Pesticide Action Network North America.

356. Kegley, S., L. Neumeister, and T. Martin, *Disrupting the Balance. Ecological Impacts of Pesticides in California (Report)*. 1999, Pesticide Action Network North America and Californians for Pesticide Reform.

357. National Center for Environmental Health, *Second National Report on Human Exposure to Environmental Chemicals*. 2004, Centers for Disease Control.

358. Longnecker, M., et al., *Association between maternal serum concentration of DDT metabolite DDE and preterm adn small-for-gestational-age babies at birth*. Lancet, 2001. **358**(9276): p. 110-4.

359. Bell, E., Hertz-Piccotto, and J. Beaumont, *A case-control study of pesticides and fetal death due to congenital anomalies*. Epidemiology, 2001. **22**(2): p. 148-156.

360. Swan, S., et al., *Semen quality in relation to biomarkers of pesticide exposure*. Environmental Health Perspectives, 2003. **111**(12): p. 1478-84.

361. Abell, A., E. Ernst, and J.P. Bonde, *High sperm density among members of organic farmers' association*. Lancet, 1994. **343**(8911): p. 1498.

362. Schwartz, N., *Latin American Banana Farmers Sue U.S. Companies Over Pesticides*, in *Business Week*. 2007: Los Angeles.

363. DiMonte, D., M. Lavaasani, and A. Manning-Bog, *Environmental factors in Parkinson's Disease*. NeuroToxicology, 2002. **23**(4-5): p. 487-502.

364. Reeves, R., A. Katten, and M. Guzman, *Fields of poison 2002. California farmworkers and pesticides*. 2002, Pesticide Action Network: San Francisco.

365. Kegley, S., *Limitations of toxicity data*. 2003, Pesticide Action Network.

366. Payne, J., M. Scholze, and A. Kortenkamp, *Mixtures of four organocholorines enhance human breast cancer cell proliferation*. Environ Health Perspect, 2001. **109**: p. 391-7.

367. Hayes, T., *There is No Denying This: Defusing the Confusion about Atrazine*. BioScience, 2004. **54**(12): p. 1138-1149.

368. Institute for Food and Development Policy, *Circle of Poison: Pesticides and People in a Hungry World*. 1981.

369. *Toxic Control Substances Act, Regulation of hazardous chemical substances and mixtures*, in *United States Code*.

370. National Resource Council, N.A.o.S., *Pesticides in the Diets of Infants and Children*. 1993.

371. National Treasury Employees Union, S.L.A. letter to Johnson, US EPA), Editor. 2006.

372. Janofsky, M., *Unions say E.P.A. bends to political pressure*, in *The New York Times*. 2006: New York.

373. Union of Concerned Scientists, *Voices of Scientists at FDA: Protecting Public Health Depends on Independant Science*. 2006.

374. Nestle, M., *The spinach fallout: Restoring trust in California produce: The E. Coli Outbreak Demonstrates Why America's Food Safety System Needs an Overhaul*, in *Mercury News*. 2006.

375. Worth, M., W. Hauter, and S. Epstein, *A Broken Record. How the FDA Legalized – and   Continues to Legalize – Food Irradiation Without Testing It for Safety*. 2000, Public Citizen's Critical Mass Energy and Environment Program, The Cancer Prevention Coalition, and Global Resource Action Center for the Environment.

376. American Medical Association, *Irradiation of Food*. 1993, Council on Scientific Affairs: Chicago.

377. Morrison, R., *Food irradiation still faces hurdles*. FoodReview, 1992. **15**(2): p. 11-15.

378. Murray, D., (: , and Inc. 1990), *Biology of Food Irradiation*. 1990, New York: John Wiley & Sons.

379. Zhu, M.J., et al., *Influence of irradiation and storage on the quality of ready-to-eat turkey breast rolls*. Poultry Science, 2004. **83**(8): p. 1462-6.

380. U.S. Environmental Protection Agency, Integration Risk Information System, National Center for Environmental Assessment, Office of Research and Development, U.S. Environmental Protection Agency.

381. Delincee, H. and B. Pool-Zobel, *Genotoxic properties of 2-dodecylcyclobutanone, a compound formed on irradiation of food containing fat*. Radiation Physics and Chemistry, 1998. **52**: p. 39-42.

382. US Government Accounting Office, *The Department of the Army's Food Irradiation Program: Is it Worth Continuing: PSAD-78-146*. 1978: Washington, D.C. p. 27-28.

383. Life Sciences Research Office and Federation of American Societies for Experimental Biology, *Evaluation of the health aspects of certain compounds found in irradiated beef*. 1979, Prepared for U.S. Army Medical Research and Development Command, Fort Detrick, Frederick, Maryland, Contract No. DAMD-17-76-C-6055. August 1977. Supplements I and II, March 1979.: Bethesda, Maryland.

384. Consumer Reports, *The truth about irradiated meat*. August, 2003.

385. Houser, T., J. Sebranek, and S. Lonergan, *Effects of irradiation on properties of cured ham*. Journal of Food Science, 2003. **68**(7): p. 2362-2365.

386. Ahn, D., *Quality characteristics of vacuum-packaged, irradiated normal, PSE, and DFD pork. Swine Research Report.* 2000, Iowa State University.

387. Ahn, D. and C. Jo, *Quality characteristics of vacuum-packaged pork patties irradiated and stored in refrigerated or frozen conditions. Swine Research Report.* 1999, Iowa State University.

388. Zhu, M. and e. al., *Control of Listeria monocytogenes contamination in ready ready-to-eat meat products.* Comprehensive Reviews in Food Science and Food Safety, 2005. **4**: p. 34-42.

389. Chen, X., et al., *Lipid Oxidation, Volatiles and Color Changes of Irradiated Pork Patties as Affected by Antioxidants.* Journal of Food Science, 1999. **64**(1): p. 16-19.

390. United States Department of Agriculture Food and Nutrition Service, *Questions and Answers on Irradiated Ground Beef.* 2003.

391. Jenkins, P. and M. Worth, *Food Irradiation: A Gross Failure.* 2006, Center For Food Safety, Food and Water Watch.

392. Post, K. and *If Beefs Don't Kill Irradiated Meat, Lean Sales Might,* in *Press of Atlantic City.* 2003.

393. *Chicken: What you don't know can't hurt you.* Consumer Reports, 1998(March): p. 12-18.

394. Zhu, L., et al., *Production of human monoclonal antibody in eggs of chimeric chickens.* Nat Biotechnol, 2005. **23**(9): p. 1159-69.

395. Lappe, F.M., *World Hunger. Twelve Myths.* 1998, New York: Grove Press.

396. Benbrook, C., *"Evidence of the Magnitude of the Roundup Ready Soybean Yield Drag from University- Based Varietal Trials in 1998.* 1999, Ag BioTech InfoNet Technical Paper Number 1.

397. Holzman, D., *Agricultural Biotechnology: Report Leads to Debate on Benefits of Transgenic Corn and Soybean Crops.* Genetic Engineering News, 1999. **19**(8).

398. Lappe, M. and B. Bailey, *Against the Grain: Biotechnology and the Corporate Takeover of Your Food.* 1998, Monroe, ME: Common Courage Press.

399. Lean, G., *Research Backs Charles: GM Crops Don't Deliver,* in *Independent.* 2000.

400. Busch, L., et al., *Plants, power and profit.* 1990, Oxford, England: Basil Blackwell.

401. Halweil, B., *Transgenic Crop Area Surges.* 2000, Vital Signs 2000, WorldWatch Institute. p. 118.

402. Benbrook, C., *Genetically Engineered Crops and Pesticide Use in the United States: The First Nine Years.* 2004, BioTech InfoNet.

403. Anderson, L., *Genetic Engineering, Food, and our Environment.* 1999, White River Junction, VT: Chelsea Green Publishing Company.

404. Pollan, M., *Playing God in the Garden,* in *New York Times Magazine.* 1998: New York.

405. Wrubel, R.P., S. Krimsky, and M.D. Anderson, *Regulatory Oversight of Genetically Engineered Microorganisms: Has Regulation Inhibited Innovation?* Environ Manage, 1997. **21**(4): p. 571-86.

406. *Statement of Policy: Foods Derived from New Plant Varieties.* Federal Register. **57**(104 at 22991).

407. Pribyl, L., *Biotechnology Draft Document, 2/27/92.*

408. Freese, W. and D. Schubert, *Safety testing and regulation of genetically engineered foods.* Biotechnol Genet Eng Rev, 2004. **21**: p. 299-324.

409. Domingo, J.L., *Health risks of GM foods: many opinions but few data.* Science, 2000. **288**(5472): p. 1748-9.

410. *Monsanto goes GMO-free in its cafeteria,* in *Ode Magazine.* 2007. p. 15.

411. Kirby, A., *Monsanto's caterers ban GM foods,* in *BBC Online.* 1999.

412. Smith, J., *Seeds of Deception. Exposing Industry and Government Lies About the Safety of the Genetically Engineered Foods You're Eating.* 2003, Fairfield, Iowa: Yes! Books.

413. *Duplicate Dinner.* New Scientist, 2001.

414. Food and Nutrition Board (FNB), et al., *Safety of Genetically Engineered Foods: Approaches to Assessing Unintended Health Effects (2004).* 2004, Washington, D.C.: The National Academies Press.

415. Commission of Genetic Resources for Food and Agriculture (United Nations Food and Agriculture Organization), *The State of Zoogenetic Global Resources for Food and Agriculture.* 2007.

416. Panarace, M., et al., *How healthy are clones and their progeny: 5 years of field experience.* Theriogenology, 2007. **67**(1): p. 142-51.

417. USDA/NASS. *Trends in US Agriculture: A 20th Century Time Capsule.* 2002 [cited 2003 January 2003]; Available from: www.usda.gov/nass/pubs/trends/index.htm.

418. Durning, A. and H. Brough, *Taking stock: Animal Farming and the Environment.* Worldwatch Paper No. 103, Worldwatch Institute, 1991.

419. United States Department of Agriculture, *Agricultural Statistics.* 1997: Washington. p. 8.

420. Union of Concerned Scientists, *World Scientists' Warning to Humanity.* 1992.

421. Union of Concerned Scientists, *World Scientists' Call for Action at the Kyoto Climate Summit.* 1997.

422. Warshall, P., *Tilth and technology: The industrial redesign of our nation's soils.*, in *The fatal harvest reader: The tragedy of industrial agriculture*, A.e. Kimbrell, Editor. 2002, The Foundation for Deep Ecology: Sausalito.

423. Goering, P., H. Norberg-Hodge, and J. Page, *From the ground up: Re-thinking industrial agriculture.* 1993, London: Zed Books.

424. Carson, R., *Silent Spring.* 1964, London: Reader's Union.

425. SCHULTHEIß, U., et al., *Heavy metal balances in livestock farming.* 2005, AROMIS – Assessment and reduction of heavy metal inputs into agro-ecosystems: Landwirtschaftsverlag Muenster Hiltrup, Germany.

426. U.S. Department of the Interior - Bureau of Land Management, *State of the Public Rangelands.* 1990, Washington, D.C.

427. Ryan, J. and A. Durning, *Stuff: The Secret Lives of Everyday Things.* 1997, Seattle: Northwest Environment Watch.

428. Lappe, F.M., *Diet for a small planet, 20th anniversary edition.* 1991, Ballantine Books: New York. p. 69, 445-6.

429. National Cattlemen's Association, *"Cattle Feeding,"* in *"Myths and Facts about Beef Production".*

430. Brower, M. and W. Leon, *The Consumer's guide to effective environmental choices.* 1999, New York: Crown Publisher's, Inc.

431. Buringh, P., *Availability of agricultural land for crop and livestock production*, in *Food and Natural Resources*, D. Pimental and C. Hall, Editors. 1989, Academic Press.

432. Myers, N., *The Primary Source: Tropical Rainforest and our Future.* 1984, New York: W.W. Norton.

433. Uhl, C. and G. Parker, *Our steak in the jungle.* BioScience, 1986. **36**: p. 642.

434. Food and Agriculture Organization of the United Nations, A.D., *Livestock and Environment, Agriculture 21.*

435. Wuerthner, G., *The price is wrong.* Sierra, 1990. **September/October**: p. 40-1.

436. Bogo, J., *Where's the beef?* E, 1999. **November/December**: p. 49.

437. Sussman, A., *Dr. Art's Guide to Planet Eart.* 2000, White River Junction, VT: Chelsea Green.

438. U.S. Environmental Protection Agency, *Reducing risk: Setting priorities and strategies for environmental protection. Report of the Science Advisory Board to William K. Reilly, Administrator (September 1990).* 1990.

439. California Comparative Risk Project, *Toward the 21st century: Planning for the protection of California's environment, Summary Report, Submitted to the California Environmental Protection Agency (May 1994).* 1994.

440. Reijnders, L. and S. Soret, *Quantification of the environmental impact of different dietary protein choices.* American Journal of Clinical Nutrition, 2003. **78**(3 Suppl): p. 664S-668S.

441. *Water Scarcity in the Twenty-First Century.* International Journal of Water Resources Development, 1999.

442. Veneman, A. *Plenary Session: State of Food and Agriculture.* in *UN Food and Agriculture Organization 31st Conference.* 2001. Rome, Italy.

443. Robbins, J., *The Food Revolution. How your diet can help save your life and our world.* 2001, York Beach: Conari Press.

444. Shulbach, H. and e. al., Soil and Water, 1978. **38**.

445. Water Education Foundation, *Water inputs in California food production.*

446. International Water Management Institute, *World water supply and demand.* 2000: Colombo, Sri Lanka.

447. Burkholder, J., et al., *Impacts of Waste from Concentrated Animal Feeding Operations (CAFOs) on Water Quality.* Environ Health Perspect:, 2006. **Online 14 November 2006**.

448. Gilchrist, M., et al., *The Potential Role of CAFOs in Infectious Disease Epidemics and Antibiotic Resistance.* Environmental Health Perspectives, 2006. **14 November 2006**.

449. Feedstuffs. **July 3, 1995**.

450. Williams, T., *Assembly Line Swine.* Audubon, 1998. **March/April**: p. 27.

451. Huffman, R. and P. Westerman, *Estimated Seepage Losses from Established Swine Waste Lagoons in the Lower Coastal Plain in North Carolina.* 1995, American Society of Agricultural Engineers. p. 449-453.

452. Environmental Protection Agency (EPA), *Revised National Pollutant Discharge Elimination System Permit Regulation and Effluent Limitation Guidelines for Concentrated Animal Feeding Operations in Response to Waterkeeper Decision.* 2006. **40 CFR Parts 122 and 412**.

453. Little, A., *Ag Reflex*, in *Muckracker.* 2006.

454. U.S. Environmental Protection Agency, *Animal Waste Management: What's the Problem?* 2005.

455. U.S. Environmental Protection Agency, O.o.W.-T., *National Water Quality Inventory - 2000 Report to Congress.* EPA 841-F-02-003. 2002: Washington, D.C.

456. National Science and Technology Council - Committee on Environment and Natural Resources, *An Integrated Assessment: Hypoxia in the Northern Gulf of Mexico.* 2000. **May**.

457. Myers, R.A. and B. Worm, *Rapid worldwide depletion of predatory fish communities.* Nature, 2003. **423**(6937): p. 280-3.

458. Food and Agriculture Organization of the United Nations, *The State of World Fisheries and Agriculture - 1996.* 1996.

459. Stokstad, E., *Global Loss of Biodiversity Harming Ocean Bounty.* Science, 2006. **314**(5800): p. 745.

460. Nellemann, C., S. Hain, and J.E. Alder, *In dead Water: Merging of climate change with pollution, over-harvest, and infestations in the world's fishing grounds.* 2008, United Nations Environment Programme: GRID-Arendal, Norway.

461. Ross, A. and S. Isaac, *The Net Effect? A review of cetacean bycatch in pelagic trawls and other fisheries in the north-east Atlantic.* 2004, Whale and Dolphin Conservation Society.

462. Horsten, M.B. and E. Kirkegaard, *Bycatch from a perspective of sustainable use. IUCN SSC Group: Comments on the European Commission green paper on the Common Fisheries Policy after 2002. IUCN, Brussels.* Science, 2002. **293**: p. 629-638.

463. Watling, L. and E.A. Norse, *Disturbance of the seabed by mobile fishing gear: a comparison with forest clear-cutting.* Conservation Biology, 1998(December).

464. Bruno, J. and E. Selig, *Regional Decline of Coral Cover in the Indo-Pacific: Timing, Extent, and Subregional Comparisons.* PloS One, 2007. **2**(8).

465. Food and Agriculture Organization of the United Nations (FAO). *FISHSTAT.* 2001 [cited; Available from: http://www.fao.org/fi/statist/FISOFT/FISHPLUS.asp.

466. Naylor, R.L., et al., *Effect of aquaculture on world fish supplies.* Nature, 2000. **405**(6790): p. 1017-24.

467. Union of Concerned Scientists, *The Hidden Cost of Fossil Fuels.* 2002.

468. WorldWatch, *The price of beef.* 1994. **July/August**: p. 39.

469. Heitschmidt, R., R. Short, and E. Grings, *Ecosystems, sustainability, and animal agriculture.* Journal of Animal Science, 1996. **74**(6): p. 1395-1405.

470. Pimental, D. and M. Pimental, *Food, Energy and Society.* 1979: p. 59.

471. Pimental, D., et al., *Energy and land constraints in food protein production.* Science, 1975. **November 21, 1975**.

472. Pimental, D., *Food, Energy and Society.* 1995?

473. Emanuel, K., *Increasing destructiveness of tropical cyclones over the past 30 years.* Nature, 2005. **436**(7051): p. 686-8.

474. Khalil, M. and R. Rasmussen, *Sources, sinks, and seasonal cycles of atmosphjeric methane.* Journal of Geophysical Research, 1983. **88**: p. 5131-5133.

475. Steinfeld, H., et al., *Livestock's Long Shadow: Environmental issues and options.* 2006, Food and Agriculture Organization of the United Nations.

476. UNESCO, U.N., et al., *Human Alteration of the Nitrogen Cycle: Threats, Benefits and Opportunities.* UNESCO-SCOPE Policy Briefs, 2007. **4**.

477. Pretty, J., et al., *Farm costs and food miles: An assessment of the full cost of the UK weekly food basket.* Food Policy, 2005. **In press, March 2005**.

478. Carlsson-Kanyama, A., *Climate change and dietary choices: How can emissions of greenhouse gases from food consumption be reduced?* Food Policy, 1998. **Fall/Winter 1998**: p. 288-9.

479. Kimbrell, A.e., *Fatal Harvest: The Tragedy of Industrial Agriculture.* 2002, Washington, DC: Island Press.

480. Fernandez-Armesto, F., *Food: A History.* 2002, London: Pan Macmillan.

481. Osorio, A., et al., *California farm survey of occupational injuries and hazards.* J Agric Safety Hlth, 1998. **1**: p. 99-108.

482. Iowa State University, *Livestock confinement dust and gases.* 1992: Iowa State University. University Extension.

483. Iowa's Center for Agricultural Health and Safety and Institute for Agriculture and Trade Policy (IATP), *Concentrated animal feeding operations: Public health and community impacts.* Vol. September. 2002.

484. Human Rights Watch, *Blood, Sweat, and Fear: Workers' Rights in U.S. Meat and Poultry Plants.* 2005.

485. USDA Economic Research Service, *U.S.-EU Food and Agriculture Comparisons.* 2004.

486. University of Tennessee - Agricultural Policy Analysis Center, *Rethinking U.S. Agricultural Policy: Changing Course to Secure Farmer Livelihoods Worldwide.* 2003.

487. WorldWatch, *Corporations on the dole.* 1996. **January/February**: p. 39.

488. Tillotson, J., Annual Review of Nutrition, 2004.

489. Grinder-Pedersen, L., et al., *Effects of diets based on foods from conventional versus organic production on intake and excretion of flavonoids and markers of antioxidant defense in humans.* Journal of Agriculture and Food Chemistry, 2003. **51**(19): p. 5458-62.

490. World Food Programme. *Reducing poverty and hunger: the critical role of financing for food, agricutlure and rural development.* in *International Conference on Financing for Development.* 2002. Monterrey, Mexico.

491. U.S. Conference of Mayors, *Hunger and Homelessness Survey 2005.* 2005.

492. Bender, W. and M. Smith, *Population, Food, and Nutrition.* 1997: p. 5.

493. UN Food and Agriculture Organization statistical database, *FAOstat.* 2002.

494. Renton, A., *How America is betraying the hungry children of Africa*, in *The Observer*. 2007: United Kingdom.

495. Dugger, C., *CARE Turns Down Federal Funds for Food Aid* in *New York Times*. 2007: New York.

496. Sengupta, S., *On India's Farms, a Plague of Suicide*, in *New York Times*. 2006: New York City.

497. CSPI Press Release, *Heinz is cheating Canada's babies*. 1996.

498. Food and Drug Administration, *Food labeling, health claims, soy protein, and coronary heart disease*. Federal Register, 1999. **57**: p. 699-733.

499. Gunther, C., et al., *Dairy products do not lead to alterations in body weight or fat mass in young women in a 1-y intervention*. American Journal of Clinical Nutrition, 2005. **81**: p. 751-6.

500. Steinman, G., *Mechanisms of Twinning: VII. Effect of Diet and Heredity on the Human Twinning Rate*. Journal of Reproductive Medicine, 2006. **51**(5): p. 405-410.

501. Bakalar, N., *Rise in rate of twins births may be tied to dairy case.*, in *New York Times*. 2006: New York City.

502. Calorie Control Council. *Low-Calorie Sweeteners*. 2007 [cited 2007 March 9, 2007]; Available from: http://www.caloriecontrol.org/aspartame.html.

503. Warner, M., *The Lowdown on Sweet?* , in *New York Times*. 2006.

504. *Lifespan Exposure to Low Doses of Aspartame Beginning During Prenatal Life Increases Cancer Effects in Rats*. Environmental Health Perspectives, 2007(accepted for publication.).

505. Soffritti, M., et al., *First experimental demonstration of the multipotential carcinogenic effects of aspartame administered in the feed to Sprague-Dawley rats*. Environmental Health Perspectives, 2006. **114**(3): p. 379-85.

506. Environmental Health Perspectives, 2001. **109**: p. 983-994.

507. Harris, J. and F. Benedict, *A biometric study of basal metabolism in man*. 1919, Washington D.C.: Carnegie Institute of Washington.

508. NRC (National Research Council), *Recommended Dietary Allowances*. Tenth ed. 1989, Washington, DC: National Academy Press.

509. Simopoulos, A.P., *Essential fatty acids in health and chronic disease*. American Journal of Clinical Nutrition, 1999. **70**(3 Suppl): p. 560S-569S.

510. Leaf, A. and P. Weber, *A new era for science in nutrition*. American Journal of Clinical Nutrition, 1987. **45**: p. 1048-1053.

511. Freese, R. and M. Mutanen, *Alpha-linolenic acid and marine long-chain fatty acids differ only slightly in their effects on hemostatic factors in healthy subjects*. American Journal of Clinical Nutrition, 1997. **66**: p. 591-8.

512. Cunnane, S., et al., *High alpha-linolenic acid flaxseed: some nutritional properties in humans*. British Journal of Nutrition, 1993. **69**: p. 443-453.

513. Consumer Reports, *Fish-oil pills*. 2003(July).

514. vom Saal, F. and C. Hughes, *An Extensive New Literature Concerning Low-Dose Effects of Bisphenol A Shows the Need for a New Risk Assessment*. Environmental Health Perspectives, 2005. **113**(8): p. 926-33.